D0761119

CHILD AND ADOLESCENT PSYCHOPATHOLOGY

There has been a substantial increase of interest in research into child and adolescent psychopathology. In this book, Cecilia Essau brings together contributions from the UK, the USA and Canada to provide a comprehensive summary of the information available on the subject.

Beginning with an introduction to general issues related to child and adolescent psychopathology, including theoretical models of normal and abnormal development, each chapter goes on to address the issues associated with specific disorders, such as:

- Oppositional Defiant Disorder and Conduct Disorder
- Attention-Deficit/Hyperactivity Disorder
- Eating Disorders
- Substance Use Disorders
- Somatoform Disorders

The contributors present a thorough overview of each disorder, including discussion of definition and classification, epidemiology, risk factors, comorbidity, course, outcome, and prevention.

Child and Adolescent Psychopathology will be welcomed by all mental health professionals seeking a reliable source of scientifically and clinically relevant information on the nature and treatment of child and adolescent disorders.

Cecilia A. Essau is Professor of Developmental Psychopathology at Roehampton University.

Contributors: Brendan F. Andrade, Judy A. Andrews, William R. Beardslee, Abigail E. Bond, Cecilia A. Essau, Debra L. Franko, Paul J. Frick, Corinna F. Grindle, Richard P. Hastings, Sara King, Hanna Kovshoff, Michael C. Lambert, Luna Muñoz, Angela D. Paradis, Daniel S. Pine, Helen Z. Reinherz, Paul Rohde, Maureen Samms-Vaughan, Ruth H. Striegel-Moore, Eva M. Szigethy, Jennifer L. Tanner, Roma Vasa, Daniel A. Waschbusch, Antonette M. Zeiss.

CHILD AND ADOLESCENT PSYCHOPATHOLOGY

Theoretical and clinical implications

Edited by Cecilia A. Essau

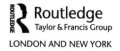

Routledge
Taylor & Francis Group

LONDON AND NEW YORK

First published 2006
by Routledge
27 Church Road, Hove, East Sussex, BN3 2FA

Simultaneously published in the USA and Canada
by Routledge
270 Madison Avenue, New York, NY 10016

Routledge is an imprint of the Taylor & Francis Group

Typeset in Times New Roman by
Keystroke, Jacaranda Lodge, Wolverhampton
Printed and bound in Great Britain by
MPG Books Ltd, Bodmin, Cornwall
Cover design by
Hannah Armstrong

This publication has been produced with paper manufactured to strict
environmental standards and with pulp derived from sustainable forests.

British Library Cataloguing in Publication Data
A catalogue record for this book is available from the British Library

Library of Congress Cataloging in Publication Data
Child and adolescent psychopathology : theoretical and
clinical implications / edited by Cecilia Essau.
p. cm.
Includes biographical references and index.
ISBN 1-58391-834-5
1. Child psychotherapy. 2. Adolescent psychotherapy.
I. Essau, Cecilia
RJ504.C465 2006
618.92′8914–dc22   2005044721

ISBN13: 978–1–58391–834–0
ISBN10: 1–58391–834–5

THIS VOLUME IS TO HONOUR THE WORK
OF PETER M. LEWINSOHN

CONTENTS

List of contributors   ix
Preface   xi

1 **Normal and abnormal development: what the child clinician should know**   1
MICHAEL C. LAMBERT

2 **Oppositional defiant disorder and conduct disorder**   26
PAUL J. FRICK AND LUNA MUÑOZ

3 **Attention-deficit/hyperactivity disorder**   52
DANIEL A. WASCHBUSCH, BRENDAN F. ANDRADE AND SARA KING

4 **Anxiety disorders**   78
ROMA A. VASA AND DANIEL S. PINE

5 **Depressive disorders**   113
HELEN Z. REINHERZ, JENNIFER L. TANNER, ANGELA D. PARADIS,
WILLIAM R. BEARDSLEE, EVA M. SZIGETHY, AND ABIGAIL E. BOND

6 **The theoretical implications of research findings on adolescent depression: implications for Lewinsohn's Integrative Model of Depression and for a lifespan developmental theory of depression**   140
ANTONETTE M. ZEISS

7 **Adolescent eating disorders**   160
RUTH H. STRIEGEL-MOORE AND DEBRA L. FRANKO

8 **Substance use disorders**   **184**
PAUL ROHDE AND JUDY A. ANDREWS

9 **Somatoform disorders**   **221**
CECILIA A. ESSAU

10 **Autism: a psychological perspective**   **246**
HANNA KOVSHOFF, CORINNA F. GRINDLE,
AND RICHARD P. HASTINGS

11 **Learning disorders**   **271**
MAUREEN SAMMS-VAUGHAN

Index   291

CONTRIBUTORS

Brendan F. Andrade, Psychology Department, Dalhousie University, Halifax, Nova Scotia

Judy A. Andrews, Oregon Research Institute, Eugene, OR

William R. Beardslee, Simmons Longitudinal Study, Simmons College, Boston, MA

Abigail E. Bond, Simmons Longitudinal Study, Simmons College, Boston, MA

Cecilia A. Essau, School of Human and Life Sciences, Roehampton University, London, UK

Debra L. Franko, Bouvé College of Health Sciences, Northeastern University, Boston, MA

Paul J. Frick, Department of Psychology, University of New Orleans, New Orleans, LA

Corinna F. Grindle, Department of Psychology, University of Southampton, Southampton, UK

Richard P. Hastings, School of Psychology, University of Wales Bangor, Bangor, UK

Sara King, Psychology Department, Dalhousie University, Halifax, Nova Scotia

Hanna Kovshoff, Department of Psychology, University of Southampton, Southampton, UK

Michael C. Lambert, Department of Human Development and Family Studies, University of Missouri-Columbia, Columbia, MO

Luna Muñoz, Department of Psychology, University of New Orleans, New Orleans, LA

Angela D. Paradis, Simmons Longitudinal Study, Simmons College, Boston, MA

Daniel S. Pine, Section on Development and Affective Neuroscience, National Institute of Mental Health, Bethesda, MD

Helen Z. Reinherz, Simmons Longitudinal Study, Simmons College, Boston, MA

Paul Rohde, Oregon Research Institute, Eugene, OR

Maureen Samms-Vaughan, Department of Child Health, University of the West Indies, Jamaica

Ruth H. Striegel-Moore, Department of Psychology, Wesleyan University, CT

Eva M. Szigethy, Simmons Longitudinal Study, Simmons College, Boston, MA

Jennifer L. Tanner, Simmons Longitudinal Study, Simmons College, Boston, MA

Roma A. Vasa, Kennedy Krieger Institute, Baltimore, MD

Daniel A. Waschbusch, Center for Children and Families, University at Buffalo, Buffalo NY

Antonette M. Zeiss, Office of Mental Health Services, VA Central Office, Washington DC

PREFACE

There has been a substantial increase of interest and research in child and adolescent psychopathology. There are numerous reasons for the amount of attention in this area. First, as many as 22 percent of those below 18 years of age have had some type of psychiatric disorder. Second, the scope of impairment among children and adolescents with psychiatric disorders is profound, including impaired educational achievement, poor social relationship, and depending on the type of disorders, may involve multiple legal systems and special education. Third, the presence of one disorder tends to increase the risk of developing comorbid disorders. Finally, some disorders which occur in childhood not only often continue into adulthood, but also have a lifelong consequence.

Given these findings, literature regarding child and adolescent psychopathology is accumulating at a fast rate. Yet, when mental health professionals need information which is scientifically and clinically relevant, their search often results in frustration. With this in mind, the aim of this volume is to provide a comprehensive summary of the state-of-the-art information on child and adolescent psychopathology.

The first chapter covers general issues related to child and adolescent psychopathology, including theoretical models of normal and abnormal development. The next ten chapters address specific child and adolescent psychopathology: oppositional defiant disorder and conduct disorder, attention-deficit/hyperactivity disorder, anxiety disorders, depressive disorders, eating disorders, substance use disorders, somatoform disorders, autism, and learning disorders. The topics covered in each chapter include: definition and classification, epidemiology, risk factors, comorbidity, course and outcome, and prevention/intervention. Given that this volume is to honor the work of Peter M. Lewinsohn, one chapter focuses on the theoretical implications of his work on depression.

This volume is conceptualized as a tool for advanced students, researchers and other professionals working in the fields of psychiatry, psychology, pediatrics, social work, and other mental health professions. Researchers and professionals working in clinical practice will find this book useful because of its wide coverage, ranging from epidemiology and risk factors through intervention, of the wide range of child and adolescent psychopathology. Advanced students will benefit from a broad review of child and adolescent psychopathology.

I wish to acknowledge the efforts of the contributors, whose expertise and dedication to the project have been outstanding. Without them, a comprehensive coverage of the various topics would not have been easily achieved. Additionally, we wish to acknowledge the support and cooperation of the staff at Routledge.

Cecilia A. Essau

1

NORMAL AND ABNORMAL DEVELOPMENT

What the child clinician should know

Michael C. Lambert

Human development is a complex process and no single theory covers this complexity. Thus, while I will address some of the major theories of development, it is important to note that such theoretical models will cover only selected portions of the developmental process. First I will discuss psychoanalytic theories then cognitive theory followed by ecological theory and behavioral and social cognitive theories. Finally, I discuss the developmental psychopathology perspective, which I view as being most critical to many clinicians who treat children with behavioral and emotional difficulties. I do have another word of caution, which is that space limitations do not permit the discussion of all major theories of development. I have therefore chosen to focus only on some of those I view as being the more dominant theories pertaining to diagnosis and treatment of children.

Psychoanalytic theories

Sigmund Freud is often referred to as the father of psychoanalytic theory. Although his theories are often thought to be more related to clinical work, they do have developmental implications. I will return to these implications near the end of my discussion of Freudian theories. Briefly described, much of Freud's theories emerged out of his work as a neurologist, where he discovered that certain psychological problems were masked in the form of neurological symptomatology. Such psychological problems, he believed, were products of experience and especially conflicts emerging in earlier life.

Freud presented two models, the topographical and structural models, which he viewed as being essential to his explanation of human behavior. The topographical model referred to the fact that virtually no experiences of the organism are lost but rest in various levels of the organism's consciousness. The conscious, according to Freud, holds current experiences of which the organism is aware. The preconscious holds material that is easily retrieved and brought to consciousness. The unconscious holds primitive material that is not easily retrievable and may emerge in dream content or that of hallucinations.

The structural model refers to the makeup of the personality, where three structures are present, the id, the ego, and the superego. Freud thought that the id was virtually unconscious and he also believed it had little contact with reality. In fact, Freud noted that the id uses primary process thought, which he viewed as being illogical and irrational. Freud further believed that as children age and as they are exposed to reality, they develop a structure that is more reality focused, which he called the ego. This structure he often referred to as the executive structure, as it constantly makes decisions within the context of reality. He therefore noted that the ego uses secondary process thought that is more logical and which also functions within the context of reality. The moral structure of the personality, Freud labeled as the superego, to which many commonly refer as being our conscience. The relationship between these three structures determines the individual's functioning, where the ego mediates between the other two structures, and where imbalance might lead to psychopathology.

Freud's theory might be considered to be dated by some. Understanding it is important not only because many clinicians continue to use it as a guiding paradigm to understanding, assessing, and treating psychopathology, but also because Freud was one of the earliest theorists to formally write about his theories of human development and also to indict faulty development as the root cause of psychological problems. To explain this process, he indicated that there were five developmental stages that he labeled the oral, anal, phallic, latency, and genital stages. The oral stage, he believed, occurred at birth through the first year and a half of life where the infant seeks gratification through, and explores the world with, the mouth. The anal stage occurs between ages 18 and 36 months, where the anus becomes the place of focus and pleasure. The phallic phase emerges and remains between ages 3 and 6, where the genitals are discovered and are sources of pleasure. Although not discussed in detail here, Freud addressed the Oedipus complex as critical in this phase, where the child desires the opposite sex parent while fearing that the same sex parent might punish the child for such impulses. Freud believed that the conflicts at this phase are resolved by the child's identification with the same sex parent. This stage is followed by latency, which emerges at age 6 and continues through puberty, where all sexual impulses are repressed and are replaced with interest in mastering social and intellectual development. The final stage, the genital stage, occurs at the time of puberty, where the sexual impulses of the child reemerge, but are focused outside the family.

It should be noted that Freud believed that developmental problems could occur if the individual does not successfully master the challenges emerging at each phase. More specifically, he believed that parts of the libido would be left at these phases, a process he labeled as fixation. Under stress, the organism would therefore return to these points of fixation and exhibit symptoms that are typical of such phases. For example, an individual who experienced difficulty during the oral phase might become needy under stress or someone who is fixated at the anal stage might become obstinate. Freud also noted that to maintain its integrity, the ego develops certain defenses. Such defenses, he believed, were often dependent on the stage of development where the individual might be fixated. Therefore he labeled some defenses as being more primitive than others. An example of a primitive defense is that of denial, whereas a higher order defense might be rationalization.

It should be noted that Freud's theories have experienced numerous criticisms and these theories have been modified by psychoanalysts to address such criticisms. Criticisms include the difficulty in testing a theory that attempts to explain just about every aspect of human behavior but in so doing explains little. The theories are believed to be culturally biased and also possess gender bias. Despite these and other criticisms, the theory must be credited for emphasizing that early experiences are important contributors to the development of the organism.

Although others (e.g., Jung) modified Freud's theory, one important variant of this modification is that of Erik Erikson. While Erikson acknowledged Freud's contributions, he was concerned that Freud only partially covered the stages of human development and focused entirely on psychosexual development. According to Erickson, Freud's theory missed other aspects of development. Erickson therefore proposed eight stages of what he labeled as psychosocial development, trust versus mistrust, autonomy versus shame and doubt, initiative versus guilt, identity versus identity confusion, intimacy versus isolation, generativity versus stagnation, and integrity versus despair. Trust versus mistrust emerges in the first year of life where trust emerges from physical comfort and a sense of security. Autonomy versus shame and doubt occurs during ages 1 to 3 where upon mastering the challenges associated with trust the organism exerts its own autonomy. Initiative versus guilt emerges in the preschool years, where the child must begin coping with the social challenges in the society. Industry versus inferiority emerges in the elementary school years where the child is required to master intellectual skills. Identity versus identity confusion emerges in adolescence, where an important task for adolescents is defining who they are. In early adulthood the challenge of intimacy versus isolation emerges, where the adult must form healthy and intimate relationships. Generativity versus stagnation emerges in middle adulthood where the adult must begin assisting the younger generation in leading useful lives. Integrity versus despair constitutes the final stage occurring in late adulthood where in evaluating one's life, one has a sense of satisfaction or despair.

It should be noted that as the case with other psychoanalytic theories Erikson's theory is criticized. One criticism that is levied against Erikson's theory, as well as many existing theories, is that it is culturally biased. That is, it is possible that the development of individuals in other cultures does not necessarily follow the stages Erikson purports. One of its strengths, however, rests in its emphasis on the effects that changes in childhood and adulthood have on the developmental functioning of the individual. For example, both Freud's and Erikson's theories underscore the need to successfully address the challenges inherent at each stage. Furthermore they underscore that lack of success in such domains can have serious consequences and thus lead to abnormal development of the organism.

Cognitive theory

The distinct field of cognitive development dates back to the early 1950s. Thus, prior to the 1950s, few specialists on cognitive development existed. As a related area, learning theory goes back to the beginning of the field of psychology and was conceptualized primarily in terms of behavioral principles (Feldman, 2003). While Piaget is credited with work on numerous areas regarding the development of reasoning in childhood, including space, time, morality, causality, and necessity, he is most regarded for being the major contributor to understanding cognitive development (Feldman, 2003). Partly as an antidote to what he considered as an unhealthy focus on individual differences among children, Piaget was interested in developing universal principles of human behavior and not individual differences (Berlin, 1992; Feldman, 2003). Piaget also viewed human development as being fundamentally continuous and that it proceeds according to an invariant sequence (Berlin, 1992; Feldman, 2003). Thus, while he did present stages of cognitive development, he pointed out the need to explain the mechanisms under which stage-like changes occur, and thus account for the transformation from one stage to the next (Berlin, 1992). Piaget's theories were both structural and functional, which he believed were closely associated. That is, he believed that there is no structure without function and no function without structure (Berlin, 1992). He also believed in constructivism, where the development of cognition emerges from the interaction of a knowing subject and reality. That is, the action of the subject on the object. Piaget saw development as the differentiation and integration of increasingly abstract structures (Berlin, 1992).

Piaget indicated that children actively construct their own cognitive world and that two processes engineer the children's construction of their world. These processes are organization and adaptation (Santrock, 2001). That is, to make sense of the world, children use their developing cognitive ability to organize it. Furthermore, he believed that continued refinement is a product of cognitive development. That is, the child goes through the process of assimilation when new information is incorporated into existing knowledge and accommodation occurs when the child is able to adjust to new information. Piaget also used the term equilibration to explain the process of children's shift from one stage of thought to the next. This process occurs when children experience cognitive dissonance in their attempt to understand their world. In resolving this conflict, Piaget noted that the child achieves equilibrium (Berlin, 1992; Santrock, 2001).

In order to understand the process of cognitive development, Piaget presented four stages of development, which he noted were gradual and continuous. First is sensorimotor intelligence, which lasts from birth through to the eighteenth month of life. The infant at this stage begins coordinating sensation and action by using reflexive behaviors (Santrock, 2001). Circular reaction is evident at this stage, where the child tries to replicate a chance event that resulted in pleasurable outcomes. Thus, repetition plays a major role at this phase where the infant increasingly refines the process of exploring objects. Also important at this phase of development is the acquisition of object permanence, where the child now acknowledges that objects out of sight continue to exist. In other words, the infant develops the capability of thinking about an object that is not present in the line of sight (Santrock, 2001).

At approximately ages 2 to 7 representational also known as preoperational thought emerges. Children at this stage are able to fantasize and in many cases ascribe characteristics of life to inanimate objects. Cognition becomes representational where the use of language emerges and where objects are represented by spoken word, drawings, and images. Children are, however, egocentric in their thought and are thus unable to take the perspectives of others. Also important at this phase is that the child develops the ability to conserve. Here the child can understand that quantity does not change despite changes in shape (Berlin, 1992). Piaget cautioned that although the child can represent parts of the world, the child lacks the ability to perform operations.

The concrete operational phase occurs approximately between the ages of 7 and 11. Achieving this developmental phase allows the child to perform logical operations that are one-way or reversible. At this phase the child also begins to understand the rules of mathematics including addition, multiplication and subtraction. More specifically, if the problems can be solved using concrete examples, the child is able to understand and apply the operation. Problems such as algebra, which require more abstract thought, present a problem that the child at the concrete operational phase is unable to solve (Berlin, 1992).

The formal operations phase is the final phase of cognitive development Piaget postulated. This phase emerges between the ages of 11 and 15 and involves propositional thought where the adolescent can think hypothetically and thus solve hypothetical problems. Because adolescents are able to think in more abstract forms, they also have the ability to contemplate the future and are also able to theorize using abstract thought. Thus, adolescents are also able to think about their own thoughts. Because of their ability to think in abstract terms, adolescents sometimes use this ability to hypothesize regarding ideal situations. Thus, many adolescents are described as being idealistic in their thinking (Santrock, 2001).

Reflecting on Piaget's contributions, he remains a dominant figure in the field of children's cognitive development. He also provided a framework for the observation and study of children. Despite these accomplishments, contemporary research has challenged the accuracy of the ages at which children achieve the different phases of cognitive development. For example, it is now believed that children achieve some cognitive competencies at earlier ages than Piaget presented while some adolescents might not achieve formal operational thought as early as once thought (Flavell et al., 1993; Santrock, 2001).

Ecological systems theory

Ecological theory is credited to Urie Bronfenbrenner. While recognizing the effects of biological factors on development, ecological theory emphasizes the effects of environmental influences (Santrock, 2001). According to Bronfenbrenner (1992) the ecology of human development is the scientific study of progressive, mutual accommodation, throughout the life course, between the active growing human being, and the changing properties of the immediate settings in which the developing person lives. This process is affected by the relations between these settings and the larger context in which the settings are embedded. Bronfenbrenner (1992) further highlighted the interaction of the person and the environment in which the person exists. Thus, he noted that the person context phenomenon indicates that the person's characteristics and those of the environment are taken into account jointly. For example, he indicated that children growing up in similar environmental contexts often develop differently. These differences he viewed as a function of particular personal characteristics.

Bronfenbrenner further theorized that no characteristic of a person exists or exerts influence on development in isolation. He viewed every human quality as being inextricably embedded. Such quality therefore finds both its meaning and fullest expression in particular environmental settings. Bronfenbrenner further noted that the family is a prime example of a system in which human qualities are embedded. Thus, within the family and other systems in which human qualities exist, there is always interplay between the psychological characteristics of the person and the specific environment. One cannot therefore be defined without the other (Bronfenbrenner, 1992).

Bronfenbrenner is also credited for his focus on human development within the context of culture and the assessment of individuals within cultural context. For example, he pointed out that differences in cognitive performance between groups from different cultures or subcultures are a function of experience in the course of growing up with the types of cognitive processes existing in a given culture or subculture at a particular time in history. Bronfenbrenner further stated that any assessment of cognitive competence of an individual or group must be interpreted in light of the culture or subculture in which the person was brought up. Furthermore, he stated that scientific progress in the study of development in context requires the increased use of contextually based measures of cognitive ability and performance (Bronfenbrenner, 1992).

Bronfenbrenner proposed five environmental systems. First is the microsystem, which includes patterns of activities, roles, and interpersonal relations experienced by a developing person in a given face-to-face setting with particular physical and material features, and containing other persons with distinctive characteristics of temperament, personality, and systems of beliefs (Bronfenbrenner, 1992). The microsystem is therefore the direct context in which the individual lives. Thus in the case of a child this system might consist of the family, peers, school, and neighborhood (Santrock, 2001).

Second, the mesosystem comprises the linkages and processes taking place between microsystems of two or more settings (e.g., between home and school and home and work). Thus, the mesosystem is a system of microsystems that might directly and indirectly influence the developing organism's well-being (Bronfenbrenner, 1992). This system might therefore be the relationship between family experiences and school experiences and also family experiences and peer experiences. Recognition of the mesosystem is evident in more recent developmental work where researchers have emphasized the necessity of assessing the child in different settings (Santrock, 2001).

Third, the exosystem encompasses the linkage and process taking place between two or more settings. At least one of these settings does not ordinarily contain the developing person. Nevertheless the events that occur within such a setting influence processes within the immediate setting that do contain the person (Bronfenbrenner, 1992). Bronfenbrenner used an example of the child within the home and the relation between the child's home and the parent's workplace as an example of this system.

Fourth, the macrosystem, according to Bronfenbrenner's ecological system is reflected in the culture in which the developing organism lives. Thus, the behavioral patterns, beliefs, and other customs that are passed from individuals of one generation to the next vary according to cultural groups.

Finally, the chronosystem involves environmental events occurring over the individual's lifetime. Also included are sociohistorical events (Santrock, 2001). For example the Civil Rights Act and desegregation of US schools have resulted in the interaction between children from different socioethnic groups. Therefore, over the years of such changes some individuals have developed more tolerance and in some cases acceptance of others from ethnic groups that are different from their own.

Although comprehensive in its approach, Bronfenbrenner's theory has been criticized. One criticism is that it has largely omitted biological effects on development. To address this concern Bronfenbrenner has included some focus on the influence of biological effects on development. The theory is, however, dominated by ecological issues and critics continue to indicate that the focus on biological effects is scanty (Santrock, 2001).

Additionally, by citing various limitations with the ecological perspective, namely the limited contextual scope of research, the resulting Eurocentric meanings associated with various risk and protective factors, and constructs of appropriate adaptation, a second perspective, the constructivist view, was advanced by Ungar (2004). The constructivist view places its emphasis on the individual interacting with his/her environment: the meaning the individual brings to his/her life and environment and the cultural context of the environment(s). Thus the constructivist view requires one to learn about the individual's culture, the environmental cultural context, and the associated values of the individual and the environment in order to understand, and accurately interpret, the influences of various factors on children's social and emotional development. For example, from the individual's perspective, a commonly noted Eurocentric risk factor such as low academic performance can be a protective factor when the attribute ensures peer group acceptance due to the cultural values of the environment.

Social cognitive theory

Albert Bandura is the architect of social cognitive theory. According to Bandura, social cognitive theory focuses on a model of causation involving a triadic reciprocal determinism. Within the social cognitive perspective social factors play an influential role on cognitive development. Thus while maturational factors and exploratory activities contribute to cognitive growth, the most valuable knowledge is imparted socially (Bandura, 1992). It is important to note that Bandura does not see the individual or the context in which such an individual lives as exerting benign influences on one another. He noted that people evoke different reactions from their social environment by their physical characteristics, such as their age, race, size, gender, and physical attractiveness. Because of the bidirectional influence between people's behavior and their environment, people are both producers and byproducts of their environment. For example aggressive persons create hostile environments whereas friendly individuals generate an amiable milieu (Bandura, 1992).

Bandura emphasizes the importance of modeling and learning, a process he labeled as observational learning. He believes that this type of learning is governed by four subfunctions. First, he believed that attentional processes determine what people observe. Second, he believed that retention involves an active process of transforming and restructuring information conveyed by the modeled events. Third, behavioral production processes are symbolic conceptions translated into appropriate courses of action. Fourth, motivational processes refer to the fact that people do not perform everything they learn. Such performance is influenced by three major types of incentive motivators, which are direct, vicarious, and self produced (Bandura, 1992).

According to Bandura, modeling can also be an abstract process. Thus, he referred to abstract modeling, which occurs when observers extract the rules embodied in specific behaviors others exhibit. From modeled information, people acquire judgmental standards, linguistic rules, styles of inquiry, information processing skills, and standards of self evaluation. In Bandura's model, behavior, cognition, other personal factors, and environmental influences all operate as interacting determinants that influence each other bidirectionally. Bandura, however, cautioned that reciprocal causation does not mean that that the different sources of influence are of equal strength or that they all occur simultaneously. Moreover he stressed that it takes time for causal factors to exert influence and to activate reciprocal influences.

Bandura highlighted the importance of language in social cognitive development by stating that children initially gain knowledge about objects in nonlinguistic fashion. He further noted that most later thought such children develop and thoughts of older humans are linguistically based. According to Bandura, modeling supplemented with semantic aids and devices is often used to focus attention on key linguistic features, which is a highly effective way of promoting language acquisition. To promote this language acquisition parents usually tailor their language to children's level of cognitive and linguistic capabilities. This process, according to Bandura, begins early in the child's life and the child begins to learn language through the process of modeling (Bandura, 1992).

Bandura believes that although limited, as early as the neonatal period children possess modeling capabilities. Mutual imitation, for example, serves as a means of conveying interest and sharing experiences. Attentional processes are, however, critical to this function, as the more attention the neonate pays to imitated activities, the more likely it is that this child will adopt them (Bandura, 1992). Performance of this imitated behavior, especially that displayed in the distant future, is dependent on symbolic memory.

Besides language acquisition, modeling fosters the acquisition of new competencies, cognitive skills, and behavior patterns and also affects the level of motivation and restraints over previously learned behavior. Modeling influences and serves as social prompts that actuate and channel behavior and social actions. Models therefore express emotional reactions and initiate emotional arousal in others. Through such arousals people acquire attitudes, values, and emotional dispositions toward people, places, and objects (Bandura, 1992).

Critical societal factors such as sex typing are promoted through a vast system of socialization practices. For example, as early as birth, certain colors are ascribed to the attire of boys versus girls. Later in childhood children learn to use certain attributes such as type of hair style to distinguish between the sexes. They also learn to gender label that not only allows them to sort people according to gender but also allows them to learn the features and activities that characterize each gender. Some of this early learning occurs with play and how parents structure such play with gender-related toys. Such socialization continues outside the home with peers and school being major players in such socialization where teaching materials depict gender roles as separate for males and females (Bandura, 1992).

Bandura also focused on self regulation by noting that theories that explain human behavior as simply the product of external rewards present a truncated view of human nature. That is, people possess self-directive capabilities that enable them to exercise some control over their thoughts, feelings, and actions by consequences they produce themselves. Therefore psychological functioning is regulated by interplay between self-produced and external influence. In the social cognitive perspective, people function as active agents in their own motivation. Self motivation varies according to the discrepancy between standards and attainments. Excessively high standards can be demotivating by promoting a sense of discouragement and inefficacy. Moderately difficult standards produce high effort and produce satisfaction through subgoal achievements. Excessively high standards can be demotivating by promoting a sense of discouragement and inefficacy.

The developmental psychopathology perspective

Defined as a "macroparadigm" (Achenbach, 1990), developmental psychopathology is a discipline of study integrated across multiple domains that aims to unify such domains as a singular theory within the developmental lifespan framework

(Cicchetti and Rogosch, 2002). It is therefore comprised of multiple fields of inquiry including the merging of developmental psychology and clinical child and adolescent psychology (Cicchetti and Rogosch, 2002; Wicks-Nelson and Israel, 2003). Thus, it integrates normative development and psychopathology and allows the identification of critical points in which children deviate from "normal" developmental course and are consequently at risk for continued problem behavior (Cicchetti and Rogosch, 2002; Keenan and Shaw, 1997). This discipline also aims to study clinical dysfunction over the lifespan, where dysfunction denotes impairment that has significant impact on everyday functioning, as reflected in aberrant behavior, maladjustment, and psychiatric disorders (Kazdin, 1989).

Developmental psychopathology provides a vocabulary to explain phenomena that are observed clinically and seeks to explain such phenomena empirically (Holmbeck and Kendall, 2002). It is therefore conceptualized as a discipline that studies the origins and examines pathways and course of maladaptive behavior, including the age of onset, the transformation of such behavior over time, and its outcome over the lifespan (Goodman and Gotlib, 1999; Sroufe and Rutter, 1984). Nevertheless its purpose is not simply the study of normal and abnormal development and symptom presentation at different developmental levels, but it also focuses on the convergence and divergence in the biological, physiological, and social contextual systems as they relate to symptom manifestation and disorder (Cicchetti and Rogosch, 2002).

Within the developmental psychopathology framework, the origins and course of individual patterns of behavioral and emotional problems over the lifespan are studied. Such study includes the age and developmental levels of onset, the individual and multiple causes of such problems, and the transformations of such behavior over time (Cicchetti and Rogosch, 2002; Sroufe and Rutter, 1984). Thus, the discipline is designed to study abnormal behavior regardless of age of onset, causes of such problems, the quality of the problems over time, the complexity of the problem, and the patterns such problems take over time (Sroufe and Rutter, 1984). Because of the complexity of the discipline's focus we have learned that childhood dysfunction varies according to multiple factors including gender, ethnicity, and geographic regions (Kazdin, 1989). Such findings are critical to our determination of the cause of abnormal behavior. For example, knowing that behavioral and emotional problems vary as a function of geographic regions might lead the researcher to determine whether variance is caused by cultural factors that might differ across such regions.

In conducting research on these phenomena researchers who subscribe to the developmental psychopathology paradigm are not bound by specific theoretical interpretations, but these researchers integrate a myriad of developmental questions in explaining human behavior (Achenbach, 1990; Cicchetti, 1993). Thus, findings from such research are interpreted within the broad contexts of both biological and psychological influences and their interaction. Such foci underscore the multi-disciplinary nature of this approach (Kazdin, 1989) and also emphasize the importance of understanding both abnormal and normal development.

Developmental pathways

Evaluation of children's functioning at any age requires a clear understanding of normal development from the time of conception throughout the lifespan (Kazdin, 1989). Such understanding should include a clear understanding of gender differences at the time of conception, throughout gestation and the lifespan. For example, we know that human development begins at conception where the chromosomes theoretically determine the gender of the child. This is more complex than is usually thought, as the developing gonads must develop and secrete the necessary hormones to influence phenotypic sexual differentiation including the development of internal and external genitals (Collaer and Hines, 1995). The complexity in this process lies in the fact that a manipulation of steroids during critical periods of development can produce a child with the chromosomal makeup of one gender but the behavioral and neuronal features of the other (Collaer and Hines, 1995).

Physical characteristics or changes can also be associated with development outcomes. Such characteristics include body type and size, attractiveness, physical and physiological changes associated with development such as puberty and old age. Also critical are demographic characteristics such as age, gender, and race (Bronfenbrenner, 1992). It should be noted that organic injury or maldevelopment can threaten psychological growth. Such anomalies include damage of brain function through accidents or degenerative processes, and physical disabilities (Bronfenbrenner, 1992). One area of maldevelopment that has garnered much focus is low birthweight. Because of the profound effects on children who were born low birthweight, I especially focus on this phenomenon within this chapter.

The problem of very low birthweight

Although other problems can occur during gestation and the neonatal period, one problematic area that has repercussions for the child's development and child psychopathology is very low birthweight (VLBW) and its sequela. It should also be noted that that the problem of low birthweight has both biological and environmental origins. Moreover the outcomes for children born with low birthweight are both biologically and environmentally based.

To elucidate the interplay of biological and environmental origins we first note that the risk for low birthweight is increased if the mother comes from a background with two or more of the following features: the mother has less than a high school education, lives in the inner city section of a large metropolitan city or is unmarried. The probability doubles if the mother is at or under age 19, and doubles again if the mother is black (Bronfenbrenner, 1992).

In understanding both the biological and environmental contributions to the consequences of low birthweight, I note that the outcomes for children are governed by not only the effects of being low in birthweight but also the effects of treatment that address the problems accompanying low birthweight. We know, for example,

11

that in developed countries such as those in North America and Europe the development of neonatal intensive care units (NICU) has increased the survival rates of low birthweight (i.e., < 2000 grams), very low birthweight (i.e., <1500 grams) and even extremely low birthweight (<1000 grams) neonates (Paneth, 1995).

Some researchers (Lorenz et al., 1998; Paneth, 1995) are, however, concerned about the long term effects of NICU intervention and its influence on biologically based developmental processes, including hearing (Aram et al., 1991; Veen et al., 1993), vision, cognitive and neurological functioning (Breslau and Chilcoat, 2000; Breslau et al., 2000; Escobar et al., 1991; Veen et al., 1991b). Thus, researchers interested in how such outcomes affect children born prematurely, have focused primarily on physical disability and mental retardation and have documented moderate or severe disabilities in 15–20 percent of VLBW infants (Escobar et al., 1991; Veen et al., 1991a).

An intriguing example of the effects of the interplay between biological and environmental factors on children born prematurely is based on some studies that my colleagues and I have done regarding children born prematurely in Jamaica (a developing country) and the United States (an industrialized nation). Because of the scientific advancement in NICUs, most children born VLBW in the United States survive. By contrast, in Jamaica, which lacks the proliferation of NICUs, approximately half of the children born VLBW perish. The physiological outcomes for children across the two nations are markedly different, where some 80 percent of surviving VLBW children born in the Unites States suffer from cerebral palsy. By contrast, because only the hardy Jamaican children survive, the rate of cerebral palsy in Jamaican children born VLBW is less than 1 percent (see Lambert et al., 2000).

Findings regarding the interplay between environmental and biological factors do not end here. Using the Child Behavior Checklist, a parent report form, we further studied the psychological adjustment of Jamaican VLBW children who are of African descent and that of African American children. African American VLBW children had more physical disabilities than Jamaican VLBW children. Nevertheless, African American parents rated their children born VLBW as having significantly fewer behavior and emotional difficulties than their Jamaican counterparts (Lambert et al., 2000). We reasoned that in spite of the higher biological-related problems that African American children born prematurely might possess, and despite less access to social programs than their white peers, they have far more access to such social, medical, and other programs of support than their Jamaican peers. Such service utilization is likely to reduce the presence of behavioral and emotional difficulties

Some investigations have revealed that despite "normal" intellectual abilities, children born prematurely have higher levels of academic underachievement than normal birthweight children (Klebanov et al., 1994a, 1994b; Ornstein et al., 1991) and that their academic underachievement is often associated with high rates of behavior and emotional problems (Schraeder et al., 1990).

Research has shown that behavior problems and especially attention deficit hyperactivity disorder (ADHD) in VLBW children may have a basis in perinatal brain injury (Whitaker et al., 1997). Many scholars of VLBW children, however, continue to focus primarily on physical disability and only intellectual development (i.e., aptitude for academic functioning). Some researchers (e.g., Whitaker et al., 1997) have begun to focus on behavioral outcomes but few investigators have begun to address the direct, indirect, and mediated effects of intellectual development and behavior problems on adjustment including academic achievement (i.e., school based learning) among the VLBW population (Pharoah et al., 1994).

Behavior and emotional problems can have severe consequences for children who exhibit them, including poor academic outcomes and disturbed interpersonal relationships (Klebanov et al., 1994a; Ornstein et al., 1991). Attention deficit hyperactivity disorder represents one of the most prevalent child behavior problem syndromes in all children (Nigg et al., 1998; Tannock, 1998) and has been repeatedly documented as more prevalent among VLBW children (Hille et al., 2001; Klebanov et al., 1994a; McCormick et al., 1990; Ornstein et al., 1991) than controls. High prevalence of ADHD in VLBW children places them at severe risk for other psychological problems because of its high comorbidity with such problems (Shelton et al., 1998; Tannock, 1998) including conduct and social problems (Hinshaw, 1992) and it also makes them vulnerable to poor adaptive functioning throughout their adolescent and adulthood years (Barkley, 1990; Klein and Mannuzza, 1991).

Although VLBW children are at risk for poor psychological adjustment, he environment in which children reside can mediate such risks (Liaw and Brooks-Gunn, 1994). For example, the effects of sociocultural factors including socioeconomic status (SES) and family functioning can mediate certain risk factors. Indicators of SES such as maternal education, parental occupation and material resources have been linked not only to physical health, but also to cognitive abilities, school achievement and emotional outcomes in most children (Barsky and Siegel, 1992; Brooks-Gunn et al., 1999; Jimerson et al., 1999; Wills et al., 1995). Therefore, some researchers who study VLBW children (Liaw and Brooks-Gunn, 1994) have begun to investigate the effects of sociocultural variables including ethnicity and SES and how such factors influence critical developmental outcomes including scholastic achievement (e.g., Ross et al., 1990), intellectual development (Liaw and Brooks-Gunn, 1994; Ross et al., 1992; Saigal et al., 1990), academic achievement (Klebanov et al., 1994a; Ornstein et al., 1991) and behavioral and emotional problems (Liaw and Brooks-Gunn, 1994; Whitaker et al., 1997).

These studies have furthered our understanding of the outcomes for VLBW and other children, but like most research the methodology used possesses limitations. Among drawbacks inherent in such methodology is the limited number of risk and protective factors one may examine in a given analysis and failure to simultaneously account for critical issues such as measurement error in addressing mediation, an issue that is important to most social scientists (Hoyle and Smith, 1994). Although methodology exists to address such limitations, studies that utilize such methodology are all but nonexistent. One study (Lambert et al., 2000) examined causal relationships existing between resources available to the family, its effect on family functioning and such functioning on the intellectual development of children ages

11 to 12 who were born very low birthweight and their peers who were born normal birthweight. It also tested the effects of intellectual ability on both sets of children's behavioral and emotional problems and achievement, with a causal pathway between child behavioral and emotional problems and achievement. Structural equation modeling revealed links between maternal education and material possessions and that both factors have direct, indirect, and mediated effects on family functioning and psychological adjustment in both VLBW and HBW children. The findings also showed that irrespective of prenatal and perinatal risk factors, paths from contributors, especially maternal education and material possessions, to psychological functioning were not only significant but also the same for children who were born low birthweight and those who were not.

It is important to note that this research project did not simply address whether children of very low birthweight differed from their higher birthweight peers. What it indicated is that the pathways to development are identical regardless of birthweight status. Thus, having adequate material resources is critical to the development of both sets of children. Clinicians who assess and treat children of varying birthweights might do well to gather information regarding the resources available to the family, as they might be important factors in children's well-being.

Genetic and environmental contributions

There is increasing consensus from multiple disciplines as diverse as family systems and biological psychiatry that there is a need to synthesize critical findings from social, genetic, and developmental research and to design studies that can rigorously test and refine competing models of psychopathology (O'Connor and Rutter, 1996). For example, we know that there is a strong genotypic and phenotypic interplay in the development of abnormal functioning, where genes might increase one's sensitivity to the environment (O'Connor and Rutter, 1996). A person with such genotypic sensitivity might therefore respond in a more maladaptive fashion to stress than one without. Thus, the differences in relationship styles, hyperactivity, conduct problems, and sociability are sustained through dynamic interchanges between the characteristics of the person and the person's social experiences (O'Connor and Rutter, 1996).

It is important to note that there is no fixed heritability for any behavioral trait, as radical changes in the environment will most likely have an effect on genetic predisposition. Moreover, the genotypic and phenotypic characteristics interplay in complementary fashion. O'Connor and Rutter (1996) point to the example of where a parent not only might pass a genetic risk factor to the child but also might provide a high risk environment for the child. This combination makes it likely that the risk factor would be realized. We should, however, be mindful that the environment provided is not only limited to the parent as parent and children have varying degrees of influence over one another (Zahn-Waxler, 1996). That is, children alter parenting styles, child rearing, and discipline practices which influence patterns of reciprocal relationships between parents and children (Zahn-Waxler, 1996).

Family and parental contributions

Family risk factors, including marital discord among parents, affectionless control, low family cohesion, and parental divorce, are often more prevalent among depressed parents. But the presence of such risk factors are associated with higher rates of major depression, conduct disorder, and any diagnosis in children from such families (Fendrich et al., 1990). Moreover, exposure to parental divorce results in a sixfold increase in the risk for conduct disorder among children of parents who were not depressed (Fendrich et al., 1990). These findings strongly implicate the quality of family functioning on the development of children.

Parental psychopathology interferes with parenting functioning, including reducing the availability of the parent, which may in turn negatively affect the parent's ability to attend to the child, such as feeding and caring for the child (Dodge, 1990). One parental characteristic that has received much recent emphasis is that of maternal depression. Despite this focus, we know very little about the mechanisms that underlie risk and outcomes for children of depressed mothers. What we do know is that maternal depression can have severe consequences for the child. Such effects are evident as early as infancy, where infants of depressed mothers are documented to be fussier, have difficult temperaments, are less securely attached to their mothers and do poorly on measures of motor and mental development (Goodman and Gotlib, 1999). We therefore address maternal depression more extensively below.

Maternal depression

Depression and other psychopathology lead to disruptions in parenting and family environment and such disruptions lead to maladaptive functioning in the child (Dodge, 1990). Additionally, children born to mothers who were depressed during pregnancy cry more frequently than those who are not and are more inconsolable during such crying episodes (Goodman and Gotlib, 1999). Depressed mothers provide low levels of stimulation to their infants. They spend less time mutually engaged with toddlers, and expose children to depressed affect and negative or maladaptive cognitions including more internal stable and global attributions for negative events (Goodman and Gotlib, 1999).

Besides creating an environment that might not be conducive to appropriate child development, children born to depressed mothers inherit their mother's DNA (Goodman and Gotlib, 1999). Additionally children of depressed mothers are born with dysfunctional neuroregulatory systems. Dysfunctions in such systems could be caused by their mothers' depression during pregnancy, which could have exposed the developing fetus to neuroendocrine alterations. For example, there is evidence to suggest that maternal cortisol, a stress-related hormone, crosses the placenta (Dodge, 1990; Goodman and Gotlib, 1999). Other contributing components include the effects of the treatments used in the treatment of mothers' depression, some of which can contribute to the neuroendocrine alterations previously mentioned and to constricted blood flow to the fetus, which in turn restricts the fetus's weight. Such weight restriction might contribute to low birthweight and the difficulties on functioning mentioned earlier.

To reemphasize, maternal psychopathology interferes with parenting, if only by reducing the availability of the parent. This in turn could also interfere with the parent attending to the basic needs of the child such as feeding, attending to, and taking care of the child (Dodge, 1990). It is also important to note that maternal depression can cascade into contributing to marital discord, low family cohesion, and parental divorce. The presence of these risk factors are associated with high rates of major depression, conduct disorder, and other types of diagnosis in children (Fendrich et al., 1990).

Effect of fathers

Despite the risk of psychopathology for a child who is born of a depressed mother, children most often have to live with other family members, including fathers. Fathers and paternal psychopathology have, however, received little attention in the literature on development psychopathology (Pheres and Compas, 1992). Fathers do interact with children differently from how mothers do but it is likely that some of the basic underlying mechanisms of the father's impact on children's functioning are similar to that of mothers (Pheres and Compas, 1992). Additionally, there are specific disorders that have been linked to fathers' psychopathology. Antisocial behavior in boys, for example, is strongly related to their fathers' antisocial behavior. Additionally, fathers of boys with attention problems differ from those of boys without, where the fathers of boys with the disorder have less favorable perceptions of their own parenting capabilities and their self confidence in being able to parent their children (Pheres and Compas, 1992).

Paternal but not maternal psychopathology is related to children's anxiety. Children of fathers who suffer from alcoholism are found to be at risk for a wide variety of behavioral and emotional difficulties (Pheres and Compas, 1992). Both fathers and mothers of girls suffering from bulimia are likely to be engaged in hostile enmeshment with their daughters while investing energies in undermining their daughter's attempts at separation and self assertion (Pheres and Compas, 1992). While sparse when compared with that on mothers' psychopathology and maternal depression in particular, the literature on fathers' contribution to psychopathology not only indicates a clear link but also underscores the need for further research in this domain.

Family's contributions to child psychopathology

Shifting focus to the family and its contributions to normal and abnormal development, we first note that biological blueprint does not provide all that is essential for normal development. The environment in which we live, including that which our family provides, shapes the quality of our lives (National Advisory Mental Health

Council (NAMHC), 1996). Family relationships are our earliest and most important social relationships. Emotional and economic links among family members stretch across households and decades influencing one's outlook on life, motivations, strategies for achievement, and styles of coping with adversity (NAMHC, 1996).

Although many families provide a caring and supportive relationship that advances positive development in their members, the effects of families are not always positive. For example a minority of families provides the context for some of the severest forms of violence in our society and long term patterns of physical and emotional abuse, which can have profound effects on the mental health of adults and children (NAMHC, 1996). Families can therefore have a profound effect on the developmental outcomes of children.

Social and emotional development

Appropriate social and emotional functioning for children as young as those who are preschoolers is critical not only for initial school readiness in preschool but also for the school-age years (Izard et al., 2001). Research indicates that children with higher levels of social and emotional development tend to have a positive developmental trajectory in overall growth and maturity, academic achievement, and social competence, whereas children who have poorer social and emotional development tend to experience scholastic dysfunction (low academic achievement, grade retention, and problematic relations with peers and teachers), antisocial behavior, and diagnosable psychiatric conditions such as conduct disorder and depression (Gershoff, 2003; Lee and Burkam, 2002; Raver and Knitzer, 2002; Zill and West, 2001).

Familial, environmental, and an individual's personal attributes are factors that influence social and emotional development. Certain risk factors can predispose young children to poor social and emotional development. Other elements which can, however, "buffer" a child from detrimental influences or serve to enhance development are often referred to as protective factors. Social and emotional strengths, for example, can buffer the presentation of social and emotional problems (Lambert et al., 2004) and might even buffer the effects of economic disadvantage (Raver, 2002). Yet a substantial number of children move from preschool to kindergarten with severe social and emotional developmental problems (Raver, 2002).

The ecological perspective allows one to categorize various familial, environmental, and personal attributes into groups and subgroups of risk and protective factors. The resulting interplay of these factors, whether they impede or enhance development, provides a causal linkage to the individual's developmental trajectory (Ungar, 2004). Citing various limitations with the ecological perspective, namely the limited contextual scope of research, the resulting Eurocentric meanings associated with various risk and protective factors, and constructs of appropriate adaptation, a second perspective, a constructivist view, was advanced by Ungar (2004).

The constructivist view places its emphasis on the individual interacting with his/her environment: the meaning the individual brings to his/her life and environment and the cultural context of the environment(s). Thus, the constructivist view requires one to learn about the individual's culture, the environmental cultural context, and the associated values of the individual and the environment in order to understand, and accurately interpret, the influences of various factors on children's social and emotional development. For example, from the individual's perspective, a commonly noted Eurocentric risk factor such as low academic performance can be a protective factor when the attribute ensures peer group acceptance due to the cultural values of the environment. We now turn to a discussion of risk and protective factors.

Protective and risk factors influencing social and emotional development

Although most clinicians recognize that protective factors are critical to a child's psychological well-being, there is a dearth in research on such factors. Existing research indicates protective factors are elements in a child's environment that promote a sense of well-being and safety as well as a child's own attributes. These include supportive relationships with others (e.g., family, peers, and adults such as teachers) and resources that meet basic needs (e.g., stability in the areas of housing, food, and a sense of routine). A child's personality attributes and competence in the areas of cognitive functioning, language, social and emotional development, and cultural belief system can also contribute as protective factors (Ladd and Burgess, 2001; Mendez et al., 2002; Raver, 2002; Ungar, 2004).

Protective factors are elements in a child's environment that promote a sense of well-being and safety as well as a child's own attributes. These include supportive relationships with others (e.g., family, peers, and adults such as teachers) and resources that meet basic needs (e.g., stability in the areas of housing, food, and a sense of routine). A child's attributes and competence in the areas of cognitive functioning, language, social and emotional development, and cultural belief system also contribute as protective factors (Ladd and Burgess, 2001; Mendez et al., 2002; Raver, 2002; Ungar, 2004).

Risk factors include aspects of family life such as living in a low-income family, a home where English is not the primary language, a single-parent home, or a home with a high level of stress or marital discord (Jones et al., 2002; Lee and Burkam, 2002; Mendez et al., 2002). Children reared in single parent families are at risk for developmental problems. Such children are likely to have depressed IQ scores and are more likely to be school dropouts. Girls in single parent families are more likely to become single mothers in their teenage years (Basic Behavioral Science Task Force, 1995).

Children with delinquent behavior are more likely to have been abused by their fathers and mothers, to have witnessed severe family violence, and to have a mother with a history of psychiatric hospitalization (Basic Behavioral Science Task Force,

1995). Rates of psychological dysfunction in children, however, vary according to age, gender, type of disorder, ethnic background and even geographical location, suggesting that these characteristics could be indicative of risk (Kazdin, 1989). For example, it is widely known that the rates of depression are virtually identical in children but that during late childhood to adolescence girls have a higher risk of depression than boys.

Parental characteristics, such as a low level of education, substance abuse, criminal history, and mental illness, are also risk factors (Gershoff, 2003; Lee and Burkam, 2002; Webster-Stratton, 1998; Zill and West, 2001). Other parent-related risk factors include overprotectiveness which is negatively associated with autonomy and is positively associated with child and adolescent depression, oppositional and other externalizing behavior (Holmbeck et al., 2002).

Environmental risk factors include living in a neighborhood with high levels of violence (e.g., witnessing violence and/or being the victim of violence), noise and crowding, limited services for children and adults, and factors unique to rural communities including isolation and limited community resources (Brody et al., 2002; Ceballo et al., 2001; Evans and English, 2002; O'Donnell et al., 2002; Zill and West, 2001).

Risk factors that are chronic and those that co-occur with others in the life of a child can jeopardize children's social and emotional development because of their cumulative impact (Duncan et al., 1994; Evans and English, 2002; Jones et al., 2002). Children who experience multiple risk factors are especially vulnerable for compromised social and emotional development (Gershoff, 2003; Raver and Knitzer, 2002; Webster-Stratton, 1998; Zill and West, 2001). That is, although it is not totally clear that risk factors are linear or exponential or that specific numbers of risk factors are needed to show negative effects, we do know that the larger the accumulation of risk factors, the higher the probability of negative outcomes (Stouthamer-Loeber et al., 2000).

To summarize, the trajectory of children's development is heavily dependent on their characteristics such as behavioral and emotional strengths, and their environment, both within and outside their families. Well functioning and supportive families are important to their social and emotional well-being. The clinicians who assess and treat the child should be cognizant of not only children and their functioning, but also the context that the family and community provide. This professional should be prepared to use the strengths within such contexts to bolster healthy child development and to address the developmental difficulties that some children encounter.

Measurement of children's functioning and developmental change

Parents' influence and perspectives are important to consider in the evaluation of children's functioning. Children seldom view their behavior and functioning as deviant. Developmental difficulties and other problems children present are therefore usually identified by parents and other significant adults who closely interact with children (Kazdin, 1989). Thus, clinicians and other professionals who assess children rely on informal parent reports in interviews or on more standardized assessment procedures that obtain parents' responses on measures such as checklists of children's behavioral and emotional problems. While it is tempting to view the ratings on such checklists as standardized measurement, it is important to note that parents' perceptions of deviance in their evaluations of their own children on such scales are related to their own symptoms of psychopathology. Such symptoms include parental depression and anxiety, marital discord, expectations of child behavior, parental self esteem, and reported stress in the home (Kazdin, 1989).

Conclusion

In addressing normal and abnormal development issues I first summarized some of the more dominant theories of development and culminated with the developmental psychopathology perspective, which today many deem as being the principal theory of addressing disorders of childhood. I then examined developmental pathways emphasizing the interplay between biological and environmental bases of such pathways. Toward this end I used the problem of low birthweight and some of the studies others and I have conducted that show linkages and interplay between biological and environmental effects in the outcomes for one of the most vexing developmental outcomes. I further underscored the interplay of biological and environmental influences on development by briefly focusing on genetic determinants of development and how the prenatal environment might influence developmental outcomes of the fetus and neonate. Finally, I examined the most recent research and other literature on the environmental influences on abnormal development such as maternal depression, and the family's contributions, including that of fathers. I acknowledge that the space this chapter affords has given me limited opportunity to address the contributors to normal and especially abnormal development. It is my hope that it will provide a springboard for the professional who desires to further explore the issues presented here.

References

Achenbach, T.M. (1990). Conceptualizations of developmental psychopathology. In M.L.S.M. Miller (Ed.), *Handbook of developmental psychopathology*. New York: Plenum.

Aram, D.M., Hack, M., Hawkins, S., Weissman, B.M., and Borawski Clark, E. (1991). Very-low-birthweight children and speech and language development. *Journal of Speech and Hearing Research*, *34*, 1169–1179.

Bandura, A. (1992). Social cognitive theory. In R. Vasta (Ed.), *Six theories of child development: Revised formulations and current issues* (pp. 1–60). Philadelphia, PA: Jessica Kingsley.

Barkley, R.A. (1990). *Attention-deficit hyperactivity disorder: A handbook for diagnosis and treatment*. New York: Guilford.

Barsky, V.E. and Siegel, L.S. (1992). Predicting future cognitive, academic and behavioral outcomes for very-low-birthweight (<1,500 grams) infants. In S.L. Friedman and M.D. Sigman (Eds.), *The psychological development of low birthweight children* (pp. 275–298). Norwood, NJ: Ablex.

Basic Behavioral Science Task Force of the National Advisory Mental Health Council (1995) Basic behavioural science research for mental health: Family processes and social networks. *American Psychologist, 51,* 622–630.

Berlin, H. (1992). Piagetian theory. In R. Vasta (Ed.), *Six theories of child development: Revised formulations and current issues* (pp. 85–131). Philadelphia, PA: Jessica Kingsley.

Breslau, N. and Chilcoat, H.D. (2000). Psychiatric sequelae of low birth weight at 11 years of age. *Biological Psychiatry, 47,* 1005–1011.

Breslau, N., Chilcoat, H.D., Johnson, E.O., Andreski, P., and Lucia, V.C. (2000). Neurologic soft signs and low birthweight: Their association and neuropsychiatric implications. *Biological Psychiatry, 47,* 71–79.

Brody, G.H., Murry, V.M., Kim, S., and Brown, A.C. (2002). Longitudinal pathways to competence and psychological adjustment among African American children living in rural single-parent households. *Child Development, 73,* 1505–1516.

Bronfenbrenner, U. (1992). Ecological systems theory. In R. Vasta (Ed.), *Six theories of child development: Revised formulations and current issues* (pp. 187–249). Philadelphia, PA: Jessica Kingsley.

Brooks-Gunn, J., Duncan, G.J., and Britto, P. (1999). Are socioeconomic gradients for children similar to those of adults. In D.P. Keating and C. Hertzman (Eds.), *Developmental health and the wealth of nations: Social, biological, and educational dynamics* (pp. 94–123). New York: Guilford.

Ceballo, R., Dahl, M., Aretakis, M.T., and Ramirez, C. (2001). Inner-city children's exposure to community violence: How much do parents know? *Journal of Marriage and the Family, 63,* 927–940.

Cicchetti, D. (1993). Developmental psychopathology: Reactions, reflections, and projections. *Developmental Review, 13,* 471–502.

Cicchetti, D. and Rogosch, F.A. (2002). A developmental psychopathology perspective on adolescence. *Journal of Consulting and Clinical Psychology, 70,* 6–20.

Collaer, M.L. and Hines, M. (1995). Human behavioral sex differences: A role for gonadal hormones during early development. *Psychological Bulletin, 118,* 55–107.

Dodge, K. (1990). Developmental psychopathology in children of depressed mothers. *Developmental Psychology, 26,* 3–6.

Duncan, G.J., Brooks-Gunn, J., and Klebanov, P.K. (1994). Economic deprivation and early childhood development. *Child Development, 65,* 296–318.

Escobar, G.J., Littenberg, B., and Petitti, D.B. (1991). Outcome among surviving very low birthweight infants: A meta-analysis. *Archives of Disease in Childhood, 66,* 204–211.

Evans, G.W. and English, K. (2002). The environments of poverty: Multiple stressors exposures, psychophysiological stress, and socioemotional adjustment. *Child Development, 73,* 1238–1248.

Feldman, D.H. (2003). Cognitive development in childhood. In R. Lerner, M.A. Easterbrooks, and J. Mistry (Eds.), *Developmental psychology* (Vol. 6, pp. 195–210). Hoboken, NJ: John Wiley.

Fendrich, M., Warner, V., and Weissman, M.M. (1990). Family risk factors, parental depression, and psychopathology in offspring. *Developmental Psychology, 26,* 40–50.

Flavell, J.H., Miller, P.H., and Miller, S.A. (1993). *Cognitive development.* Englewood Cliffs, NJ: Prentice Hall.

Gershoff, E. (2003). *Low income and the development of America's kindergartners* (Living at the Edge Research Brief no. 4). Retrieved May 10, 2004, from Columbia University, National Center for Children in Poverty website: http://www.nccp.org

Goodman, S.H. and Gotlib, I.H. (1999). Risk for psychopathology in the children of depressed mothers: A developmental model for understanding mechanisms of transmission. *Psychological Review, 106,* 458–490.

Hille, E.T.M., den Ouden, A.L., Saigal, S., Wolke, D., Meyer, R., Lambert, M.C., et al. (2001). Behavior in very and extremely low birthweight infants at school age: Is outcome different in different countries. *Lancet, 357,* 1641–1643.

Hinshaw, S.P. (1992). Externalizing behavior problems and academic underachievement in childhood and adolescence: Causal relationships and underlying mechanisms. *Psychological Bulletin, 111,* 127–155.

Holmbeck, G.N. and Kendall, P.C. (2002). Introduction to the special section on clinical adolescent psychology: Developmental psychopathology and treatment. *Journal of Consulting and Clinical Psychology, 21,* 3–5.

Holmbeck, G.N., Johnson, S.Z., Wils, K.E., McKernon, W., Rose, B., Erklin, S., et al. (2002). Observed and perceived overprotectiveness in relation to psychological adjustment in preadolescents with a physical disability: Mediational role of behavioral autonomy. *Journal of Consulting and Clinical Psychology, 70,* 96–110.

Hoyle, R.H. and Smith, G.T. (1994). Formulating clinical research hypotheses as structural equation models: A conceptual overview. *Journal of Consulting and Clinical Psychology, 62,* 429–440.

Izard, C., Fine, S., Schultz, D., Mostow, A., Ackerman, B., and Youngstrom, E. (2001). Emotion knowledge as a predictor of social behavior and academic competence in children at risk. *Psychological Science, 12,* 18–23.

Jimerson, S., Egeland, B., and Teo, A. (1999). A longitudinal study of achievement trajectories: Factors associated with change. *Journal of Educational Psychology, 91,* 116–126.

Jones, D.J., Forehand, R., Brody, G., and Armistead, L. (2002). Psychosocial adjustment of African American children in single-mother families: A test of three risk models. *Journal of Marriage and Family, 64,* 105–115.

Kazdin, A.E. (1989). Developmental psychopathology: Research, issues, and directions. *American Psychologist, 44,* 180–187.

Keenan, K. and Shaw, D. (1997). Developmental and social influences on young girls. *Psychological Bulletin, 121,* 95–113.

Klebanov, P.K., Brooks-Gunn, J., and McCormick, M.C. (1994a). Classroom behavior of very low birth weight elementary school children. *Pediatrics, 94,* 700–708.

Klebanov, P.K., Brooks-Gunn, J., and McCormick, M.C. (1994b). School achievement and failure in very low birth weight children. *Journal of Developmental and Behavioral Pediatrics, 15,* 248–256.

Klein, R.G. and Mannuzza, S. (1991). Long-term outcome of hyperactive children: A review. *Journal of the American Academy of Child and Adolescent Psychiatry, 30,* 383–387.

Ladd, G.W. and Burgess, K.B. (2001). Do relational risks and protective factors moderate the linkages between childhood aggression and early psychological and school adjustment? *Child Development, 72,* 1579–1601.

Lambert, M.C., Samms-Vaughan, M.E., Bellas, V.F., and Russ, C.M. (2000). Problems in very lowbirthweight Jamaican children. Paper presented at the Second International Conference on Child and Adolescent Mental Health, Kuala Lumpur, Malaysia.

Lambert, M.C., Rowan, G.T., Kirsch, E.A., Rowan, S.A., Mount, D., Kim, S., et al. (2004). Factors that contribute directly and indirectly to academic achievement in African American children: A causal modeling approach. Paper presented at the Roundtable on Addressing the Education Needs of At Risk Children, Oriel College in the University of Oxford, Oxford, UK.

Lee, V.E. and Burkam, D.T. (2002). *Inequality at the starting gate: Social background differences in achievement as children begin school.* Washington, DC: Economic Policy Institute.

Liaw, F.R. and Brooks-Gunn, J. (1994). Cumulative familial risks and low-birthweight children's cognitive and behavioral development. *Journal of Clinical Child Psychology, 23,* 360–372.

Lorenz, J.M., Wooliever, D.E., Jetton, J.R., and Paneth, N. (1998). A quantitative review of mortality and developmental disability in extremely premature newborns. *Archives of Pediatrics and Adolescent Medicine, 152,* 425–435.

McCormick, M.C., Gortmaker, S.L., and Sobol, A.M. (1990). Very low birth weight children: behavior problems and school difficulty in a national sample [see comments]. *Journal of Pediatrics, 117,* 687–693.

Mendez, J.L., Fantuzzo, J., and Cicchetti, D. (2002). Profiles of social competence among low-income African American preschool children. *Child Development, 73,* 1085–1100.

National Advisory Mental Health Council (NAMHC) (1996). Basic behavioral science research for mental health. *American Psychologist, 51,* 622–630.

Nigg, J.T., Hinshaw, S.P., Carte, E.T., and Treuting, J.J. (1998). Neuropsychological correlates of childhood attention-deficit/hyperactivity disorder: Explainable by comorbid disruptive behavior or reading problems? *Journal of Abnormal Psychology, 107,* 468–480.

O'Connor, T.G. and Rutter, M. (1996). Risk mechanisms in development: Some conceptual and methodological considerations. *Developmental Psychology, 32,* 748–795.

O'Donnell, D.A., Schwab-Stone, M.E., and Muyeed, A.Z. (2002). Multidimensional resilience in urban children exposed to community violence. *Child Development, 73,* 1265–1282.

Ornstein, M., Ohlsson, A., Edmonds, J., and Asztalos, E. (1991). Neonatal follow-up of very low birthweight/extremely low birthweight infants to school age: A critical overview. *Acta Paediatrica Scandinaica, 80,* 741–748.

Paneth, N.S. (1995). The problem of low birth weight. *The Future of Children, 5,* 19–34.

Pharoah, P.O., Stevenson, C.J., Cooke, R.W., and Stevenson, R.C. (1994). Prevalence of behaviour disorders in low birthweight infants [see comments]. *Archives of Disease in Childhood, 70,* 271–274.

Pheres, V. and Compas, B.E. (1992). The role of fathers in child and adolescent psychopathology: Make room for daddy. *Psychological Bulletin, 111,* 384–412.

Raver, C.C. (2002). Emotions matter: Making the case for the role of young children's emotional development for early school readiness. *Social Policy Report, 16,* 3–18.

Raver, C.C. and Knitzer, J. (2002). *Ready to enter: What research tells policymakers about strategies to promote social and emotional school readiness among three- and four-year olds.* Retrieved May 10, 2004, from Columbia University, National Center for Children in Poverty website: http://www.nccp.org

Ross, G., Lipper, E.G., and Auld, P.A. (1990). Growth achievement of very low birth weight premature children at school age. *Journal of Pediatrics, 117*(2 Pt 1), 307–309.

Ross, G., Lipper, E.G., and Auld, P.A. (1992). Hand preference, prematurity and developmental outcome at school age. *Neuropsychologia, 30*, 483–494.

Saigal, S., Szatmari, P., Rosenbaum, P., Campbell, D., and King, S. (1990). Intellectual and functional status at school entry of children who weighed 1000 grams or less at birth: A regional perspective of births in the 1980s. *Journal of Pediatrics, 116*, 409–416.

Santrock, J.W. (2001). *Child Development*, 9th edn. New York: McGraw-Hill.

Schraeder, B. D., Heverly, M. A., and Rappaport, J. (1990). Temperament, behavior problems, and learning skills in very low birth weight preschoolers. *Research in Nursing and Health, 13*, 27–34.

Shelton, T.L., Barkley, R.A., Crosswait, C., Moorehouse, M., Fletcher, K., Barrett, S., et al. (1998). Psychiatric and psychological morbidity as a function of adaptive disability in preschool children with aggressive and hyperactive-impulsive-inattentive behavior. *Journal of Abnormal Child Psychology, 26*, 475–494.

Sroufe, L.A. and Rutter, M. (1984). The domain of developmental psychopathology. *Child Development, 55*, 17–29.

Stouthamer-Loeber, M., Farrington, D.P., Loeber, R., Wikstrom, P.H., and Wei, E. (2000). Risk and promotive effects in the explanation of persistent serious delinquency in boys. *Journal of Consulting and Clinical Psychology, 70*, 111–123.

Tannock, R. (1998). Attention deficit hyperactivity disorder: Advances in cognitive, neurobiological, and genetic research. *Journal of Child Psychology and Psychiatry and Allied Disciplines, 39*, 65–99.

Ungar, M. (2004). A constructionist discourse on resilience: Multiple contexts, multiple realities among at-risk children and youth. *Youth and Society, 35*, 341–365.

Veen, S., Ens Dokkum, M.H., Schreuder, A.M., Brand, R., Verloove Vanhorick, S.P., and Ruys, J.H. (1991a). Impairments, disabilities, and handicaps in low-birthweight babies [letter; comment]. *Lancet, 338*, 1011–1012.

Veen, S., Ens Dokkum, M.H., Schreuder, A.M., Verloove Vanhorick, S.P., Brand, R., and Ruys, J.H. (1991b). Impairments, disabilities, and handicaps of very preterm and very-low-birthweight infants at five years of age. The Collaborative Project on Preterm and Small for Gestational Age Infants (POPS) in The Netherlands [see comments]. *Lancet, 338*, 33–36.

Veen, S., Sassen, M.L., Schreuder, A.M., Ens Dokkum, M.H., Verloove Vanhorick, S.P., Brand, R., et al. (1993). Hearing loss in very preterm and very low birthweight infants at the age of 5 years in a nationwide cohort. *International Journal of Pediatric Otorhinolaryngology, 26*, 11–28.

Webster-Stratton, C. (1998). Preventing conduct problems in Head Start children: Strengthening parenting competencies. *Journal of Consulting and Clinical Psychology, 66*, 715–730.

Whitaker, A.H., Van Rossem, R., Feldman, J.F., Schonfeld, I.S., Pinto Martin, J.A., Tore, C., et al. (1997). Psychiatric outcomes in low-birth-weight children at age 6 years: relation to neonatal cranial ultrasound abnormalities [see comments]. *Archives of General Psychiatry, 54*, 847–856.

Wicks-Nelson, R. and Israel, A.C. (2003). *Behavior disorders of childhood*, 5th edn. Upper Saddle River, NJ: Prentice Hall.

Wills, T.A., McNamara, G., and Vaccaro, D. (1995). Parental education related to adolescent stress-coping and substance use: Development of a mediational model. *Health Psychology, 14*, 464–478.

Zahn-Waxler, C. (1996). Environment, biology, and culture: Implications for adolescent development. *Developmental Psychology, 32*, 571–573.

Zill, W. and West, J. (2001). *Entering kindergarten: A portrait of American children when they begin school: Findings from the Condition of Education 2000* (US Department of Education, National Center for Education Statistics, NCES 2001–035). Washington, DC: US Government Printing Office.

2

OPPOSITIONAL DEFIANT DISORDER AND CONDUCT DISORDER

Paul J. Frick and Luna Muñoz

The study of conduct problems in children has been a major focus of research in child psychology for a number of reasons. First, conduct problems are one of the most common reasons that children and adolescents are referred to mental health clinics (Frick and Silverthorn, 2001) or to residential treatment centers (Lyman and Campbell, 1996). This high rate of referral for children with conduct problems is likely due to the significant disruptions caused by these problems to both the child's family (Frick, 1998) and the child's school (Gottfredson and Gottfredson, 2001). Second, severe conduct problems are the form of psychopathology that has been most strongly associated with delinquency (Moffitt, 1993). There has been increased recognition in recent years of the societal costs associated with juvenile crime, including the direct harm to victims, the decrease in quality of life associated with high crime neighborhoods, and the costs of incarceration or other forms of responding to delinquent youth (Loeber and Farrington, 2000; Zigler et al., 1992). Third, severe conduct problems can also be quite stable, leading to problems in the child's adjustment across the life span (Frick and Loney, 1999). This stability adds to the societal costs associated with juvenile antisocial behavior. For example, the estimated cost to society of a single youth engaging in four years of offending as a juvenile and ten years of offending as adult ranges from $1.7 million to $2.3 million in 1997 US dollars (Cohen, 1998).

Definition

There have been a number of different methods used to define serious conduct problems in research (see Frick and Ellis, 1999, for a review). Perhaps the most widely used classification system is the diagnostic criteria published in the *Diagnostic and statistical manual of mental disorders – Fourth edition/text revision* (DSM-IV/TR; American Psychiatric Association (APA), 2000). This manual specifies two primary disorders involving conduct problem behavior. The first disorder is Oppositional Defiant Disorder (ODD), which is defined as a recurrent pattern of negativistic, defiant, disobedient and hostile behavior toward authority figures that persists for at least six months (APA, 2000). The characteristic symptoms include losing temper, arguing with adults, actively defying or refusing to comply with requests or rules of adults, deliberately doing things that will annoy other people, blaming others for own mistakes or misbehavior, being touchy or easily annoyed by others, being angry and resentful, or being spiteful or vindictive (APA, 2000).

The second conduct problem diagnosis defined by the DSM-IV/TR is Conduct Disorder (CD). This disorder is defined as a repetitive and persistent pattern of behavior which violates the rights of others or which violates major age appropriate societal norms or rules. These behaviors fall into four main groupings: aggressive conduct that threatens physical harm to other people or animals, nonaggressive conduct that causes property loss or damage, deceitfulness and theft, and serious violations of rules (APA, 2000). The DSM-IV/TR also makes the distinction between children who begin showing severe antisocial and aggressive behaviors before age 10 (i.e., childhood-onset) and those who do not show severe conduct problems before age 10 (i.e., adolescent-onset). This distinction between childhood and adolescent onset to severe conduct problems has proven to be very important for defining subgroups of youth who differ on their childhood and adolescent behavior and who differ in their adjustments as young adults (Frick and Loney, 1999). Most importantly, however, children in these groups show a number of distinct characteristics suggesting that different causal processes are operating in the development of conduct problems for the two groups of youth (Frick, 1998; Moffitt, 1993). This research on the different prognosis and the unique causal processes for these two groups of youth with CD is summarized in more detail later in the chapter.

Epidemiology

Prevalence estimates for severe conduct problems in community samples of youth generally range from between 6 percent and 10 percent (Anderson et al., 1987; Costello et al., 1988; Offord et al., 1987; Rayfield et al., 1999). When broken down by type of conduct disorder diagnoses and when using current diagnostic criteria, ODD seems to be present in 3 percent to 5 percent of youth and CD is found in about 1 percent to 4 percent of youth (Loeber et al., 2000). Importantly, prevalence rates of conduct problems can be influenced by a number of factors, such as the exact criteria used to define the disorder (Anderson et al., 1987; Offord et al., 1987) and the method used to assess these criteria (Costello et al., 1988). For example, Costello et al. (1988) reported that prevalence estimates for oppositional behaviors were somewhat higher when using parental report to assess the problem behavior, whereas the use of child report resulted in somewhat higher rates of CD (Costello et al., 1988). Differences in prevalence rates across ethnic groups have not been found consistently. For example, higher rates of conduct problems in African-American youth have been found in some samples (Fabrega et al., 1993; Lahey et al., 1995) but not others (McCoy et al., 2000). More importantly, it is unclear whether any association with minority status and conduct problems is independent of the fact that ethnic minorities are more likely to experience economic hardships and live in urban neighborhoods with higher concentrations of crime than non-minority individuals (Lahey et al., 1999; Peeples and Loeber, 1994).

There is consistent evidence for differences in prevalence rates of severe conduct problems for children of different ages. For example, aggression and oppositional behaviors tend to decrease in prevalence from the pre-school to school-age years (Keenan and Shaw, 1997), whereas the prevalence rates for ODD and CD increase in adolescence (Loeber et al., 2000). For example, Loeber et al. (2000) reported prevalence rates for CD of 5.6, 5.4, and 8.3 for boys aged 7, 11, and 13 respectively, and prevalence rates for ODD of 2.2, 4.8, and 5.0 for boys of the same age in a sample of 1517 youth in a large urban area. However, the increase in the prevalence of conduct problems from childhood to adolescence may not be consistent for all types of conduct problems. Specifically, there is evidence that mild forms of physical aggression (e.g., fighting) show a decrease in prevalence rates across development, whereas non-aggressive and covert forms of antisocial behavior (e.g., lying, stealing) and serious aggression (e.g., armed robbery, sexual assault) show an increase in prevalence rates from childhood to adolescence (Loeber and Hay, 1997).

There also appears to be clear sex differences in the prevalence rates of conduct problems. Overall estimates of the sex ratio for boys and girls with severe conduct problems range from 2:1 to 4:1 (Cohen et al., 1993; Loeber et al., 2000; Offord et al., 1987; Shaffer et al., 1996). However, this overall ratio hides several important developmental differences in the sex ratio. Specifically, there are few sex differences between boys and girls in the prevalence rate of most types of conduct problems prior to age 5 (Keenan and Shaw, 1997). However, after age 4 the rate of girls' behavior problems decreases while the rate of behavioral problems for boys either increases or stays at the same rate, leading to a male predominance of conduct problems throughout much of childhood. Numerous studies have also noted that the sex ratio between girls and boys with CD narrows dramatically from about 4:1 in childhood to about 2:1 in adolescence (see Silverthorn and Frick, 1999, for a review). This decrease appears to be due to the dramatic increase in the number of girls engaging in antisocial behaviors in adolescence combined with a much less dramatic increase in the rate of antisocial behavior in boys.

There is some controversy as to whether the differences in prevalence rates in childhood and adolescence for girls and boys are real differences or whether they may be an artifact of diagnostic criteria that are not sensitive to sex differences in how conduct problems are expressed. For example, it has been argued that girls are less often diagnosed with severe conduct problems than boys because they manifest more indirect or relational aggression (i.e., spreading rumors, hurting others in the context of a relationship), rather than physical aggression (e.g., Crick and Grotpeter, 1995). Others have argued that girls manifest similar types of behaviors as boys, but that they should be diagnosed using a more lenient criteria that compares girls to other girls rather than to mixed samples of girls and boys (e.g., Zoccolillo, 1993). Still others have argued that girls manifest antisocial behaviors that are similar to those of boys but are less likely than boys to experience many of the risk factors for conduct problems (Moffitt and Caspi, 2001; Silverthorn and Frick, 1999).

Comorbidity

As mentioned previously, conduct problems can be very impairing for the child and can lead to a host of other problems in adjustment. Further, the same factors that cause conduct problems can lead to other problems in adjustment (Frick, 1998). Therefore, it is not surprising that there are high rates of comorbidity between conduct problem diagnoses and many other forms of childhood psychopathology. Perhaps the most common comorbid disorder, and the one on which there is the largest amount of research, is Attention Deficit Hyperactivity Disorder (Frick, 1998; Lilienfeld and Waldman, 1990; Lynam, 1996). Specifically, between 65 percent and 90 percent of children with either ODD or CD exhibit the significant attentional problems, impulsivity, and hyperactivity associated with a diagnosis of ADHD (Abikoff and Klein, 1992). Importantly, the comorbidity between ADHD and CD/ODD predicts a more chronic course of conduct problems (Barkley et al., 2002; Frick and Loney, 1999). For example, children with both ADHD and CD seem to show a greater variety of delinquent acts in adolescence (Loeber et al., 1990), a greater number of aggressive acts in adolescence (Moffitt, 1993), and more violent offending in adulthood (Klinteberg et al., 1993).

Another frequent comorbidity in children with severe conduct problems is learning disabilities (Cantwell and Baker, 1992). There are many explanations for this link and there is some evidence that the learning problems are more related to ADHD which is frequently comorbid with conduct problems, rather than to the conduct problems themselves (Frick et al., 1991; Maughan et al., 1996). However, this explanation seems to largely apply to children in the childhood-onset group, with some children with learning disabilities developing conduct problems in adolescence without an early history of ADHD or other behavior problems (Hinshaw, 1992).

Children with severe conduct problems also show high rates of emotional disorders, such as depression and anxiety. Between 15 percent and 31 percent of children with CD have comorbid depression and between 22 percent and 33 percent of children with CD in community samples and between 60 percent and 75 percent in clinic samples have a comorbid anxiety disorder (Russo and Beidel, 1994; Zoccolillo, 1993). One important finding from this research is that children with CD and depression appear to be at increased risk for suicidal ideation. For example, in a community sample of seventh and eighth grade students, 31 percent of the children with CD and depression reported suicidal ideation compared to only 12 percent of the students with CD only (Capaldi, 1992). Also, for many children with CD, the presence of anxiety and depression seems to be largely a result of the interpersonal conflicts (e.g., with peers, teachers, and police) and other stressors (e.g., family dysfunction, school failure) that often are experienced by children with severe conduct problems (Capaldi, 1992; Frick et al., 1999; Panak and Garber, 1992). As a result, the anxiety and depression experienced by children with ODD or CD is often best conceptualized as emotional distress or negative affectivity that results from their impaired psychosocial functioning.

Severe conduct problems are also associated with alcohol and drug use. The comorbidity between CD and substance abuse is important because, when children with conduct problems also abuse substances, they tend to show an early onset of substance use and they are more likely to abuse multiple substances (Lynskey and Fergusson, 1995). Although most of the research on the association between CD and substance abuse prior to adulthood has been conducted with adolescents, the association between conduct problems and substance use may begin very early in development. In an urban community sample (N = 2573) of children in the first, fourth and seventh grades, substance use was fairly rare in first and fourth grade children (Van Kammen et al., 1991). When it did occur in these early grades, however, it was usually associated with the presence of significant conduct problems. In the seventh grade, substance use became more common, especially the use of milder substances like alcohol. However, the use of harder drugs and the use of multiple drugs were associated with conduct problems in this older age group. Therefore, conduct problems appear to be associated with *non-normative substance use* throughout childhood and adolescence.

Course and outcome

The developmental association between ODD and CD

Research seems to suggest that the less severe ODD symptoms are linked to the more severe CD symptoms both hierarchically and developmentally (Lahey and Loeber, 1994). For example, research has found that pre-adolescent children rarely begin showing the severe conduct problem behaviors associated with CD without first showing the milder ODD behaviors earlier in development. Instead, the typical developmental progression is for a child to start showing oppositional and argumentative behaviors early in life (e.g., between the ages of 3 and 8) and then gradually progress into increasingly more severe patterns of conduct problem behavior over the course of childhood (Loeber et al., 1992). However, there are three important aspects to this developmental trajectory. First, although most children who show the more severe conduct problems of CD start by showing the less severe ODD symptoms, a large number of children with ODD do not progress on to show more severe conduct problems (Lahey and Loeber, 1994). Second, most children who progress on to CD do not change the types of behaviors they display but instead add the more severe conduct problem behaviors to their behavioral repertoire (Lahey and Loeber, 1994). Third, this progression from ODD to CD seems to be characteristic only of the childhood-onset pattern of CD (Hinshaw et al., 1993; Moffitt, 1993). Specifically, youth who show the adolescent onset of their severe conduct problems do not typically show the less severe conduct problems earlier in development but begin to show a range of both ODD and CD behaviors coinciding with the onset of puberty.

Multiple casual pathways to conduct disorder

It is important to note that there has been little research conducted on children with ODD who do not go on to develop CD. However, for children who do go on to show the more severe problems of CD, there has been a substantial amount of research documenting a number of potentially important correlates. The common theme of recent comprehensive reviews of this research is that there are a large number of risk factors associated with CD (Dodge and Pettit, 2003; Frick, 1998; Loeber and Farrington, 2000; Raine, 2002). These risk factors include factors that are dispositional involving characteristics located within the child (e.g., biological abnormalities, predisposing personality traits, cognitive deficits), as well as factors involving the child's social context (e.g., dysfunctional parenting practices, peer rejection, impoverished living conditions). The first implication of this research is that it is very unlikely that the focus on any single risk factor will adequately account for the development of severe conduct problems. As a result, causal theories need to somehow integrate multiple factors in trying to explain CD. For example, Loeber and Farrington (2000) demonstrated that the risk for serious conduct problems was a function of the number of risk factors present, with risk increasing in a linear manner from the presence of no risk factors to the presence of six or more risk factors.

Research has also suggested that is important to recognize that not all children with CD develop their behavioral difficulties due to the same causal factors (Frick et al., 2003b; Frick and Morris, 2004). As a result, there have been a number of attempts to define meaningful subgroups of children with CD who differ on the causal processes that lead to the child's aggressive and antisocial behavior (see Frick and Ellis, 1999, for a review). As noted previously, current diagnostic definitions of CD distinguish between the childhood-onset and adolescent-onset subtypes of the disorder (APA, 2000). This distinction is supported by a substantial amount of research documenting important differences between these two groups of youth with CD (see Moffitt, 2003, for a review). Specifically, children in the childhood-onset group are more likely to show aggressive behaviors in childhood and adolescence and are more likely to continue to show antisocial and criminal behavior into adulthood (Frick and Loney, 1999; Moffitt and Caspi, 2001). More relevant to causal theory, most of the dispositional (e.g., temperamental risk, low intelligence) and contextual (e.g., family dysfunction) correlates that have been associated with CD seem primarily associated with the childhood-onset subtype. In contrast, the youth in the adolescent-onset subtype do not consistently show these same risk factors. If they do differ from other children, it seems primarily to be in showing greater affiliation with delinquent peers and scoring higher on measures of rebelliousness and authority conflict (Moffitt and Caspi, 2001; Moffitt et al., 1996).

The different characteristics of children in the two subtypes of CD have led to theoretical models that propose very different causal mechanisms operating across the two groups. For example, Moffitt (1993, 2003) has proposed that children in the childhood-onset group develop their problem behavior through a transactional process involving a difficult and vulnerable child (e.g., impulsive, with verbal deficits, and a difficult temperament) who experiences an inadequate rearing environment (e.g., poor parental supervision, a poor quality school; a neighborhood with a high rate of violence; see also Hinshaw et al., 1993). This dysfunctional transactional process disrupts the child's socialization leading to poor social relations with persons both inside (e.g., parents and siblings) and outside the family (e.g., peers and teachers) which further disrupts the child's socialization. These disruptions lead to enduring vulnerabilities that can negatively affect the child's psychosocial adjustment across multiple developmental stages. In contrast, Moffitt (1993, 2003) views children in the adolescent-onset pathway as showing an exaggeration of the normative developmental process of identity formation that takes place in adolescence. Their engagement in antisocial and delinquent behaviors is conceptualized as a misguided attempt to obtain a subjective sense of maturity and adult status in a way that is maladaptive but that is encouraged by an antisocial peer group.

This distinction between childhood-onset and adolescent-onset trajectories to CD is a very influential model for explaining the different pathways through which children may develop severe conduct problems. However, it is important to note that clear differences between children in the two pathways are not always found (Lahey et al., 2000) and the applicability of this model to girls requires further testing (Silverthorn and Frick, 1999). Also, research has begun extending this conceptualization in a number of important ways. Specifically, it has begun to test whether additional distinctions can be made within children who follow the childhood-onset pathway to (a) differentiate groups based on the severity, type, and stability of conduct problems exhibited, (b) differentiate groups that have distinct vulnerabilities that can make them more difficult to socialize by parents, teachers, and other important socializing agents, and (c) more clearly specify the developmental processes that can be disrupted by the transaction between a vulnerable child and a non-optimal socializing environment.

To illustrate such an extension, one line of research has uncovered a subgroup of antisocial youth in juvenile forensic facilities (Caputo et al., 1999; Silverthorn et al., 2001), outpatient mental health clinics (Christian et al., 1997; Frick et al., 1994), and school-based samples (Frick et al., 2000) who show high rates of callous and unemotional (CU) traits (e.g., lacking empathy and guilt). Importantly, youth with conduct problems who also show CU traits seem to show a more severe and aggressive pattern of conduct problems than other youth with CD (Christian et al., 1997; Frick et al., 2003a; Kruh et al., 2005). Even more specifically, they are more likely to show a pattern of behavior that includes reactive (e.g., aggression that is in response to real or perceived provocation) aggressive acts, as well as instrumental (e.g., aggression to gain a desired outcome) and premeditated aggressive acts (Caputo et al., 1999; Frick et al., 2003a; Kruh et al., 2005). In addition to showing a more severe and aggressive pattern of conduct problems, children within the childhood-onset group who also show CU traits seem to have a stronger genetic basis to their conduct problems. Specifically, Viding et al. (2004) reported data from a study of 6330 7-year-old twins (3165 twin pairs). In this study, children scoring in the top 10 percent of the sample on a measure of conduct problems were further divided into those with (N = 359) and without (N = 333) significant levels of CU traits. Estimates of the genetic and environmental effects on variations in conduct problems were very different for the two groups. Specifically, the heritability estimate for the group high on both conduct problems and CU traits (0.81) was over twice that for the group low on CU traits (0.30).

While this finding suggests that genetic factors may play a larger role in the development of conduct problems for children with CU traits, it does not provide clues as to the mechanism by which heredity may exert its effects. There is, however, a growing body of research to suggest that children with conduct problems and CU traits exhibit a temperamental style that is distinct from other conduct problem youth. For example, children with conduct problems who also show CU traits show a preference for novel, exciting, and dangerous activities (Frick et al., 2003b; Frick et al., 1999). Additionally, children with CU traits are less sensitive to cues of punishment, especially when a reward-oriented response set is primed (Barry et al., 2000; Fisher and Blair, 1998; Frick et al., 2003b; O'Brien and Frick, 1996). This reward-oriented response set appears not only in computerized laboratory tests but also in social situations in which children with CU traits show a tendency to emphasize the positive aspects (e.g., obtaining rewards, gaining dominance) of solving peer conflicts with aggression and to de-emphasize the negative aspects (e.g., getting punished; hurting others) of aggressive acts (Pardini et al., 2003). And finally, children with CU traits and conduct problems have been shown to be less reactive to threatening and emotionally distressing stimuli than other antisocial youth (Blair, 1999; Frick et al., 2003b; Loney et al., 2003).

This preference for novel and dangerous activities, the lack of sensitivity to cues to punishment, and the lack of emotional responsiveness to negative emotional material are all consistent with a temperamental style that has been labeled as low fearfulness (Rothbart and Bates, 1998) or low behavioral inhibition (Kagan and Snidman, 1991). Importantly, several studies of normally developing children have linked this temperament with lower scores on measures of conscience development in both concurrent (Asendorf and Nunner-Winkler, 1992; Kochanska et al., 2002) and prospective studies (Rothbart et al., 1994). These findings have led to a number of theories as to how this temperament may be involved in conscience development (see Frick and Morris, 2004, for a more comprehensive review). For example, some developmental theories suggest that moral socialization and the internalization of parental and societal norms are partly dependent on the negative arousal evoked by potential punishment for misbehavior (e.g., Kagan, 1998; Kochanska, 1993). Guilt and anxiety associated with actual or anticipated wrongdoing can be impaired, if the child has a temperament in which the negative arousal to cues of punishment is too low (Kagan, 1998; Kochanska, 1993). Similarly, this temperament could place a child at risk for missing some of the early precursors to empathetic concern which involves emotional arousal evoked by the misfortune and distress of others (Blair, 1995; Blair et al., 2001; Blair et al., 1997). Consistent with these theories, children with conduct problems and CU traits are less distressed by the negative effects of their behavior on others (Blair et al., 1997; Frick et al., 1999; Pardini et al., 2003), are more impaired in their moral reasoning and empathic concern towards others (Blair, 1999; Fisher and Blair, 1998; Pardini et al., 2003), and are less able to recognize expressions of sadness in the faces and vocalizations of other children (Blair et al., 2001; Stevens et al., 2001).

However, it is important to note that not all children in the childhood-onset pathway show CU traits. In fact, it appears to be only a minority of children who do so (Christian et al., 1997; Frick et al., 2000). Therefore, it is important to also consider what processes may be operating for children with a childhood-onset to CD but without CU traits. As reviewed previously, children with conduct problems who are not elevated on CU traits are less likely to be aggressive than those who are high on these traits. However, when they do act aggressively, it is more likely to be reactive in nature and in response to real or perceived provocation by others (Frick et al., 2003b). Also, antisocial children who do not show CU traits have conduct problems that are more strongly associated with dysfunctional parenting practices (Oxford et al., 2003; Wootton et al., 1997) and with deficits in verbal intelligence (Loney et al., 1998). Finally, antisocial youth who do not show CU traits also show problems in their emotional functioning. However, unlike the group of children with CU traits who seem to show deficiencies in their experience of certain emotions, children with conduct problems without CU traits seem to show problems in regulating negative emotions. Specifically, they exhibit high levels of emotional distress (Frick et al., 2003b; Frick et al., 1999), are more reactive to the distress of others in social situations (Pardini et al., 2003), and are highly reactive to negative emotional stimuli (Loney et al., 2003).

Overall, these findings suggest that different mechanisms are operating in the development of conduct problems for children who do not show high rates of CU traits compared to those with these traits. Further, a large number of children with CD but without CU traits seem to have problems regulating their emotions (Frick and Morris, 2004). These problems in emotional regulation can lead to very impulsive and unplanned aggressive and antisocial acts for which the child may be remorseful afterwards but may still have difficulty controlling in the future (Pardini et al., 2003). The problems in emotional regulation can also make a child particularly susceptible to becoming angry due to perceived provocations from peers leading to violent and aggressive acts within the context of high emotional arousal (Hubbard et al., 2002; Kruh et al., 2005; Loney et al., 2003; Shields and Cicchetti, 1998).

Although problems with regulating emotion can lead directly to conduct problems and aggression, there are a number of mechanisms through which they can have indirect effects on the development of conduct problems as well. For example, emotional dysregulation can impair the development of social cognitive skills that allow a child to effectively process information and effectively respond to this information in social situations (Dodge and Pettit, 2003). In addition to disruptions in the child's peer context, problems in emotional regulation can disrupt other aspects of the child's socialization. For example, Kochanska (1993, 1995) has proposed that children who are susceptible to strong negative affect can have difficulties internalizing parental norms because their intense emotional arousal to discipline encounters prevents them effectively processing the parental message. Also, Patterson and colleagues (Patterson et al., 1992; Snyder and Patterson, 1995) have proposed that antisocial and aggressive youth often are involved in coercive cycles with their parents in which both parent and child attempt to control each other through increasingly aversive behaviors (e.g., parental harsh discipline, child's temper outburst). A child with problems in emotional regulation can be more likely to elicit and maintain such coercive cycles in parent–child interactions and to have this pattern of behavior generalize to other settings, such as at school and with peers (Gauvain and Fagot, 1995).

Taken together, this research suggests that there appear to be a number of different pathways through which children may develop CD, each involving somewhat different causal mechanisms. The presence of distinct developmental pathways to conduct problems has important treatment implications, which are discussed later in the chapter. Given these very different subgroups of children with CD, it is not surprising that there is substantial variability in the stability of conduct problems across groups of youth with this disorder.

Stability and prognosis of CD

When studying the lifespan course of antisocial behavior retrospectively, research has consistently found that most adults who show severe patterns of antisocial behavior have childhood histories of CD (Robins et al., 1991). When viewed prospectively, research has documented less strong, but still substantial, stability in antisocial behavior across the lifespan. Frick and Loney (1999) reviewed twelve prospective longitudinal studies of the stability of conduct problems over short periods of time (from eight months to five years) and found that the correlations between initial and follow-up assessments generally fell between 0.42 and 0.64. In studies that estimated the degree of stability in diagnoses of CD, about 50 percent of the children diagnosed with CD at an initial assessment were rediagnosed with CD at a follow-up assessment.

Frick and Loney (1999) also summarized the results of nine prospective longitudinal studies that investigated the stability of conduct problems over longer periods of time (i.e., > six years). Although lower than those found for shorter follow-up periods, these studies still documented fairly substantial stability in conduct problems. Specifically, the correlation coefficients for the long-term follow-up studies generally fell between 0.20 and 0.40. Several studies specifically estimated the stability within samples of youth with CD. For example, Kratzer and Hodgins (1997) found that about 64 percent of boys and 17 percent of girls (ages 12–16) with CD had committed a crime during a sixteen-year follow-up period. Similarly, Robins (1966) reported that 43 percent of boys and 12 percent of girls who had been referred for a significant number of CD symptoms were later imprisoned at least once as an adult. These longitudinal studies suggest that girls with CD do not show as high a rate of antisocial outcomes as boys. However, follow-up studies of girls with CD suggest that they are at high risk for other adjustment problems as adults, such as (1) showing high rates of somatization disorders and other emotional disorders, (2) making suicide attempts, and (3) having severe impairments in their occupational and social adjustment (see Robins et al., 1991; Silverthorn and Frick, 1999; Zoccolillo, 1993).

One of the more consistent predictors of poor outcome for children with CD is the severity of the initial disorder. Importantly, the frequency and intensity of the behavior exhibited, the variety of different types of symptoms displayed, and the presence of symptoms in more than one setting have all been related to a more severe and persistent form of CD (Loeber, 1982). For example, Mitchell and Rosa (1981) found that boys rated by both parents and teachers as evidencing stealing or lying were between two and six times more likely to show chronic criminal behavior as adults than boys rated by only one of these informants as showing these symptoms. As mentioned previously, children with the childhood-onset form of CD are more likely to show a chronic and stable pattern of behavior than children in the adolescent-onset group (Moffitt, 2003; Patterson, 1993; Robins, 1966). For example, in a prospective study of the adult outcomes of a birth cohort in New Zealand, Moffitt et al. (2002) reported that the adolescent-onset group was 50 percent to 60 percent less likely to be convicted of an offense and their offenses tended to be less serious (e.g., minor theft, public drunkenness) and less violent (e.g., property offenses) than children whose chronic conduct problems started prior to adolescence.

There is much less research on whether the distinction between children in the childhood-onset group with and without CU traits predict differences in later antisocial behavior (Edens et al., 2001). There are several notable exceptions in which the predictive utility of these traits has been tested in samples of institutionalized adolescents. These studies have documented that CU traits predict subsequent delinquency, aggression, number of violent offenses, and a shorter length of time to violent reoffending in antisocial youth (Brandt et al., 1997; Forth et al., 1990; Toupin et al., 1995). In a community sample of non-referred children, children with conduct problems who also showed CU traits showed more severe and more instrumental aggression one year later compared to children with conduct problems but without these features (Frick et al., 2003a), and the group with CU traits showed more stable conduct problems, higher rates of self-reported delinquency, and more parent-reported police contacts across a four-year study period (Frick et al., 2005).

In their review of longitudinal studies investigating the outcome of youth with severe conduct problems, Frick and Loney (1999) documented several other predictors of stability that have consistently emerged across studies. As noted previously, the presence of a comorbid diagnosis of ADHD has been associated with a more severe and chronic form of CD. Low intelligence, especially low verbal intelligence, a family history of antisocial behavior, other aspects of the family functioning (e.g., the quality of supervision that the child's parent provided, harsh discipline, parental conflict, low maternal affection), and low socioeconomic status of the family all have predicted later antisocial behavior in longitudinal studies of children with conduct problems.

Clinical implications

Effective treatments

Reviews of the treatment outcome literature have documented four treatments with proven effectiveness for reducing conduct problems in youth in controlled treatment trials (see Brestan and Eyberg, 1998; Frick, 1998; Kazdin, 1995). The first intervention with proven efficacy involves the use of contingency management programs. The theoretical rationale for this type of treatment has typically focused on the contention that many children with ODD or CD come from families in which they have not been exposed to a consistent and contingent environment and this poor socialization experience plays a major role in their inability to modulate behavior (e.g., delay gratification, conform to parental and societal expectations: Patterson, 1986). A structured behavior management system is designed to overcome these deficiencies in socialization. However, another rationale that is also consistent with existing research is that some children with conduct problems have a temperamental vulnerability that leads them to be more susceptible to a non-contingent environment, such as being overfocused on the potential positive consequences of their behavior (e.g., obtaining a stereo) at the expense of considering the potential negative consequences (e.g., being arrested for stealing, affecting the livelihood of the store owner: Barry et al., 2000; Pardini et al., 2003).

The basic structure of contingency management programs is deceptively simple. These programs all involve (a) establishing clear behavioral goals that gradually shape more prosocial behavior, (b) developing a system of monitoring whether the child is reaching these goals, (c) having a system of reinforcing appropriate steps toward reaching these goals, and (d) providing consequences for inappropriate behavior. These programs have proven to bring about behavioral changes for children with conduct problems in a number of different settings such as at home (Ross, 1981), at school (Abramowitz and O'Leary, 1991), and in residential treatment centers (Lyman and Campbell, 1996). Although they appear quite simple and straightforward, many behavioral management programs are not used in a way that makes them effective. For example, these programs need to be individualized for children both in terms of the selection of appropriate goals for the child and in terms of the types of reinforcers and punishment that will motivate the child. In addition, many programs do not define goals in a way that allows for systematic monitoring of whether the child is meeting them. Further, many of these systems are typically used solely for behavioral control, in which negative consequences for inappropriate behavior are provided (e.g., loss of points for misbehavior) without a method for systematically encouraging positive behavioral changes (e.g., gaining points for appropriate expression of anger). Finally, it has been very difficult to find methods for having the behavioral changes brought about by the contingency management programs generalize to situations in which the consistent and structured contingencies are not operating.

The second treatment that has proven to be effective for many children with conduct problems is Parent Management Training (PMT). A critical focus of PMT programs is to teach parents how to develop and implement very structured contingency management programs in the home. However, PMT programs also focus on (a) improving the quality of parent–child interactions (e.g., having parents more involved in their children's activities, improving parent–child communication, increasing parental warmth and responsiveness), (b) changing antecedents to behavior that enhance the likelihood that positive prosocial behaviors will be displayed by children (e.g., how to time and present requests, providing clear and explicit rules and expectations), (c) improving parents' ability to monitor and supervise their children, and (d) using more effective discipline strategies (e.g., being more consistent in discipline, using a variety of approaches to discipline).

Of all of the interventions used to treat children with conduct problems, the effectiveness of PMT interventions has been the most consistently documented of any technique (Kazdin, 1995). However, a key limitation in these approaches to treatment has been the large number of parents who do not complete these programs and the lack of effectiveness for the most dysfunctional families (Kazdin, 1995; Miller and Prinz, 1990). As a result, to increase the effectiveness of these interventions, it is important to focus on methods of engaging families in the intervention and to consider the broader family context, which may include factors that could prevent parents from utilizing the techniques taught in the PMT programs (e.g., parental depression, high rates of marital conflict: Miller and Prinz, 1990). A useful guide for enhancing parental engagement and determining how parenting issues are embedded in the broader family context is an approach to family therapy called Functional Family Therapy (Alexander and Parsons, 1982). This approach to treatment has been shown to be effective in treating older children and adolescents with CD in severely distressed families from a diversity of ethnic and socio-economic backgrounds (Alexander et al., 1994; Gordon et al., 1995).

The third type of intervention that has proven effective in treating children with conduct problems is a cognitive-behavioral approach designed to overcome deficits in social cognition and deficits in social problem-solving experienced by many children and adolescents with CD. Research on children with conduct problems has consistently documented deficits in the way these children process social information, including the way they encode social cues, interpret these cues, develop social goals, develop appropriate responses, decide on appropriate responses, and enact appropriate responses (see Dodge and Pettit, 2003, for a review). For example, some severely aggressive children tend to attribute hostile intent to ambiguous provocation situations with peers making them more likely to act aggressively towards peers (Frick et al., 2003b). Other aggressive children tend to associate more positive outcomes for their aggressive behavior making them more likely to select aggressive alternatives to solving peer conflict (Pardini et al., 2003).

Most cognitive-behavioral programs include some method of having a child inhibit impulsive or angry responding. This allows the child to go through a series of problem-solving steps (e.g., how to recognize problems, how to consider alternative responses and select the most adaptive one) to deal more effectively with problems encountered in peer interactions. Also, these cognitive-behavior programs are explicitly skills-building approaches to intervention. The therapist plays a very active role in these programs, such as modeling the skills being taught, role-playing social situations with the child, prompting the use of the skills being taught, and delivering feedback and praise for the appropriate use of the skills. Most of the programs are designed to be provided in a group format. However, given the potential dangers in having antisocial individuals interact in groups (Dishion et al., 1999), the groups are kept very small, the group interactions are very structured in content, and contingency management programs are typically used to promote the use of skills and limit inappropriate behaviors. A key limitation in the effectiveness of most cognitive behavioral programs is the difficulty in getting children to use the skills learned in the program outside of the therapeutic setting (Kendall et al., 1990) and to maintain the skills over extended periods of time after the intervention has ended (Lochman, 1992). To enhance generalization, several programs have been designed to be implemented outside of the typical mental health delivery setting, such as in schools (Bierman and Greenberg, 1996), so that the skills are taught in an environment in which they will be used. Also, most programs include the practice of skills in a variety of settings to also promote generalization. Most importantly, however, all of the programs involve people in the child's natural environment, such as parents and teachers, to prompt and encourage use of these skills outside of the therapeutic context.

The final intervention that has proven to be effective for reducing conduct problems is the use of stimulant medication. As mentioned previously, a large proportion (between 60 percent and 90 percent) of clinic-referred children with conduct problems also show ADHD. The impulsivity associated with ADHD may directly lead to some of the aggressive and other poorly regulated behaviors of children with conduct problems (Frick and Morris, 2004). In addition, the presence of ADHD may indirectly contribute to the development of conduct problems through its effect on children's interactions with peers and significant others (e.g., parents and teachers), or through its effect on the parents' ability to use effective socialization strategies, or through its effect on a child's ability to perform academically (Dodge and Pettit, 2003; Frick, 1998). Therefore, for many children and adolescents with conduct problems, reducing ADHD symptoms is an important treatment goal.

One of the more successful treatments for ADHD is the use of stimulant medication (Pelham, 1993). The effectiveness of stimulants for reducing conduct problems in children with both ADHD and CD has been shown in several controlled medication trials (Hinshaw, 1991; Hinshaw et al., 1992; Pelham et al., 1993). For example, in a very structured classroom setting, Ritalin significantly decreased the rate of disruptive classroom behaviors, which included verbal and physical aggression, teasing, destruction of property, and cheating (Hinshaw et al., 1992). In fact, medication was somewhat more effective in reducing the level of these conduct problems than a very intensive contingency management system. This positive effect for medication in reducing conduct problem behavior has been replicated in a large treatment trial of 579 children rigorously diagnosed with ADHD (Jensen et al., 2001; Swanson et al., 2001). Importantly, this trial also suggested that combining stimulant medication with psychosocial treatments, including PMT and contingency management systems, leads to somewhat better outcomes in reducing conduct problem behavior than the use of medication alone.

Limitations in existing treatment approaches

Although each of the four interventions summarized above has proven to be effective in reducing the conduct problems associated with diagnoses of either ODD or CD, even these efficacious treatments have a number of substantial limitations (Kazdin, 1995). First, a significant proportion of children with CD do not show a significant response to these interventions and, for those that do respond, their behavior problems are often not reduced to a normative level. Second, the greatest degree of improvement seems to be in the treatment of younger children (prior to age 8) with less severe behavioral disturbances. Although this finding highlights the need to focus on the prevention of CD in young children who are beginning to show problematic behaviors, it also suggests that there is a need for better interventions for older children and adolescents with more severe conduct problems. Third, with some notable exceptions (McNeil et al., 1991), the generalizability of treatment effects across settings tends to be poor. That is, treatments that are effective in changing a child's behavior in one setting (e.g., mental health clinics) often do not bring about changes in the child's behavior in other settings (e.g., schools). Fourth, and also with some notable exceptions (Long et al., 1994), improvements brought about in the behavior of children with CD are often difficult to maintain over time. This seems to be particularly true of older children with severe conduct problems (Lochman, 1992) and for children from very dysfunctional family environments (Kazdin, 1995; Serketich and Dumas, 1996).

Given these rather substantial limitations, there has been an increasing focus on comparing how well these existing treatments match what we know about how conduct problems develop and using this research base to guide the development of innovative approaches to intervention (Frick, 1998, 2001). Each of the four treatments described above target basic processes that research has shown to be important in the development of conduct problems. However, these treatments have ignored two important additional characteristics of children with ODD or CD. First, they ignore the multi-determined nature of conduct problems. As noted previously, for most children and adolescents who develop ODD or CD, the conduct problems are associated with a number of different types of risk factors. As a result, interventions that target only one type of risk factor (e.g., parenting, impulsivity) will address only one of a myriad of potential factors contributing to the child's behavioral problems. Second, as also noted previously, research suggests that there are multiple pathways, each with somewhat unique causal processes, underlying the development of conduct problems. As a result, any single intervention, even if it is comprehensive, is not likely to be effective for all children with ODD or CD.

The overarching implication is that there is not likely to be any single "best" treatment for children with conduct problems. Instead, interventions must be tailored to the individual needs of a child with ODD or CD and these needs will likely differ depending on the specific mechanisms underlying the child's behavioral disturbance. As noted previously, children with an adolescent-onset to their conduct problem behavior seem to have very different causal processes leading to their behavioral difficulties than those with a childhood-onset. Further, within the childhood-onset group, there appear to be important differences between those who show a callous-unemotional interpersonal style and those who do not. As a result, different interventions are likely needed for children in these various groups (see Frick, 1998, 2001, for specific examples).

Comprehensive and individualized approaches to treatment

By integrating research on developmental models of conduct problems with empirically supported treatments, several general principles for designing and implementing interventions for children with severe conduct problems appear important. First, one must understand the multiple causal processes that can be involved in the development of conduct problems. For example, by recognizing the developmental progressions that often characterize children and adolescents with CD, interventions can be implemented as early as possible in the developmental sequence. In addition, this knowledge base can help in determining which processes may be involved in the development of CD for a particular child and can guide decisions as to the most important targets of interventions. Second, this flexible approach to treatment requires a clear, comprehensive, and individualized case conceptualization that guides the design of a focused and integrated approach to treatment (Frick and McCoy, 2001). A case conceptualization is a "theory" about the factors most likely involved in the development, exacerbation, and maintenance of conduct problems for an individual child or adolescent. It uses the research on developmental pathways to conduct problems and attempts to apply it to an individual child with ODD or CD. Third, successful intervention for children and adolescents with severe conduct problems typically involves multiple professionals and multiple community agencies all working together to provide a comprehensive and integrated intervention.

This comprehensive and individualized approach to intervention outlined here and elsewhere (Frick, 1998, 2001) has not been subjected to controlled outcome evaluations. However, one approach to treatment that incorporates many of the features of this developmental approach to treatment and that has been tested in controlled outcome studies is Multi-Systemic Therapy (MST). MST was originally developed as a general approach to intervention for psychopathological conditions (Henggeler and Borduin, 1990) but has been applied extensively to the treatment of severe antisocial behavior in children and adolescents (Henggeler et al., 1998). The orientation of MST is an expansion of a systems orientation to family therapy. In systemic family therapy, problems in children's adjustment are viewed as being embedded within the larger family context. MST expands this notion to include other contexts, such as the child's peer group, school and neighborhood. MST is not explicitly developmental in orientation. For example, it does not emphasize the individual child's characteristics that may contribute to the development of severe conduct problems and that may play a role in shaping his or her psychosocial contexts (e.g., the influence of the child on his or her family environment). Nonetheless, MST does emphasize a comprehensive and individualized approach to intervention.

MST involves an initial comprehensive assessment that seeks to understand the level and severity of the child or adolescent's presenting problems and to understand how these problems may be related to factors in the child's familial, peer, and cultural environment. The information from this assessment is used to outline an individualized treatment plan based on the specific needs of the child and his or her family. A critical component of MST is a system of intensive supervision for the therapists implementing the treatment to determine how the basic components of the intervention should be implemented to meet the needs of each family (Henggeler et al., 1998).

One of the important contributions of MST to the treatment outcome literature is its demonstration that individualized interventions can be rigorously evaluated through controlled treatment outcome studies. The initial findings on the effectiveness of MST suggest that it is one of the most successful interventions for reducing severe antisocial and aggressive behavior among older youth (Henggeler et al., 1992). For example, in a controlled treatment outcome study of MST at a university-based outpatient clinic, 88 adolescent repeat juvenile offenders underwent MST. To illustrate the individualized nature of the treatment, the length of treatment with MST ranged from 5 to 54 hours (mean of 23 hours). In addition to this variation in intensity, the way in which these hours were utilized varied depending on the needs of the clients: 83 percent of the MST group participated in family therapy, 60 percent participated in some form of school intervention (e.g., facilitation of parent–teacher communication, academic remediation, or help in classroom behavior management), 57 percent received some form of peer intervention, and 28 percent received individual therapy which typically involved some form of cognitive-behavioral skills building intervention. Additionally, in 26 percent of the cases, the adolescent's parents became involved in marital therapy. The outcomes of the group of offenders receiving MST were compared to a control group of 68 offenders who received traditional outpatient services, typically involving individual psychotherapy

(Borduin et al., 1995). At a four-year follow-up, only 26 percent of the youth who underwent MST were rearrested compared to 71 percent of the control adolescents.

Summary and conclusion

As mentioned previously, externalizing disorders of children constitute one of the most common reasons that children are referred to mental health clinics for treatment (Frick and Silverthorn, 2001). This fact is not surprising given the disruptions that children with these disorders often cause to those around them, especially to parents and teachers who are most likely to refer a child for treatment. Further, given the association between externalizing disorders and many costly and impairing outcomes (e.g., substance abuse, delinquency), understanding and effectively treating children with these disorders is an important endeavor for psychologists and other mental health professionals.

Fortunately, there is a large body of research on children with severe conduct problems. As summarized in this chapter, research has led to great advances in our understanding of the causes of these disorders and the development of effective interventions to prevent and treat them. Unfortunately, this research is often not translated well into practice and, as a result, many children with these disorders do not receive state-of-the-art treatment. This gap between research and practice can be the result of a number of factors (Frick, 2000). For example, it can be the result of practitioners not being trained on the most current theories and approaches to treatment or not remaining current on this research. Alternatively, the gap between research and practice can be the result of research not being conducted or presented in a way that is useful to the practicing psychologist. In either case, the quality of services provided to children with ODD or CD depends heavily on advances in research and in our ability to translate these findings into widely used applications. The focus of this chapter was to summarize research on children with conduct problems in a way that promotes such a translation.

Perhaps the most important advance in recent research is the recognition that severe conduct problems, such as those displayed by children with ODD and CD, are (a) often the result of multiple interacting risk factors and (b) these interacting factors may be very different for various groups of children with conduct problems. Further, research has begun to identify some of the important causal pathways that can lead to severe conduct problems. To summarize, there appears to be one group of children with CD who begin showing serious antisocial behaviors coinciding with the onset of adolescence and these youth seem to show an exaggeration of the normal developmental process of adolescent rebellion. In contrast, there is another group of children with CD who begin by showing oppositional behaviors early in life and whose behavior worsens into more and more severe conduct problems over the course of development. These children with childhood-onset CD seem to have a more characterological disturbance that transcends a single developmental stage. Further, they can be divided into (a) those who seem to show a deficit in conscience development and are characterized by a callous and unemotional interpersonal style and (b) those who show very impulsive and emotionally dysregulated behaviors without this callous and unemotional style.

Additional research on youth with severe conduct problems is needed to clarify even further the developmental mechanisms that lead to the problem behaviors for children in each of these groups. Also, other pathways may be uncovered that better explain the development of conduct problems for some children. Most importantly, however, there is the urgent need for this research to inform prevention and treatment programs for severely aggressive and antisocial youth. It clearly suggests that treatments that focus on a single process or that attempt to provide the same intervention to all youth with ODD or CD are not likely to be highly successful. There are a number of promising models of comprehensive and individualized approaches to treatment being developed and tested. Such programs provide great hope and optimism that effective treatments for this very chronic, impairing, and costly form of psychopathology are on the immediate horizon.

References

Abikoff, H. and Klein, R.G. (1992). Attention-deficit hyperactivity and conduct disorder: Comorbidity and implications for treatment. *Journal of Consulting and Clinical Psychology, 60,* 881–892.

Abramowitz, A.J. and O'Leary, S.G. (1991). Behavioral interventions for the classroom: Implications for students with ADHD. *School Psychology Review, 20,* 220–234.

Alexander, J.F. and Parsons, B.V. (1982). *Functional family therapy.* Monterey, CA: Brooks-Cole.

Alexander, J.F., Hotzworth-Munroe, A., and Jameson, P.B. (1994). The process and outcome of marital and family therapy research: Review and evaluation. In A.E. Bergin and S.L. Garfield (Eds.), *Handbook of psychotherapy and behavior change,* 4th edn (pp. 595–630). New York: Wiley.

American Psychiatric Association (APA) (2000). *Diagnostic and statistical manual of mental disorders,* 4th edn, text revision. Washington, DC: APA.

Anderson, J.C., Williams, S., McGee, R., and Silva, P.A. (1987). DSM-III disorders in preadolescent children. *Archives of General Psychiatry, 44,* 69–76.

Asendorf, J.B. and Nunner-Winkler, G. (1992). Children's moral motive strength and temperamental inhibition reduce their egoistic behavior in real moral conflicts. *Child Development, 63,* 1223–1235.

Barkley, R.A., Fischer, M., Smallish, L., and Fletcher, K. (2002). The persistence of attention-deficit/hyperactivity disorder into young adulthood as a function of reporting source and definition of disorder. *Journal of Abnormal Psychology, 111,* 279–289.

Barry, C.T., Frick, P.J., Grooms, T., McCoy, M.G., Ellis, M.L., and Loney, B.R. (2000). The importance of callous-unemotional traits for extending the concept of psychopathy to children. *Journal of Abnormal Psychology, 109,* 335–340.

Bierman, K.L. and Greenberg, M.T. (1996). Social skills training in the FAST Track program. In R.D. Peters and R.J. McMahon (Eds.), *Preventing childhood disorders, substance abuse, and delinquency* (pp. 65–89). Thousand Oaks, CA: Sage.

Blair, R.J.R. (1995). A cognitive developmental approach to morality: Investigating the psychopath. *Cognition, 57,* 1–29.

Blair, R.J.R. (1999). Responsiveness to distress cues in the child with psychopathic tendencies. *Personality and Individual Differences*, *27*, 135–145.

Blair, R.J.R., Jones, L., Clark, F., and Smith, M. (1997). The psychopathic individual: A lack of responsiveness to distress cues? *Psychophysiology*, *34*, 192–198.

Blair, R.J.R., Colledge, E., Murray, L., and Mitchell, D.G.V. (2001). A selective impairment in the processing of sad and fearful expressions in children with psychopathic tendencies. *Journal of Abnormal Child Psychology*, *29*, 491–498.

Borduin, C.M., Mann, B.J., Cone, L.T., Henggeler, S.W., Fucci, B.R., Blaske, D.M., et al. (1995). Multisystemic treatment of serious juvenile offenders: Long term prevention of criminality and violence. *Journal of Consulting and Clinical Psychology*, *63*, 569–578.

Brandt, J.R., Kennedy, W.A., Patrick, C.J., and Curtin, J.J. (1997). Assessment of psychopathy in a population of incarcerated adolescent offenders. *Psychological Assessment*, *9*, 429–435.

Brestan, E.V. and Eyberg, S.M. (1998). Effective psychosocial treatments conduct disordered children and adolescents. *Journal of Clinical Child Psychology*, *27*, 180–189.

Cantwell, D.P. and Baker, L. (1992). Attention deficit disorder with and without hyperactivity: A review and comparison of matched groups. *Journal of the American Academy of Child and Adolescent Psychiatry*, *31*, 432–438.

Capaldi, D.M. (1992). The co-occurrence of conduct problems and depressive symptoms in early adolescent boys, II: A 2-year follow-up at grade 8. *Development and Psychopathology*, *4*, 125–144.

Caputo, A.A., Frick, P.J., and Brodsky, S.L. (1999). Family violence and juvenile sex offending: Potential mediating roles of psychopathic traits and negative attitudes toward women. *Criminal Justice and Behavior*, *26*, 338–356.

Christian, R., Frick, P.J., Hill, N., Tyler, L.A., and Frazer, D. (1997). Psychopathy and conduct problems in children: II. Subtyping children with conduct problems based on their interpersonal and affective style. *Journal of the American Academy of Child and Adolescent Psychiatry*, *36*, 233–241.

Cohen, M.A. (1998). The monetary value of saving a high-risk youth. *Journal of Quantitative Criminology*, *14*, 5–33.

Cohen, P., Cohen, J., Kasen, S., Velez, C.N., Hartmark, C., Johnson, J., et al. (1993). An epidemiological study of disorders in late childhood and adolescence, I: age and gender-specific prevalence. *Journal of Child Psychology and Psychiatry*, *34*, 851–867.

Costello, E.J., Costello, A.J., Edelbrock, C., Burns, B.J., Dulcan, M.K., Brent, D., et al. (1988). Psychiatric disorders in pediatric primary care. *Archives of General Psychiatry*, *45*, 1107–1116.

Crick, N.R. and Grotpeter, J.K. (1995). Relational aggression, gender, and social-psychological adjustment. *Child Development*, *66*, 710–722.

Dishion, T.J., McCord, J., and Poulin, F. (1999). When interventions harm: Peer groups and problem behavior. *American Psychologist*, *54*, 755–764.

Dodge, K.A. and Pettit, G.S. (2003). A biopsychosocial model of the development of chronic conduct problems in adolescence. *Developmental Psychology*, *39*, 349–371.

Edens, J., Skeem, J., Cruise, K., and Cauffman, E. (2001). The assessment of juvenile psychopathy and its association with violence: A critical review. *Behavioral Sciences and the Law*, *19*, 53–80.

Fabrega, J.H., Ulrich, R., and Mezzich, J.E. (1993). Do Caucasian and Black adolescents differ at psychiatric intake? *Journal of the American Academy of Child and Adolescent Psychiatry*, *32*, 407–413.

Fisher, L. and Blair, R.J.R. (1998). Cognitive impairment and its relationship to psychopathic tendencies in children with emotional and behavioral difficulties. *Journal of Abnormal Child Psychology, 26,* 511–519.

Forth, A.E., Hart, S.D., and Hare, R.D. (1990). Assessment of psychopathy in male young offenders. *Psychological Assessment, 2,* 342–344.

Frick, P.J. (1998). *Conduct disorders and severe antisocial behavior.* New York: Plenum.

Frick, P.J. (2000). Laboratory and performance-based measures of childhood disorders. *Journal of Clinical Child Psychology, 29,* 475–478.

Frick, P.J. (2001). Effective interventions for children and adolescents with conduct disorder. *Canadian Journal of Psychiatry, 46,* 26–37.

Frick, P.J. and Ellis, M.L. (1999). Callous-unemotional traits and subtypes of conduct disorder. *Clinical Child and Family Psychology Review, 2,* 149–168.

Frick, P.J. and Loney, B.R. (1999). Outcomes of children and adolescents with conduct disorder and oppositional defiant disorder. In H.C. Quay and A. Hogan (Eds.), *Handbook of disruptive behavior disorders* (pp. 507–524). New York: Plenum.

Frick, P.J. and McCoy, M.G. (2001). Conduct disorder. In H. Orvaschel, J. Faust, and M. Hersen (Eds.), *Handbook of conceptualization and treatment of child psychopathology* (pp. 57–76). Oxford: Elsevier Science.

Frick, P.J. and Morris, A.S. (2004). Temperament and developmental pathways to conduct problems. *Journal of Clinical Child and Adolescent Psychology, 33,* 54–68.

Frick, P.J. and Silverthorn, P. (2001). Psychopathology in children. In P.B. Sutker and H.E. Adams (Eds.), *Comprehensive handbook of psychopathology,* 3rd edn (pp. 881–920). New York: Kluwer.

Frick, P.J., Lahey, B., Christ, M.A.G., Loeber, R., and Green, S. (1991). History of childhood behavior problems in biological parents of boys with attention-deficit hyperactivity disorder and conduct disorder. *Journal of Clinical Child Psychology, 20,* 445–451.

Frick, P.J., O'Brien, B.S., Wootton, J.M., and McBurnett, K. (1994). Psychopathy and conduct problems in children. *Journal of Abnormal Psychology, 103,* 700–707.

Frick, P.J., Lilienfeld, S.O., Ellis, M.L., Loney, B.R., and Silverthorn, P. (1999). The association between anxiety and psychopathy dimensions in children. *Journal of Abnormal Child Psychology, 27,* 381–390.

Frick, P.J., Bodin, S.D., and Barry, C.T. (2000). Psychopathic traits and conduct problems in community and clinic-referred samples of children: Further development of the Psychopathy Screening Device. *Psychological Assessment, 12,* 382–393.

Frick, P.J., Cornell, A.H., Barry, C.T., Bodin, S.D., and Dane, H.A. (2003a). Callous-unemotional traits and conduct problems in the prediction of conduct problem severity, aggression, and self-report of delinquency. *Journal of Abnormal Child Psychology, 31,* 457–470.

Frick, P.J., Cornell, A.H., Bodin, S.D., Dane, H.A., Barry, C.T., and Loney, B.R. (2003b). Callous-unemotional traits and developmental pathways to severe conduct problems. *Developmental Psychology, 39,* 246–260.

Frick, P.J., Stickle, T.R., Dandreaux, D.M., Farrell, J.M., and Kimonis, E.R. (2005). Callous-unemotional traits in predicting the severity and stability of conduct problems and delinquency. *Journal of Abnormal Child Psychology, 33,* 471–487.

Gauvain, M. and Fagot, B.I. (1995). Child temperament as a mediator of mother–toddler problem-solving. *Social Development, 4,* 257–276.

Gordon, D.A., Graves, K., and Arbuthnot, J. (1995). The effect of functional family therapy for delinquents on adult criminal behavior. *Criminal Justice and Behavior, 22*, 60–73.

Gottfredson, G.D. and Gottfredson, D.C. (2001). What schools do to prevent problem behavior and promote safe environments. *Journal of Educational and Psychological Consultation, 12*, 313–344.

Henggeler, S.W. and Borduin, C.M. (1990). *Family therapy and beyond: A multisystemic approach to treating the behavior problems of children and adolescents*. Pacific Grove, CA: Brooks/Cole.

Henggeler, S.W., Melton, G.B., and Smith, L.A. (1992). Family preservation using multisystemic therapy: An effective alternative to incarcerating juvenile offenders. *Journal of Consulting and Clinical Psychology, 60*, 953–961.

Henggeler, S.W., Schoenwald, S.K., Borduin, C.M., Rowland, M.D., and Cunningham, P.B. (1998). *Multisytemic treatment of antisocial behavior in children and adolescents*. New York: Guilford.

Hinshaw, S.P. (1991). Stimulant medication and the treatment of aggression in children with attention deficits. *Journal of Clinical Child Psychology, 20*, 301–312.

Hinshaw, S.P. (1992). Externalizing behavior problems and academic underachievement in childhood and adolescence: Causal relationships and underlying mechanisms. *Psychological Bulletin, 111*, 127–155.

Hinshaw, S.P., Heller, T., and McHale, J.P. (1992). Covert antisocial behavior in boys with attention-deficit hyperactivity disorder: External validation and effects of methylphenidate. *Journal of Consulting and Clinical Psychology, 60*, 274–281.

Hinshaw, S.P., Lahey, B.B., and Hart, E.L. (1993). Issues of taxonomy and co-morbidity in the development of conduct disorder. *Development and Psychopathology, 5*, 31–50.

Hubbard, J.A., Smithmyer, C.M., Ramsden, S.R., Parker, E.H., Flanagan, K.D., Dearing, K.F., et al. (2002). Observational, physiological, and self-report measures of children's anger: Relations to reactive versus proactive aggression. *Child Development, 73*, 1101–1118.

Jensen, P.S., Hinshaw, S.P., Swanson, J.M., Greenhill, L.L., Conners, C.K., Arnold, L.E., et al. (2001). Findings from the NIMH Multimodal Treatment Study of ADHD (MTA): Implications and applications for primary care providers. *Journal of Developmental and Behavioral Pediatrics, 22*, 60–73.

Kagan, J. (1998). Biology and the child. In N. Eisenberg (Ed.), *Handbook of child psychology: Vol. 3. Social, emotional, and personality development* (pp. 177–235). New York: Wiley.

Kagan, J. and Snidman, N. (1991). Temperamental factors in human development. *American Psychologist, 46*, 856–862.

Kazdin, A.E. (1995). *Conduct disorders in childhood and adolescence*, 2nd edn. Thousand Oaks, CA: Sage.

Keenan, K. and Shaw, D.S. (1997). Developmental and social influences on young girls' behavioral and emotional problems. *Psychological Bulletin, 121*, 95–113.

Kendall, P.C., Reber, M., McLeer, S., Epps, J., and Ronan, K.R. (1990). Cognitive-behavioral treatment of conduct disordered children. *Cognitive Therapy and Research, 14*, 279–297.

Klinteberg, B.A., Andersson, T., Magnusson, D., and Stattin, H. (1993). Hyperactive behavior childhood as related to subsequent alcohol problems and violent offending: A longitudinal study of male subjects. *Personality and Individual Differences, 15*, 381–388.

Kochanska, G. (1993). Toward a synthesis of parental socialization and child temperament in early development of conscience. *Child Development, 64*, 325–347.

Kochanska, G. (1995). Children's temperament, mothers' discipline, and security of attachment: Multiple pathways to emerging internalization. *Child Development, 66*, 597–615.

Kochanska, G., Gross, J.N., Lin, M.H., and Nichols, K.E. (2002). Guilt in young children: Development, determinants, and relations with a broader system of standards. *Child Development, 73*, 461–482.

Kratzer, L. and Hodgins, S. (1997). Adult outcomes of child conduct problems: A cohort study. *Journal of Abnormal Child Psychology, 25*, 65–81.

Kruh, I.P., Frick, P.J., and Clements, C.B. (2005). Historical and personality correlates to the violence patterns of juveniles tried as adults. *Criminal Justice and Behavior, 32*, 69–96.

Lahey, B.B. and Loeber, R. (1994). Framework for a developmental model of oppositional defiant disorder and conduct disorder. In D.K. Routh (Ed.), *Disruptive behavior disorders in childhood* (pp. 139–180). New York: Plenum.

Lahey, B., Loeber, R., Hart, E., Frick, P.J., Applegate, B., Zhang, Q., et al. (1995). Four-year longitudinal study of conduct disorder in boys: Patterns and predictors of persistence. *Journal of Abnormal Psychology, 104*, 83–93.

Lahey, B.B., Miller, T.L., Gordon, R.A., and Riley, A. (1999). Developmental epidemiology of the disruptive behavior disorders. In H. Quay and A. Hogan (Eds.), *Handbook of the disruptive behavior disorders* (pp. 23–48). New York: Plenum.

Lahey, B.B., Schwab-Stone, M., Goodman, S.H., Waldman, I.D., Canino, G., Rathouz, P.J., et al. (2000). Age and gender differences in oppositional behavior and conduct problems: A cross-sectional household study of middle childhood and adolescence. *Journal of Abnormal Psychology, 109*, 488–503.

Lilienfeld, S.O. and Waldman, I.D. (1990). The relation between childhood attention-deficit hyperactivity disorder and adult antisocial behavior reexamined: The problem of heterogeneity. *Clinical Psychology Review, 10*, 699–725.

Lochman, J.E. (1992). Cognitive-behavior intervention with aggressive boys: Three-year follow-up and preventive effects. *Journal of Consulting and Clinical Psychology, 60*, 426–432.

Loeber, R. (1982). The stability of antisocial and delinquent child behavior: A review. *Child Development, 53*, 1431–1446.

Loeber, R. and Farrington, D.P. (2000). Young children who commit crime: Epidemiology, developmental origins, risk factors, early interventions, and policy implications. *Development and Psychopathology, 12*, 737–762.

Loeber, R. and Hay, D.F. (1997). Key issues in the development of aggressive and violence from childhood to early adulthood. *Annual Revue of Psychology, 48*, 371–410.

Loeber, R., Brinthaupt, V.P., and Green, S.M. (1990). Attention deficits, impulsivity, and hyperactivity with or without conduct problems: Relationships to delinquency and unique contextual factors. In R.J. McMahon and R.D. Peters (Eds.), *Behavior disorders of adolescence: Research, intervention, and policy in clinical and school setting* (pp. 39–61). New York: Plenum.

Loeber, R., Green, S.M., Lahey, B.B., Christ, M.A.G., and Frick, P.J. (1992). Developmental sequences in the age of onset of disruptive child behaviors. *Journal of Child and Family Studies, 1*, 21–41.

Loeber, R., Burke, J.D., Lahey, B.B., Winters, A., and Zera, M. (2000). Oppositional defiant and conduct disorder: A review of the past 10 years, part I. *Journal of the American Academy of Child and Adolescent Psychiatry*, *39*, 1468–1482.

Loney, B. R., Frick, P.J., Ellis, M., and McCoy, M. G. (1998). Intelligence, psychopathy, and antisocial behavior. *Journal of Psychopathology and Behavioral Assessment*, *20*, 231–247.

Loney, B.R., Frick, P.J., Clements, C.B., Ellis, M.L., and Kerlin, K. (2003). Callous-unemotional traits, impulsivity, and emotional processing in antisocial adolescents. *Journal of Clinical Child and Adolescent Psychology*, *32*, 139–152.

Long, P., Forehand, R., Wierson, M., and Morgan, A. (1994). Does parent training with young noncompliant children have long-term effects? *Behavior Research and Therapy*, *32*, 101–107.

Lyman, R.D. and Campbell, N.R. (1996). *Treating children and adolescents in residential and inpatient settings*. Thousand Oaks, CA: Sage.

Lynam, D.R. (1996). The early identification of chronic offenders: Who is the fledgling psychopath? *Psychological Bulletin*, *120*, 209–234.

Lynskey, M.T. and Fergusson, D.M. (1995). Childhood conduct problems, attention deficit behaviors, and adolescent alcohol, tobacco, and illicit drug use. *Journal of Abnormal Child Psychology*, *23*, 281–302.

McCoy, M.G., Frick, P.J., Loney, B.R., and Ellis, M.L. (2000). The potential mediating role of parenting practices in the development of conduct problems in a clinic-referred sample. *Journal of Child and Family Studies*, *8*, 477–494.

McNeil, C.B., Eyberg, S., Eisenstadt, T.H., Newcomb, K., and Funderburk, B.W. (1991). Parent–child interaction therapy with behavior problem children: Generalization of treatment effects to the school setting. *Journal of Clinical Child Psychology*, *20*, 140–151.

Maughan, B., Pickles, A., Hagell, A., Rutter, M., and Yule, W. (1996). Reading problems and antisocial behaviour: Developmental trends in comorbidity. *Journal of Child Psychology and Psychiatry and Allied Disciplines*, *37*, 408–415.

Miller, G.E. and Prinz, R.J. (1990). Enhancement of social learning family interventions for childhood conduct disorder. *Psychological Bulletin*, *108*, 291–307.

Mitchell, S. and Rosa, P. (1981). Boyhood behavior problems as precursors of criminality: A fifteen year follow-up study. *Journal of Child Psychology and Psychiatry*, *22*, 19–33.

Moffitt, T.E. (1993). Adolescence-limited and life-course persistent antisocial behavior: A developmental taxonomy. *Psychological Review*, *100*, 674–701.

Moffitt, T.E. (2003). Life-course persistent and adolescence-limited antisocial behavior: A 10-year research review and research agenda. In B.B. Lahey, T.E. Moffitt and A. Caspi (Eds.), *Causes of conduct disorder and juvenile delinquency* (pp. 49–75). New York: Guilford.

Moffitt, T.E. and Caspi, A. (2001). Childhood predictors differentiate life-course persistent and adolescence-limited antisocial pathways among males and females. *Development and Psychopathology*, *13*, 355–375.

Moffitt, T.E., Caspi, A., Dickson, N., Silva, P., and Stanton, W. (1996). Childhood-onset versus adolescent-onset antisocial conduct problems in males: Natural history from ages 3 to 18 years. *Development and Psychopathology*, *8*, 399–424.

Moffitt, T.E., Caspi, A., Harrington, H., and Milne, B.J. (2002). Males on the life-course persistent and adolescent-limited antisocial pathways: Follow-up at age 26 years. *Development and Psychopathology*, *14*, 179–207.

O'Brien, B.S. and Frick, P.J. (1996). Reward dominance: Associations with anxiety, conduct problems and psychopathy in children. *Journal of Abnormal Child Psychology*, *24*, 223–240.

Offord, D.R., Boyle, M.H., Szatmari, P., Rae-Grant, N.I., Links, P.S., Cadman, D.T., et al. (1987). Ontario Child Health Study: II. Six-month prevalence of disorder and rates of service utilization. *Archives of General Psychiatry*, *44*, 832–836.

Oxford, M., Cavell, T.A., and Hughes, J.N. (2003). Callous-unemotional traits moderate the relation between ineffective parenting and child externalizing problems: A partial replication and extension. *Journal of Clinical Child and Adolescent Psychology*, *32*, 577–585.

Panak, W.F. and Garber, J. (1992). Role of aggression, rejection, and attributions in the prediction of depression in children. *Development and Psychopathology*, *4*, 145–165.

Pardini, D.A., Lochman, J.E., and Frick, P.J. (2003). Callous/unemotional traits and social cognitive processes in adjudicated youth. *Journal of the American Academy of Child and Adolescent Psychiatry*, *42*, 364–371.

Patterson, G.R. (1986). Performance models for antisocial boys. *American Psychologist*, *41*, 432–444.

Patterson, G.R. (1993). Orderly change in a stable world: The antisocial trait as a chimera. *Journal of Consulting and Clinical Psychology*, *61*, 911–919.

Patterson, G.R., Reid, J.B., and Dishion, T.J. (1992). *Antisocial boys*. Eugene, OR: Castilia.

Peeples, F. and Loeber, R. (1994). Do individual factors and neighborhood context explain ethnic differences in juvenile delinquency? *Journal of Quantitative Criminology*, *10*, 141–158.

Pelham, W.E. (1993). Pharmacotherapy for children with attention-deficit hyperactivity disorder. *School Psychology Review*, *22*, 199–227.

Pelham, W.E., Carlson, C., Sams, S.E., Vallan, G., Dixon, M.J., and Hoza, B. (1993). Separate and combined effects of methylphenidate and behavior modification on boys with attention deficit-hyperactivity disorder in the classroom. *Journal of Consulting and Clinical Psychology*, *61*, 506–515.

Raine, A. (2002). Biosocial studies of antisocial and violent behavior in children and adults: A review. *Journal of Abnormal Child Psychology*, *30*, 311–326.

Rayfield, A., Monaco, L., and Eyberg, S. M. (1999). Parent–child interaction therapy with oppositional children: Review and clinical strategies. In S.W. Russ and T.H. Ollendick (Eds.), *Handbook of psychotherapies with children and families*. New York: Kluwer Academic/Plenum.

Robins, L.N. (1966). *Deviant children grown up*. Baltimore, MD: Williams and Wilkins.

Robins, L.N., Tipp, J., and Pryzbeck, T. (1991). Antisocial personality. In L.N. Robins and D.A. Regier (Eds.), *Psychiatric disorders in America* (pp. 224–271). New York: Free Press.

Ross, A.O. (1981). *Child behavior therapy: Principles, procedures, and empirical basis*. New York: Wiley.

Rothbart, M.K. and Bates, J.E. (1998). Temperament. In W. Damon (Ed.), *Handbook of child psychology: Vol. 3, Social, emotional, and personality development* (pp. 105–176). New York: Wiley.

Rothbart, M.K., Ahadi, S.A., and Hershey, K. (1994). Temperament and social behavior in childhood. *Merrill-Palmer Quarterly*, *40*, 21–39.

Russo, M.F. and Beidel, D.C. (1994). Comorbidity of childhood anxiety and externalizing disorders: Prevalence, associated characteristics, and validation issues. *Clinical Psychology Review, 14*, 199–221.

Serketich, W.J. and Dumas, J.E. (1996). The effectiveness of behavioral parent training to modify antisocial behavior in children: A meta-analysis. *Behavior Therapy, 27*, 159–170.

Shaffer, D., Fisher, P., Dulcan, M., and Davies, M. (1996). The NIMH Diagnostic Interview Schedule for Children Version 2.3 (DISC-2.3): Description, acceptability, prevalence rates, and performance in the MECA study. *Journal of the American Academy of Child and Adolescent Psychiatry, 35*, 865–877.

Shields, A. and Cicchetti, D. (1998). Reactive aggression among maltreated children: The contributions of attention and emotion dysregulation. *Journal of Clinical Child Psychology, 27*, 381–395.

Silverthorn, P. and Frick, P.J. (1999). Developmental pathways to antisocial behavior: The delayed-onset pathway in girls. *Development and Psychopathology, 11*, 101–126.

Silverthorn, P., Frick, P.J., and Reynolds, R. (2001). Timing of onset and correlates of severe conduct problems in adjudicated girls and boys. *Journal of Psychopathology and Behavioral Assessment, 23*, 171–181.

Snyder, J.J. and Patterson, G.R. (1995). Individual differences in social aggression: A test of a reinforcement model of socialization in the natural environment. *Behavior Therapy, 26*, 371–391.

Stevens, D., Charman, T., and Blair, R.J.R. (2001). Recognition of emotion in facial expressions and vocal tones in children with psychopathic tendencies. *Journal of Genetic Psychology, 16*, 201–211.

Swanson, J.M., Kraemer, H.C., Hinshaw, S.P., Arnold, L.E., Conners, C.K., Abikoff, H.B., et al. (2001). Clinical relevance of the primary findings of the MTA: Success rates based on severity of ADHD and ODD symptoms at the end of treatment. *Journal of the American Academy of Child and Adolescent Psychiatry, 40*, 168–179.

Toupin, J., Mercier, H., Dery, M., Cote, G., and Hodgins, S. (1995). Validity of the PCL-R for adolescents. *Issues in Criminological and Legal Psychology, 24*, 143–145.

Van Kammen, W.B., Loeber, R., and Stouthamer-Loeber, M. (1991). Substance use and its relationship to conduct problems and delinquency in young boys. *Journal of Youth and Adolescence, 20*, 399–413.

Viding, E., Blair, R.J.R., Moffitt, T.E., and Plomin, R. (2004). Evidence for substantial genetic risk for psychopathy in 7-year-olds. *Journal of Child Psychology and Psychiatry, 45*, 1–6.

Wootton, J.M., Frick, P.J., Shelton, K.K., and Silverthorn, P. (1997). Ineffective parenting and childhood conduct problems: The moderating role of callous-unemotional traits. *Journal of Consulting and Clinical Psychology, 65*, 301–308.

Zigler, E., Taussig, C., and Black, K. (1992). Early childhood intervention: A promising preventative for juvenile delinquency. *American Psychologist, 47*, 997–1006.

Zoccolillo, M. (1993). Gender and the development of conduct disorder. *Development and Psychopathology, 5*, 65–78.

3

ATTENTION-DEFICIT/ HYPERACTIVITY DISORDER

Daniel A. Waschbusch, Brendan F. Andrade, and Sara King

Attention-deficit/hyperactivity disorder (ADHD) is a serious mental health problem of childhood characterized by inattention, hyperactivity, and impulsivity. The term ADD, which later became ADHD, was first coined in the mid 1980s as part of the development of the *Diagnostic and statistical manual of mental disorders* (DSM) by the American Psychiatric Association (APA, 1980, 1987, 1994, 2000). There is a common sentiment among lay audiences and some health professionals that ADHD is a creation of the late twentieth century. However, ADHD actually has a long history. In the late 1700s Dr. Alexander Crichton identified individuals who had problems with "mental restlessness," which he then described as having characteristics that we currently refer to as ADHD (Palmer and Finger, 2001). Similarly, in the early 1900s Dr. George Still described a group of children who had poor inhibition, a lack of self control, excessive activity, high distractibility, and difficulty sustaining attention (Barkley, 1990). In each of these writings, the features of ADHD are clearly present despite the fact that the term ADHD was not applied. This same theme re-emerges throughout the twentieth century: problems with inattention, hyperactivity, and/or impulsivity have been referred to as brain damage, minimal brain damage, minimal brain dysfunction in the 1940s and 1950s; hyperkinetic, hyperkinesis, hyperactive in the 1960s and 1970s; attention-deficit, attention-deficit disorder with or without hyperactivity, and attention deficit/ hyperactive disorder in the 1970s through the present time. Clearly, there is a long history of children who have problems with inattention, hyperactivity and/or impulsivity, despite the fact that the phrase ADHD has only recently been applied to these children.

The purpose of this chapter is to provide an overview of attention-deficit/ hyperactivity disorder in children. We will review: (1) defining features; (2) epidemiology; (3) associated features (family functioning and peer functioning); (4) etiology; (5) developmental course; (6) assessment; (7) intervention, and (8) future directions. In all of these areas it was necessary to conduct a selective rather than comprehensive review because the extant literature on ADHD is enormous. In conducting the selected review we focused on the most up-to-date information available.

Defining features

Children with ADHD are challenged by a number of observable behavioural symptoms comprising two major categories: inattention, and hyperactivity-impulsivity (American Psychiatric Association, 2000). The diagnosis of ADHD is based on the observance of these symptoms occurring in multiple areas of the child's life and causing the child "real life" problems, referred to as impairment.

Inattention

Children with ADHD have difficulty with tasks that require sustained mental effort (Sergeant et al., 1999). Children with ADHD are also more disorganized, easily distracted and forgetful compared to their same age peers. These symptoms cause them serious difficulties at home and at school and have been found using both laboratory-based measures (Nichols and Waschbusch, 2004) and applied measures (Pelham et al., 1992b).

Hyperactive-impulsive behaviour

Children with ADHD are more fidgety, restless, and squirmy compared to typically developing children. Research has shown children with ADHD, as compared to other children, have a higher activity level (Swanson et al., 2003), difficulty with inhibiting ongoing behaviour (Oosterlaan et al., 1998), and difficulty inhibiting immediate gratification (Douglas and Parry, 1983). As with attention problems, these difficulties lead to serious problems in home and school functioning.

Impact of contextual factors

The extent to which symptoms of ADHD are observable typically varies across tasks and settings. Factors such as the time of day, level of environmental stim-ulation, task demands, presence of consequences and rewards, and presence of adult supervision frequently impact the performance and behaviour of children with ADHD, just as these same factors influence children without ADHD. For example, research suggests that children with ADHD behave differently around their fathers as compared to mothers (Barkley et al., 1990). Numerous possible explanations for this pattern have been suggested, but one is that fathers use different discipline styles and therefore offer different consequences to the child. Similarly, research shows that when children with ADHD are engaging in intrinsically rewarding tasks such as television, their behaviour improves even though their attention-deficits continue (Milich and Lorch, 1994). Thus, children with ADHD do not "lose" their behavioural symptomatology in different contexts; rather, like other children, the behaviour of children with ADHD is influenced by environmental and task variables which either increase or reduce levels of behavioural disturbance.

Epidemiology

Prevalence

There is growing consensus that ADHD occurs in 3 percent to 5 percent of elementary age children (Lahey et al., 1999) and that this is true across cultures (Esser et al., 1990). However, this consensus masks the fact that prevalence estimates for ADHD diverge widely across studies. This divergence is to be expected, given that age, definition of disorder, and assessment method all influence prevalence rates. For example, more stringent definitions (e.g., clinical diagnosis to define ADHD versus elevated scores on a behaviour checklist) and more stringent assessment criteria result in fewer cases of ADHD. Because the definition of ADHD continues to evolve, and because there is no "gold standard" assessment method for evaluating ADHD, there is as yet no clear answer to how many "true" cases of ADHD actually exist.

Gender differences

One finding in the ADHD literature that is consistent across sample type (clinical or community) and culture is that the disorder is observed more often in boys than it is in girls (Gaub and Carlson, 1997; Lahey et al., 1999). The ratios of boys to girls range from 2:1 to 9:1 (Anderson et al., 1987b). The high ratio of boys to girls observed in ADHD has historically resulted in a paucity of studies of girls with the disorder, as many studies limited their samples to boys; however, more recent studies have attempted to include more girls and our knowledge has increased.

The patterns of familial transmission seen in boys with ADHD are also observed in girls in that relatives of girls with ADHD have been found to be at greater risk of developing ADHD and other disruptive behaviour disorders compared to control subjects (Faraone et al., 2000). Similarly, girls with ADHD appear to respond to treatment in much the same way as boys with ADHD (Pelham et al., 1989b), although research is limited. Interestingly, some research suggests that boys tend to show more overt and severe disruptive behaviours in the classroom, whereas girls appear to exhibit more cognitive and academic problems (Gaub and Carlson, 1997). However, this data must be interpreted with caution as other research suggests no differences (Breen, 1989).

ADHD may actually be under-recognized in girls due to the fact that ADHD rating scales typically use norms based on boys and girls rather than single-sex norms. Girls also tend to have lower levels of inattention, hyperactivity, and oppositional/defiant behaviour when compared to boys, meaning that they must show especially severe symptoms to match the level of disruptive behaviour seen in boys, an observation that has been termed a "gender paradox" (Eme, 1992;

Hartung and Widiger, 1998). However, research has shown that when teachers and parents are asked to rate ADHD symptoms in boys and girls using same sex comparisons, the gender difference remains (Waschbusch et al., in press). This suggests one of three alternatives: (1) there actually is a gender difference in ADHD; (2) the criteria used to evaluate ADHD may be more applicable to boys than to girls; or (3) ADHD develops later in girls than in boys.

Comorbidity

ADHD frequently occurs in conjunction with other disorders. It has long been established that many children with ADHD also have conduct problems (CP) such as oppositional defiant disorder (ODD) or conduct disorder (CD), and that many children with CP also have ADHD. In fact, the overlap, or comorbidity, between ADHD and CP is more common than uncommon; that is, it is more likely for a child to meet criteria for multiple disruptive behaviour disorders than it is for the child to meet criteria for just one (Hinshaw and Park, 1999; Waschbusch, 2002). The rate of comorbidity between ADHD and CP has been found to range from 30 percent to 50 percent (Jensen et al., 1997). Similarly, there appears to be an overlap between ADHD and internalizing disorder (i.e., mood and anxiety problems), with prevalence rates ranging from 15 percent to 75 percent in both community and clinical samples (Biederman et al., 1991). These patterns are robust with respect to culture, sample type (community versus clinical), age, and gender (Angold et al., 1999). For example, one study (Bird et al., 1993) examined comorbidity in a community sample of 222 Puerto Rican children between the ages of 9 and 16 using the Diagnostic Interview Schedule for Children (DISC). Results indicated that among children with a DSM-III diagnosis of ADD, 93 percent met the criteria for comorbid CD or ODD. In addition, children with a diagnosis of ADD had high rates of comorbid internalizing disorders such as anxiety disorders (58 percent) and depression (26.8 percent). Conversely, of children who met the criteria for DSM-III CD or ODD, 35.7 percent also met the criteria for ADD. Rates of comorbidity among the diagnostic groupings used to classify children in this study were higher than those expected to occur by chance. Other studies have found similar patterns (Anderson et al., 1987a; Offord et al., 1987, 1989).

A key question is why ADHD overlaps so highly with other disorders. Factors such as overlapping diagnostic criteria, artificial subdivision of syndromes, and cases where one disorder may be a precursor to another are all possible explanations (Caron and Rutter, 1991). Similarly, halo effects may contribute to high estimates of comorbidity among the disruptive behaviour disorders (Abikoff et al., 1993; Stevens et al., 1998). On the other hand, it may be that the comorbid conditions represent a distinct group of children who experience different outcomes than children with ADHD alone. For example, research shows that children with comorbid ADHD + ODD/CD tend to experience greater family adversity and have lower verbal abilities than do children with ADHD-only or CP-only (Moffitt, 1990). Similarly, children with ADHD and conduct problems exhibit more antisocial behaviours throughout childhood than do children with conduct problems alone (Moffitt, 1990; Moffitt and Silva, 1988). These and other findings have been interpreted as evidence that children with both ADHD and conduct problems are best conceptualized as a diagnostically distinct group (Jensen et al., 1997), although not all evidence is consistent with this perspective (see Waschbusch, 2002, for a review).

Associated features

Family functioning

Numerous theoretical arguments suggest that families are likely to play an important role in the development and maintenance of ADHD. First, there is now solid evidence that ADHD tends to run within families (see p. 59), suggesting that the parents of children with ADHD are more likely to have similar symptoms than parents of other children. Second, irritability, low frustration tolerance, extreme motor activity, intrusiveness, and being demanding are all associated with ADHD and these are likely to elicit negative behaviours from parents. In fact, experimental studies demonstrate that these behaviours in children elicit negative moods and behaviour from adults (Pelham and Lang, 1993; Pelham et al., 1997). Third, behaviours that co-occur with ADHD, such as conduct problems, have well-established links to parenting and family factors (Patterson et al., 1989).

Based on these and other arguments, numerous researchers have examined the families of children with ADHD (see Johnston and Mash, 2001, for a review). These studies show that parents of children with ADHD, as compared to parents of non-disordered children, are more stressed and conflicted, use worse parenting practices, and have more authoritative parenting attitudes (Whalen and Henker, 1999). For instance, observational studies show that the interactions between parents and children with ADHD are more controlling and negative than are interactions between parents and non-ADHD children (e.g., Barkley et al., 1985; Campbell et al., 1986; e.g., Johnston and Pelham, 1990). Other studies show that mothers of children with ADHD tend to have higher rates of depression than do mothers of control children (Johnston and Mash, 2001). However, it is only recently that the role of paternal mood in ADHD has been examined, and there is currently insufficient evidence to draw firm conclusions. A critical question in many of these studies is whether co-occurring conduct problems plays a role as most existing studies fail to take conduct problems into account. Those that do take conduct problems into account suggest that the combination of ADHD and conduct problems is associated with the most impaired family functioning and parenting.

Some research has examined whether parenting is causally related to ADHD. In one set of studies (Pelham and Lang, 1993; Pelham et al., 1997), adults and children who did not know each other interacted in a laboratory setting to complete challenging tasks. The adults were led to believe that the child was randomly selected from a group of children. In reality, the child was a confederate who was taught to exhibit specific disruptive behaviours and to do so in the same way across all participants. This manipulation allowed for an evaluation of whether child disruptive behaviour had a causal effect on adult behaviour towards the child. Multiple studies using this (or similar) protocol showed that severely impulsive, inattentive, hyperactive and otherwise disruptive behaviour in children was causally associated with more negative parenting skills, higher alcohol consumption, and more stress and depression in the adults (Pelham and Lang, 1993; Pelham et al., 1997).

Other research has used longitudinal designs to examine the link between ADHD and parenting. A four-year longitudinal study found that elevations in maternal depressed mood preceded elevations in children's depressed mood, but maternal depressed mood followed children's aggression and hyperactivity (Elgar et al., 2003). Thus, deviant child behaviour appears to be a precursor to depression on the part of the parent. A second study examined this same topic using daily reports of maternal mood and disruptive child behaviour, with reports gathered over approximately thirty days (Elgar et al., 2004). Pooled time-series analyses showed that the link between maternal mood and child behaviour varied as a function of both the type of maternal mood and the type of child behaviour. Specifically, when children expressed ADHD behaviours, the mother's level of anger and fatigue subsequently increased. Similarly, when children expressed conduct problems (oppositional, defiant behaviour), the mother's level of confusion subsequently increased. On the other hand, when the mothers reported feeling depression, low vigour, anger, and anxiety, their children's level of ADHD behaviours subsequently increased, and when mothers reported feeling confused and anxious, their child's level of conduct problems subsequently increased.

Overall, research on family functioning of children with ADHD seems to show that (1) their families exhibit a number of negative characteristics, such as more negative and hostile parenting styles, (2) mothers of children with ADHD experience greater stress and depression, and (3) the "common-sense" belief that parenting shapes child development should be qualified to include the notion that children's behaviour also influences the type of parenting they experience, and does so in complex ways.

Peer functioning

Much research has demonstrated that children with ADHD tend to be actively rejected by their peers. This has been found using laboratory based measures of social functioning and using measures gathered from the natural peer group (see Henker and Whalen, 1999; Milich and Landau, 1989, for a review). In fact, a number of studies have shown that children with ADHD become unpopular with peers within a few minutes of first meeting them (Hoza et al., 2000; Landau and Milich, 1988; Pelham and Bender, 1982; Whalen et al., 1979).

There are a number of possible reasons for this well-established pattern. First, there is considerable evidence that children with ADHD tend to exhibit high rates of negative behaviour with peers, including bossiness, intrusiveness, and aggression (Cunningham and Siegel, 1987). Interestingly, the primary features of ADHD – hyperactive, impulsive and inattentive behaviour – seem to each make a unique contribution to peer rejection (Henker and Whalen, 1999; Pelham and Bender, 1982), suggesting that peer problems expressed by children with ADHD are multidimensional. This may, in part, explain the disappointing results of efforts aimed at ameliorating peer relationship problems in children with ADHD (Pelham and Bender, 1982; Pelham et al., 1988).

Second, children with ADHD may have deviant social cognitive abilities. Theoretically, the symptoms of ADHD are likely to impair children's ability to accurately perceive social situations. Dodge and colleagues have argued that attending to cues is the first step in evaluating a social situation (Crick and Dodge, 1994; Dodge et al., 1986). Given that inattention is a core deficit of ADHD, children with ADHD may have an impaired ability to attend to social cues. Similarly, Dodge and colleagues have argued that generation, selection, and enactment of social responses requires deliberation. This ability is also likely to be impaired by the cognitive and behavioural impulsivity that is associated with ADHD (Milich and Kramer, 1984). Research examining social cognition in children with ADHD is in its infancy, but the little empirical data that does exist suggests that that children with ADHD have impaired social cognitive abilities and that this is true even after potential confounds (such as co-occurring conduct problems) are taken into account (Matthys et al., 1999; Milch-Reich et al., 1999; Milich and Dodge, 1984; Murphy et al., 1992; Waschbusch, 2004).

Third, ADHD may be linked to peer problems due to impaired social skills. Research shows that children with ADHD have social skills deficits, but some have suggested this is because children with ADHD possess appropriate knowledge of social skills but have difficulties putting this knowledge into practice when in social situations (Milich and Landau, 1982; Whalen and Henker, 1985). Current research seems to support this position, as there is little evidence that children with ADHD lack social skills knowledge (Bullis et al., 2001; Grenell et al., 1987), but there is ample evidence that children with ADHD use less effective strategies when joining ongoing activities (Hoza et al., 2000; Milich et al., 1982a; Pelham and Bender, 1982), have impaired social communication styles (Landau and Milich, 1988; Whalen et al., 1979), and are more often more critical of their peers in problem solving situations (Diener and Milich, 1997). All of these behaviours make the maintenance and initiation of peer relationships difficult.

Finally, some research has suggested that inattention may be an understudied but particularly important aspect of peer relationship problems. Numerous studies have found that inattention is highly and uniquely associated with peer problems, with evidence that the association is stronger than between peer problems and aggressive, hyperactive, impulsive behavior (Andrade et al., in press; Atkins et al., 1989; Bierman et al., 1993; Bierman and Wargo, 1995; Pelham and Bender, 1982; Pope and Bierman, 1999; Pope et al., 1991). One hypothesis to explain these findings is that children with inattentive symptoms do not attend to the positive behaviours of peers to the same extent that others do and are therefore perceived by peers as uncaring or unsupportive. If so, then over time peers may not initiate prosocial behaviours to inattentive children, which would ultimately lower their opportunities to learn and practice the social skills necessary to foster peer relationships. At the same time, their lack of attention may cause them to be "out of sync" with peers, which has been shown to be related to peer relationship problems (Dodge et al., 1986).

Etiology

Overview

Numerous causal factors have been postulated for ADHD, but in recent years biological causes have become prominent. Even so, virtually every influential conceptualization of ADHD emphasizes that ADHD is multiply determined, with both biological and environmental contributions to the disorder.

Genetics

There is ever-increasing evidence that genetics play an important role in the development of ADHD (Cook, 1999; Stevenson, 1992; Tannock, 1998). Approximately 25 percent of siblings and fathers of children with ADHD have ADHD themselves, and approximately 15 percent to 20 percent of mothers of children with ADHD have ADHD themselves. Conversely, rates of ADHD in offspring of adults with ADHD range from 20 percent to nearly 60 percent. In each case, these rates are significantly higher than in matched controls, indicating that ADHD tends to run within families.

Twin studies have also been used to examine the role of genetics in ADHD. Twin studies suggest that 55 percent to 92 percent of identical (monozygotic) twins are concordant for ADHD, whereas the same rates for fraternal (dizygotic) twins are no different than between any other siblings. For example, one study found a concordance rate of ADHD was 81 percent for identical twins and 29 percent for fraternal twins (Gillis et al., 1992). Application of behaviour genetic methods to studies such as this one suggest that the heritability of ADHD (i.e., the amount of population variance in ADHD that can be explained by genetic factors) averages 80 percent and may be higher when more stringent definitions of ADHD are used. In contrast, estimates of the role of non-shared environmental factors are about 15 percent, and estimates of the role of shared environmental factors are non-significant. Thus, twin studies indicate that genetics are an extremely important etiological factor in the development of ADHD, followed by unique environmental experiences.

Having solid evidence that genetics are implicated in the development of ADHD, investigators have begun to turn their attention to deciphering a specific pathway using molecular genetic methods (Stevenson, 1992). Two preliminary conclusions can be drawn from this research. First, it is increasingly clear that ADHD is a polygenetic disorder. There is no evidence to date that a single gene or genetic abnormality can account for ADHD (Rutter et al., 1999a, 1999b). Second, dopamine systems, and especially dopamine receptors, are likely implicated in ADHD (Kuntsi and Stevenson, 2000). However, other pathways are also likely to emerge, as evidenced by recent efforts suggesting that medications acting primarily through serotonin pathways are effective for treating ADHD.

Environmental factors

Although genetics play an important role in ADHD, genes alone do not account for ADHD. Numerous claims have been made about environmental factors causing ADHD. Some examples include dietary factors, allergies, socio-economic variables, poor parenting, excessive television or video games, the culture or school climate of the twentieth century, and parent/teacher intolerance. There is little to no evidence to support such simple causal explanations. For instance, one widely held belief is that ADHD is caused by sugar. Indeed, sugar leading to hyperactive behaviour has become almost a cultural truism. However, careful scientific examination of this issue suggests that sugar does not alter children's behaviour but instead alters adult perceptions of children's behaviour (Milich et al., 1986). That is, when adults believe that children have been given sugar, they evaluate those children as more hyperactive regardless of whether or not sugar actually was administered.

On the other hand, a number of environmental factors have been demonstrated to be significantly associated with ADHD. As noted earlier, family dysfunction has often been found to contribute to the development and exacerbation of ADHD. For example, parents who use an exceptionally harsh and punitive style of parenting may not attend effectively to children's needs, resulting in more disinhibited behaviour in their children. Alternatively, a lack of synchronization between children and parents may result in the development of poorly regulated behaviour in children (Barkley and Cunningham, 1979; Barkley et al., 1985).

Other environmental factors have also been implicated in the development of ADHD. Most notable are prenatal exposure to alcohol, cigarettes and other drugs, serious complications during prenatal development or delivery, postnatal head trauma, and exposure to lead and other toxins (Samudra and Cantwell, 1999). These factors are significant and important risk factors, but two points must be made when considering them. First, virtually all evidence to date indicates that these types of environmental risks account for only a small portion of the variance associated with ADHD. Second, these same risk factors are associated with nearly every area of child psychopathology, suggesting that their association with ADHD is non-specific.

Developmental course

Historically, ADHD was thought to impact childhood, but have little or no effect in adolescence or adulthood (Willoughby, 2003). For instance, one early description describes the developmental trajectory of ADHD as "disappear[ing] with maturation, anywhere between 12 and 18 years of age, so that it may no longer be present, though its unfortunate educational and emotional sequelae may persist" (Laufer, 1962, p. 504). In contrast to these historical conceptualizations, modern conceptualizations of ADHD emphasize that ADHD persists over development and is best conceptualized as a chronic disorder (e.g., Barkley, 1990; Hinshaw, 1994; Pelham, 1999a). There are numerous reasons for this dramatic change in perspective (see Willoughby, 2003, for a review), but probably the most important reason is that longitudinal studies make it clear that children with ADHD have negative outcomes when they become adolescents and adults.

The two most well-known outcome studies of children with ADHD are the Montreal study (Weiss and Hechtman, 1993) and the New York study (Gittelman-Klein and Mannuzza, 1989; Mannuzza et al., 1993). These studies found clear evidence that children with ADHD experience a number of negative outcomes in late adolescence (ages 16 to 19) and adulthood (ages 20 and over). As adolescents, individuals with ADHD received lower grades and lower achievement test scores, had higher rates of failing courses, and were more likely to drop out or be expelled from school. By the late teenage years, they had fewer friends and worse social skills and were more likely to exhibit antisocial behaviour and mental health problems. The situation does not improve in adulthood, as both studies found that the individuals with ADHD had significantly lower occupational attainment and job performance (i.e., rated by employers and low on work adequacy, working independently, getting along with supervisors, and completing tasks), were somewhat more likely to get fired, and had worse social skills.

Data from newer longitudinal studies mirror these results; children with ADHD have a greater risk of becoming teenagers who fail courses, repeat grades, have worse social skills, fewer friends, and engage in risky behaviours such as poor driving and substance use (Barkley et al., 1990; Biederman et al., 1996; Molina and Pelham, 2003).

Numerous aspects of the developmental course of ADHD remain to be addressed. First, the vast majority of existing studies examine boys only. Next to nothing is known about the developmental course of girls with ADHD. Along the same lines, follow-up research to date has not differentiated children based on types of symptoms, and the majority of studies have selected primarily based on hyperactivity. Very little is known about the role of childhood inattention in predicting developmental outcomes of children with ADHD, although there are some intriguing findings that inattention in childhood may be uniquely associated with substance abuse as a teenager (Molina and Pelham, 2003).

Second, studies have largely failed to take into account problems that go along with ADHD. Thus, it is unclear which negative outcomes are the result of ADHD and which are the result of co-occurring problems. In fact, there has been considerable debate about whether antisocial outcomes found in studies of children with ADHD are actually associated with ADHD or whether they are actually the result of unaccounted for conduct problems that frequently accompany ADHD

(Hinshaw et al., 1993; Lilienfeld and Waldman, 1990). On the one hand, a number of studies have shown that when conduct problems are taken into account, the association between ADHD symptoms and antisocial behaviour largely disappears (Lahey et al., 2002; Nagin and Tremblay, 1999; Stouthamer-Loeber et al., 2002). In contrast, other studies have found that ADHD predicts antisocial behaviour even after taking co-occurring conduct problems into account (Burns and Walsh, 2002; Farrington et al., 1990; Magnusson et al., 1992; Moffitt, 1990; Molina and Pelham, 2003). Thus, there is general agreement that ADHD in the presence of conduct problems is especially highly associated with antisocial behaviour over the course of development (Lynam, 1996; Waschbusch, 2002), but whether ADHD independently predicts antisocial behaviour remains unclear and in need of further research.

Third, little is known about the development of the symptoms of ADHD (Willoughby, 2003). Existing longitudinal studies of ADHD have focused almost exclusively on evaluating whether children with ADHD have worse functioning on measures of daily adjustment (e.g. peer relationships, academic performance, employment, etc.) when they become adolescents and adults. Very little research has examined whether the symptoms of ADHD themselves persist over time, and if so, whether they are responsible for the negative outcomes associated with ADHD. This research is challenging to conduct because the same symptoms may be expressed in very different ways in children, teenagers, and adults. However, without research examining both the developmental outcomes of ADHD and the development of symptoms of ADHD, it remains unclear whether modern concep-tualizations of ADHD as a chronic disorder are any more accurate than earlier conceptualizations of ADHD as a childhood-limited disorder (Willoughby, 2003). One could easily argue that, consistent with early formulations of ADHD, the peer problems, academic problems, and family problems associated with ADHD in childhood may be sufficient to account for negative developmental outcomes even if ADHD symptoms were to disappear with the onset of adolescence.

Regardless of whether ADHD symptoms persist or remit with the onset of adolescence, there is near universal agreement that children with ADHD are much more likely to experience a more negative developmental trajectory than are other children and that the costs of these negative outcomes are substantial. Data from an adolescent follow-up study suggest that children with ADHD are more than twice as likely as other children to be arrested in the teenage years, resulting in judicial costs that are 25 times higher as compared to non-ADHD children (Barkley, 1997). Similarly, children with ADHD are more likely to access primary health care systems, resulting in health care costs that are about three times higher than those for other children (Leibson et al., 2001).

Assessment

Components of an accurate assessment of ADHD include: (1) evaluating the defining features of ADHD (i.e., inattention, impulsivity and hyperactivity), and

(2) evaluating the functional deficits (or associated features) associated with ADHD. Assessing the defining features of ADHD provides a link to a considerable body of knowledge on treatments for ADHD, whereas assessment of the functional deficits associated with ADHD leads to the development of effective treatment for a particular child.

Assessment of defining features

Rating scales

Rating scales are one of the, if not the most, widely used measures of children's adjustment. Ratings offer a number of advantages as an assessment method. First, they are among the least expensive assessments to gather in terms of both cost and time. Second, rating scales have been developed to measure a large variety of constructs, providing researchers and clinicians ready-made measures for almost any area of children's development and adjustment, including ADHD.

Two types of ratings have been developed for assessing ADHD. The first type is based on the clinical psychology literature and consists of the symptoms of ADHD, as specified in the current DSM diagnostic nomenclature. Typically, these items are rated on Likert scales anchored by the degree to which they are present in a child (e.g., "not at all present" to "very much present"). These provide an estimate of whether a particular child meets symptomatic criteria consistent with an ADHD diagnosis. Examples include the Disruptive Behaviour Disorder (DBD) Rating Scale (Pelham et al., 1992a), the Swanson Nolan and Pelham-IV (Swanson, 1996), the Child and Adolescent Disruptive Behaviour Inventory (Burns et al., 1997), the ADHD rating scale (DuPaul, 1991), the Vanderbilt Rating Scale (Wolraich et al., 1998) and many others. These DSM-based ratings are widely used with parents and teachers and are typically normed for both groups. Some of these must be purchased, while others are available at no charge.

A second type of rating scale selects items using empirical methods, such as factor analysis or receiver operating characteristics. The main advantage to these types of rating scales is increased confidence in the psychometric properties of the scales. One of the most widely used and well known empirically based rating scales for ADHD is the IOWA Conners Rating Scale (Loney and Milich, 1982; Milich et al., 1982a, 1982b). The IOWA, which stands for Inattentive-Overactive With Aggression, was developed to address research findings that the original Abbreviated Conners Teacher Rating Scale (Conners, 1969), which was a rationally developed scale, confounded ADHD behaviours with conduct problem behaviours. The IOWA Conners has been empirically demonstrated to discriminate ADHD behaviours from conduct problem behaviours (Loney et al., 1978; Milich et al., 1982b). Further research has validated the IOWA (Atkins et al., 1985, 1989), provided normative information (Pelham et al., 1989a), and demonstrated sensitivity to treatment effects (Pelham et al., 2001). The parent version of the IOWA Conners has also been shown to be sensitive to treatment effects (Pelham et al., 2001), but unfortunately, normative information for the parent version of the IOWA Conners has not been established and is sorely needed.

Interviews

Another measure of ADHD symptoms is an interview with an adult in the child's life. Parent interviews are always employed in clinic settings. Typically these are unstructured or semi-structured clinical interviews designed to gather information about the child's history and presenting problems. Less commonly used are structured clinical interviews with parents that ask in a structured manner questions regarding DSM symptoms and are designed to yield DSM diagnoses. Several of these are available for downloading over the internet, some without charge (www.summertreatmentprogram.com; www.wpic.pitt.edu/ksads) and others for a fee (www.c-disc.com). Interviews with teachers can be accomplished on the phone or in person, but these are typically focused on the child's referring problems and contribute information towards deriving a diagnosis.

The advantage of a structured interview regarding symptoms over a rating scale is that the mental health professional is able to probe the adult's knowledge of the child, which may lead to a more accurate (that is, valid) determination of whether the behaviour in question meets diagnostic criteria. The degree to which the interview allows for exchange between the adult and the interviewer (within the structure of the interview) and clinical judgment on the part of the clinician is the aspect of the interview that putatively produces enhanced validity of diagnosis. Interviews also provide the "human touch" that is missing from questionnaire administration. Parents and teachers often prefer speaking to a clinician as opposed to completing a questionnaire.

The main disadvantage of the structured interviews is that they require considerably more time (for both the parent/teacher and the mental health professional) to complete than do rating scales, especially if they allow for exchange between the adult and the interviewer. For example, it is not uncommon for a diagnostic interview to take 60 to 90 minutes to complete, whereas rating scales typically take 10 or 15 minutes. Furthermore, recent research suggests that behaviour ratings of ADHD may be more valid than a structured interview measure of ADHD, based on the fact that behaviour ratings were more highly associated with observations of ADHD behaviours in children (Wright et al., under review). Unless additional research clearly demonstrates that such interviews yield more accurate diagnoses than rating scales – and that has not yet been demonstrated – then rating scales would be preferred based on both time/cost considerations and validity considerations.

Assessment of functional deficits

Functional analysis of ADHD involves gathering information from parents and teachers to determine what impairment the child with ADHD is exhibiting. Most functional analyses includes an evaluation of the child's referring problems and the possible controlling environmental variables (antecedents and consequences), as well as the classroom and home management practices that have been employed with the target child and with other children. Evaluation of the effectiveness (if tried) of various interventions is also important to assess as well as the parent and teacher preferences regarding possible interventions that might be employed, and his or her opinion regarding the possible functions of the target behaviours (e.g., to gain peer attention, self stimulation, to avoid tasks, etc.).

The clinician, along with parents and teachers, then formulates hypotheses regarding the functions of the target behaviours. Four primary functions have been suggested for behaviours expressed by children with ADHD (DuPaul and Eckert, 1997). First, ADHD behaviours may serve an escape or avoidance function. For example, when presented with a challenging academic task, the child may get out of his/her seat to avoid the task. Second, the behaviour may function as a means of gaining attention from adults or peers. If parents and teachers unknowingly attend more to disruptive behaviour than to non-disruptive, positive behaviour, the child may gain attention from them by drawing on this pattern. Third, ADHD behaviours may function as a means to obtain a desired object or activity. A typical example of this would be a parent who allows a child to watch TV in order to calm them down, or a teacher who does the same with a computer task. Fourth, ADHD behaviour may serve to regulate sensory stimulation. There is at least some evidence for individual differences in how children with ADHD respond to low, average, and high levels of surrounding stimuli (Pelham et al., 1994), suggesting that behaviours such as inattention or impulsivity may serve to increase stimulation to reach an optimal level for some children, whereas behaviours such as daydreaming may serve to decrease stimulation to reach an optimal level for other children.

Based on the functional assessment, the consultant then assists the parent or teacher in manipulating antecedents or consequences to investigate whether the hypotheses regarding functions were correct. If such manipulations confirm the function of a given target behaviour (e.g., peer attention is maintaining classroom clowning), then an intervention can be developed (e.g., a classwide positive consequence for ignoring class clowning) (Boyajian et al., 2001; Northup and Gulley, 2001; Sterling-Turner et al., 2001).

We should note that there are some commonly employed assessment procedures that are not useful for diagnosis/evaluation of ADHD. These include subscales on IQ tests such as the Freedom from Distractibility Index on the Wechsler scales, and such cognitive measures as continuous performance tasks. Careful research has failed to support the validity of such indices for the diagnosis and assessment of ADHD, and they are not recommended for use in school or clinical settings (American Academy of Pediatrics, 2001a). The same conclusion holds for the extensive list of neuropsychological tests that have been advocated for diagnosis of ADHD (Barkley, 1991; Nichols and Waschbusch, 2004). In other words, standardized tests are useful only to rule in or out other difficulties – not to diagnose ADHD – and neuropsychological and other cognitive tests are not useful in diagnosis.

Intervention

The chronic and serious nature of ADHD has led to considerable research on the treatment of ADHD. The majority of this research has evaluated specific treatments for managing ADHD symptoms. Several treatment approaches have been repeatedly evaluated, such as behaviour therapy, cognitive-behaviour therapy, and stimulant medication, but many others have also been evaluated, such as play therapy, relaxation training, and numerous non-stimulant medications. Much of this research was reviewed as part of the task force on empirically supported treatments for children's mental health (Lonigan et al., 1998), and the results of this review suggest that, at present, only behaviour therapy (BT) and stimulant medication (the most common of which is methylphenidate – MPH) are empirically supported treatments for ADHD (Pelham et al., 1998). In contrast, other approaches, such as cognitive therapies, biofeedback, and play therapy, have little empirical support (Waschbusch and Hill, 2003).

More recently, researchers have turned their attention to evaluating the relative effects of MPH and BT on ADHD when delivered alone and in combination. A number of findings from these efforts suggest that the combination of behaviour therapy and stimulant medication is the optimal approach for treating ADHD (American Academy of Pediatrics, 2001b; NIH Consensus Statement, 1998; Pliszka et al., 2000). First, evidence suggests that behaviour therapy and stimulant medication have complementary effects. For instance, one study of elementary school children with ADHD found that stimulant medication improved children's mood and certain negative behaviours, whereas behaviour therapy improved other negative behaviours (Kolko et al., 1999).

Second, evidence suggests that combining behaviour therapy and stimulant medication makes each more effective. Children with ADHD have been shown to respond to reward and punishment in a manner that is more similar to non-ADHD children when they receive stimulant medication (Douglas, 1999; Murray and Kollins, 2000; Tripp and Alsop, 1999). Likewise, lower doses of stimulants administered in the presence of ongoing behaviour therapy have similar effects as higher doses of stimulants delivered in the absence of BT (Pelham et al., 1980, 1993; Reitman et al., 2001).

Third, and perhaps most important, numerous studies have directly compared the combination of behaviour therapy and stimulant medication (BT+MED) to behaviour therapy alone (BT-only) and to medication only (MED-only), and these studies showed that the combined treatment is superior. A review of this question found that BT+Med was superior to BT-only and MED-only in approximately 70 percent of studies (Pelham and Waschbusch, 1999). Another literature review computed effect sizes to examine the same issue and drew the same conclusion – namely, that behavior therapy plus medication is more effective than either treatment alone (Fabiano et al., 2000).

Also noteworthy are the results of the Multi-modal Treatment of ADHD (MTA) study funded by the National Institutes of Mental Health. The primary purpose of the MTA study was to evaluate whether there is an incremental benefit of combining

BT+MPH treatments over either alone. The results of this study are especially important to consider because it enrolled a large number of participants (N = 579), used comprehensive measurement, and was implemented exceptionally well. To date, results have been published using data collected 14 months after the start of treatment (MTA Cooperative Group, 1999a, 1999b) and 24 months after the start of treatment (MTA Cooperative Group, 2004a, 2004b). These data have been widely interpreted as showing that MED was superior to BT, with no incremental effects of BT+MED. However, this interpretation is incorrect. In fact, results actually showed: (1) the MED-only and BT+MED were equally effective in reducing ADHD symptoms (both superior to BT-only and community-treated controls), but the BT+MED group was superior to the MED-only on measures of positive functioning (MTA Cooperative Group, 1999a); (2) BT+MED produced a larger number of "excellent treatment responders" (Swanson et al., 2001); (3) BT+MED was superior on 12 of the 19 outcome measures (Cunningham, 1999); (4) BT+MED was superior on an overall treatment outcome measure (Conners et al., 2001); (5) BT+MED resulted in less medication than MED-only (Pelham, 1999b); and (6) parents preferred the BT+MED over the other treatments (Pelham et al., under review).

Summary and future directions

Great progress has been made in understanding the etiology, development, and outcome associated with ADHD. The disorder that was once thought by sceptics to be caused by sugar, bad parenting, and too much television is now recognized as a legitimate mental health condition that is likely caused by a complex interplay of biological and environmental factors. Empirically valid assessment tools and evidence-based treatments have been developed, and there is a growing awareness that these should be used as standard clinical practice.

Despite the progress made in this field, there remains much research to be done to fully elucidate the development, course, outcome, and treatment of ADHD. First, more research is needed to address the impact of comorbidity on ADHD, and especially the impact of comorbid conduct problems. For instance, it has been suggested that children who have both ADHD and conduct problems should be included in their own diagnostic category that is separate from ADHD alone and from conduct problems alone. Further research evaluating this assertion is important for understanding the nature and interplay among disruptive behaviour.

Second, the role of gender in ADHD requires better examination. The lack of research on girls with ADHD is striking; nearly all research on ADHD has been on elementary age boys. As a result, it remains unclear whether girls exhibit the same types of behaviours and developmental course of ADHD as do boys with ADHD. The presence of the gender paradox in ADHD suggests that girls may not be identified as having the disorder unless the symptoms are especially severe. Research evaluating this issue would be useful.

Third, further research is needed regarding the developmental course of ADHD symptoms, an area that has not been well researched in the past. Such research would allow for a more accurate conceptualization of the nature of the disorder and would help clarify the long-term effects (or lack thereof) of treatment on ameliorating ADHD.

Fourth, determining the most appropriate treatments for ADHD and families of children with ADHD is essential. Behaviour therapy and stimulant medication have been shown to be effective in treating ADHD symptoms, but the evidence supporting these treatments has all been short term. That is, there is currently no research that shows either behaviour therapy or stimulant medication has a significant positive impact on children with ADHD over the long term. Further, even though children with ADHD show short term improvement in response to behaviour therapy, stimulant medication and their combination, these improvements typically do not lead to normalization. Instead, children with ADHD continue to be distinguished from their peers on numerous measures. This is especially true on measures of social functioning, which have proven to be difficult to improve. Research on these topics is not only important for advancing science, but also important for helping improve the lives of children, their families, and the societies in which they live.

References

Abikoff, H.B., Courtney, M., Pelham, W.E., and Koplewicz, H.S. (1993). Teachers' ratings of disruptive behaviors: The influence of halo effects. *Journal of Abnormal Child Psychology, 21*, 519–533.

American Academy of Pediatrics (AAP) (2001a). *Clinical practice guideline: Diagnosis and evaluation of a child with attention-deficit/hyperactivity disorder.* Elk Grove Village, IL: AAP.

American Academy of Pediatrics (2001b). Clinical practice guideline: Treatment of the school-aged child with attention-deficit/hyperactivity disorder. *Pediatrics, 105,* 1033–1044.

American Psychiatric Association (1980). *Diagnostic and statistical manual of mental disorders*, 3rd edn. Washington, DC: APA.

American Psychiatric Association (1987). *Diagnostic and statistical manual of mental disorders*, 3rd revised edn. Washington, DC: APA.

American Psychiatric Association (1994). *Diagnostic and statistical manual of mental disorders*, 4th edn. Washington, DC: APA.

American Psychiatric Association (2000). *Diagnostic and statistical manual of mental disorders*, 4th edn, text revision. Washington, DC: APA.

Anderson, J.C., Williams, S., McGee, R., and Silva, P.A. (1987a). DSM-III disorders in preadolescent children. *Archives of General Psychiatry, 44*, 69–76.

Anderson, J.C., Williams, S., McGee, R., and Silva, P.A. (1987b). DSM-III disorders in preadolescent children: Prevalence in a large sample from the general population. *Archives of General Psychiatry, 44*, 69–76.

Andrade, B.F., Waschbusch, D.A., King, S., and Northern Region Partners in Action for Children and Youth (in press). Adult reported peer social status: Preliminary validation and examination of potential mediators. *Journal of Psychoeducational Assessment.*

Angold, A., Costello, E.J., and Erkanli, A. (1999). Comorbidity. *Journal of Child Psychology and Psychiatry*, *40*, 57–87.

Atkins, M.S., Pelham, W.E., and Licht, M.H. (1985). A comparison of objective classroom measures and teacher ratings of attention deficit disorders. *Journal of Abnormal Child Psychology*, *13*, 155–167.

Atkins, M.S., Pelham, W.E., and Licht, M.H. (1989). The differential validity of teacher ratings of inattention/overactivity and aggression. *Journal of Abnormal Child Psychology*, *17*, 423–435.

Barkley, R.A. (1990). *Attention deficit hyperactivity disorder: A handbook for diagnosis and treatment*. New York: Guilford.

Barkley, R.A. (1991). The ecological validity of laboratory and analogue assessment methods of ADHD symptoms. *Journal of Abnormal Child Psychology*, *19*, 149–178.

Barkley, R.A. (1997). Virtual symposium on ADHD. Paper presented at the Early Career Preventionist Network, http://www.oslc.org/Ecpn/intro.html.

Barkley, R.A. and Cunningham, C.E. (1979). The effects of methylphenidate on the mother-child interactions of hyperactive children. *Archives of General Psychiatry*, *36*, 201–211.

Barkley, R.A., Karlsson, J., Pollard, S., and Murphy, J. (1985). Developmental changes in the mother-child interactions of hyperactive boys: Effects of two doses of Ritalin. *Journal of Child Psychology and Psychiatry*, *26*, 705–715.

Barkley, R.A., Fischer, M., Edelbrock, C.S., and Smallish, L. (1990). The adolescent outcome of hyperactive children diagnosed by research criteria: I. An 8-year prospective follow-up study. *Journal of the American Academy of Child and Adolescent Psychiatry*, *29*, 546–557.

Biederman, J., Newcorn, J., and Sprich, S. (1991). Comorbidity of attention deficit hyperactivity disorder with conduct, depressive, anxiety, and other disorders. *American Journal of Psychiatry*, *148*, 564–577.

Biederman, J., Faraone, S.V., Milberger, S., Jetton, J.G., Chen, L., Mick, E., et al. (1996). Is childhood oppositional defiant disorder a precursor to adolescent conduct disorder? Findings from a four-year follow-up study of children with ADHD. *Journal of the American Academy of Child and Adolescent Psychiatry*, *35*, 1193–1204.

Bierman, K.L. and Wargo, J.B. (1995). Predicting the longitudinal course associated with aggressive-rejected, aggressive (nonrejected), and rejected (nonaggressive) status. *Development and Psychopathology*, *7*, 669–682.

Bierman, K.L., Smoot, D.L., and Aumiller, K. (1993). Characteristics of aggressive-rejected, aggressive (nonrejected), and rejected (nonaggressive) boys. *Child Development*, *64*, 139–151.

Bird, H.R., Gould, M.S., and Staghezza, B.M. (1993). Patterns of diagnostic comorbidity in a community sample of children aged 9 through 16 years. *Journal of the American Academy of Child and Adolescent Psychiatry*, *32*, 361–368.

Boyajian, A.E., DuPaul, G.J., Handler, M.W., Eckert, T.L., and McGoey, K.E. (2001). The use of classroom-based brief functional analysis with preschoolers at-risk for attention-deficit hyperactivity disorder (ADHD). *School Psychology Review*, *30*, 278–293.

Breen, M.J. (1989). Cognitive and behavioral differences in ADHD boys and girls. *Journal of Child Psychology and Psychiatry*, *30*, 711–716.

Bullis, M., Walker, H.M., and Sprague, J.R. (2001). A promise unfulfilled: Social skills training with at-risk and antisocial children and youth. *Exceptionality*, *9*, 67–90.

Burns, G.L. and Walsh, J.A. (2002). The influence of ADHD-hyperactivity/impulsivity symptoms on the development of oppositional defiant disorder symptoms in a 2-year longitudinal study. *Journal of Abnormal Child Psychology, 30*, 245–256.

Burns, G.L., Walsh, J.A., Patterson, D.R., Holte, C.S., Sommers-Flanagan, R., and Parker, C.M. (1997). Internal validity of the disruptive behavior disorder symptoms: Implications from parent ratings for a dimensional approach to symptom validity. *Journal of Abnormal Child Psychology, 25*, 307–319.

Campbell, S.B., Breaux, A.M., Ewing, L.J., and Szumowski, E.K. (1986). Correlates and predictors of hyperactivity and aggression: A longitudinal study of parent-referred problem preschoolers. *Journal of Abnormal Child Psychology, 14*, 217–234.

Caron, C. and Rutter, M. (1991). Comorbidity in child psychopathology: Concepts, issues, and research strategies. *Journal of Child Psychology and Psychiatry, 32*, 1063–1080.

Conners, C.K. (1969). A teacher rating scale for use in drug studies with children. *American Journal of Psychiatry, 126*, 884–888.

Conners, C.K., Epstein, J.N., March, J.S., Angold, A., Wells, K.C., Klaric, J., et al. (2001). Multimodal treatment of ADHD in the MTA: An alternative outcome analysis. *Journal of the American Academy of Child and Adolescent Psychiatry, 40*, 159–167.

Cook, E.H.J. (1999). Genetics of attention-deficit hyperactivity disorder. *Mental Retardation and Developmental Disabilities Research Reviews, 5*, 191–198.

Crick, N.R. and Dodge, K.A. (1994). A review and reformulation of social information-processing mechanisms in children's social adjustment. *Psychological Bulletin, 115*, 74–101.

Cunningham, C.E. (1999). In the wake of the MTA: Charting a new course for the study and treatment of children with attention-deficit/hyperactivity disorder. *Canadian Journal of Psychiatry, 44*, 999–1006.

Cunningham, C.E. and Siegel, L.S. (1987). Peer interactions of normal and attention-deficit-disordered boys during free play, cooperative task, and simulated classroom situations. *Journal of Abnormal Child Psychology, 15*, 247–268.

Diener, M.B. and Milich, R. (1997). Effects of positive feedback on the social interactions of boys with attention deficit hyperactivity disorder: A test of the self-protective hypothesis. *Journal of Clinical Child Psychology, 26*, 256–265.

Dodge, K.A., Pettit, G.S., McClasky, C.L., and Brown, M.M. (1986). A social information processing model of social competence in children. With commentary by John M. Gottman. *Monographs of the Society for Research in Child Development, 51*, 1–85.

Douglas, V.I. (1999). Cognitive control processes in attention-deficit/hyperactivity disorder. In H.C. Quay and A.E. Hogan (Eds.), *Handbook of disruptive behavior disorders* (pp. 105–138). New York: Kluwer Academic/Plenum.

Douglas, V.I. and Parry, P.A. (1983). Effects of reward on delayed reaction time task performance of hyperactive children. *Journal of Abnormal Child Psychology, 11*, 313–326.

DuPaul, G.J. (1991). Parent and teacher ratings of ADHD symptoms: Psychometric properties in a community-based sample. *Journal of Clinical Child Psychology, 20*, 245–253.

DuPaul, G.J. and Eckert, T.L. (1997). Interventions for students with attention-deficit/hyperactivity disorder: One size does not fit all. *School Psychology Review, 26*, 369–372.

Elgar, F.J., Curtis, L.J., McGrath, P.J., Waschbusch, D.A., and Stewart, S.H. (2003). Antecedent-consequence conditions in maternal mood and child behavioural problems:

A four-year cross-lagged study. *Journal of Clinical Child and Adolescent Psychology*, *32*, 362–374.

Elgar, F.J., Waschbusch, D.A., McGrath, P.J., Stewart, S.H., and Curtis, L.J. (2004). Temporal relations in daily-reported maternal mood and disruptive child behaviour. *Journal of Abnormal Child Psychology*, *32*, 237–247.

Eme, R.F. (1992). Selective female affliction in the developmental disorders of childhood: A literature review. *Journal of Clinical Child Psychology*, *21*, 354–364.

Esser, G., Schmidt, M.H., and Woerner, W. (1990). Epidemiology of course of psychiatric disorders in school-age children: Results of a longitudinal study. *Journal of Child and Psychology and Psychiatry and Allied Disciplines*, *31*, 243–263.

Fabiano, G.A., Pelham, W.E., Gnagy, E.M., Coles, E.K., and Wheeler-Cox, T. (2000). *A meta-analysis of behavioral and combined treatments for ADHD*. Washington, DC: American Psychological Association.

Faraone, S.V., Biederman, J., and Monuteaux, M.C. (2000). Attention-deficit disorder and conduct disorder in girls: Evidence for a familial subtype. *Biological Psychiatry, 48*, 21–29.

Farrington, D.P., Loeber, R., and van Kammen, W.B. (1990). Long-term criminal outcomes of hyperactivity-impulsivity-attention deficit and conduct problems in childhood. In L.N. Robins and M. Rutter (Eds.), Straight and devious pathways from childhood to adulthood (pp. 62–81). Cambridge: Cambridge University Press.

Gaub, M. and Carlson, C.L. (1997). Gender differences in ADHD: A meta-analysis and critical review. *Journal of the American Academy of Child and Adolescent Psychiatry, 36*, 1036–1045.

Gillis, J.J., Gilger, J.W., Pennington, B.F., and DeFries, J.C. (1992). Attention deficit disorder in reading disabled twins: Evidence for a genetic etiology. *Journal of Abnormal Child Psychology, 20*, 303–315.

Gittelman-Klein, R.G. and Mannuzza, S. (1989). The long-term outcome of the attention deficit disorder/hyperkinetic syndrome. In T. Sagvolden and T. Archer (Eds.), *Attention deficit disorder: Clinical and basic research* (pp. 71–91). Hillsdale, NJ: Lawrence Erlebaum Associates.

Grenell, M.M., Glass, C.R., and Katz, K.S. (1987). Hyperactive children and peer interaction: Knowledge and performance of social skills. *Journal of Abnormal Child Psychology, 15*, 1–13.

Hartung, C.M. and Widiger, T.A. (1998). Gender differences in the diagnosis of mental disorders: Conclusions and controversies of the DSM-IV. *Psychological Bulletin, 123*, 260–278.

Henker, B. and Whalen, C.K. (1999). The child with attention-deficit/hyperactivity disorder in school and peer settings. In H.C. Quay and A.E. Hogan (Eds.), *Handbook of disruptive behavior disorders* (pp. 157–178). New York: Kluwer Academic/Plenum.

Hinshaw, S.P. (1994). *Attention deficits and hyperactivity in children* (Vol. 29). Thousand Oaks, CA: Sage.

Hinshaw, S.P. and Park, T. (1999). Research problems and issues: Toward a more definitive science of disruptive behavior disorders. In H.C. Quay and A.E. Hogan (Eds.), *Handbook of disruptive behavior disorders* (pp. 593–620). New York: Plenum.

Hinshaw, S.P., Lahey, B.B., and Hart, E.L. (1993). Issues of taxonomy and comorbidity in the development of conduct disorder. *Development and Psychopathology, 3*, 31–50.

Hoza, B., Waschbusch, D.A., Pelham, W.E., Molina, B., and Milich, R. (2000). Attention-deficit/hyperactivity disordered and control boys' responses to social success and failure. *Child Development, 71*, 432–446.

Jensen, P.S., Martin, D., and Cantwell, D.P. (1997). Comorbidity in ADHD: Implications for research, practice, and DSM-V. *Journal of the American Academy of Child and Adolescent Psychiatry, 36*, 1065–1079.

Johnston, C. and Mash, E.J. (2001). Families of children with attention-deficit/ hyperactivity disorder: Review and recommendations for future research. *Clinical Child and Adolescent Psychology Newsletter, 4*, 183–208.

Johnston, C. and Pelham, W.E. (1990). Maternal characteristics, ratings of child behavior, and mother-child interactions in families of children with externalizing disorders. *Journal of Abnormal Child Psychology, 18*, 407–417.

Kolko, D.J., Buckstein, O.G., and Barron, J. (1999). Methylphenidate and behavior modification in children with ADHD and comorbid ODD or CD: Main and incremental effects across settings. *Journal of the American Academcy of Child and Adolescent Psychiatry, 38*, 578–586.

Kuntsi, J. and Stevenson, J. (2000). Hyperactivity in children: A focus on genetic research and psychological theories. *Clinical Child and Family Psychology Review, 3*, 1–23.

Lahey, B.B., Miller, T.I., Gordon, R.A., and Riley, A.W. (1999). Developmental epidemiology of the disruptive behavior disorders. In H.C. Quay and A.E. Hogan (Eds.), *Handbook of disruptive behavior disorders* (pp. 23–48). New York: Kluwer Academic/ Plenum.

Lahey, B.B., Loeber, R., Burke, J.D., Rathouz, P.J., and McBurnett, K. (2002). Waxing and waning in concert: Dynamic comorbidity of conduct disorder with other disruptive and emotional problems over 17 years among clinic-referred boys. *Journal of Abnormal Psychology, 111*, 556–567.

Landau, S. and Milich, R. (1988). Social communication patterns of attention deficit disordered boys. *Journal of Abnormal Child Psychology, 16*, 69–81.

Laufer, M.W. (1962). Cerebral dysfunction and behavior disorders in adolescents. *American Journal of Orthopsychiatry, 32*, 501–506.

Leibson, C.L., Katusic, S.K., Barbaresi, W.J., Ransom, J., and O'Brien, P.C. (2001). Use and costs of medical care for children and adolescents with and without attention-deficit/hyperactivity disorder. *Journal of the American Medical Association, 285*, 60–66.

Lilienfeld, S.O. and Waldman, I.D. (1990). The relation between childhood attention-deficit hyperactivity disorder and adult antisocial behavior reexamined: The problem of heterogeneity. *Clinical Psychology Review, 10*, 699–725.

Loney, J. and Milich, R. (1982). Hyperactivity, inattention, and aggression in clinical practice. In M. Wolraich and D.K. Routh (Eds.), *Advances in developmental and behavioral pediatrics* (Vol. 3, pp. 113–147). Greenwich, CT: JAI.

Loney, J., Langhorne, J.E., and Paternite, C.E. (1978). An empirical basis for subgrouping the hyperkinetic/MBD syndrome. *Journal of Abnormal Psychology, 87*, 431–441.

Lonigan, C., Elbert, J.C., and Johnson, S.B. (1998). Empirically supported psychosocial interventions for children: An overview. *Journal of Clinical Child Psychology, 27*, 138–145.

Lynam, D.R. (1996). The early identification of chronic offenders: Who is the fledgling psychopath? *Psychological Bulletin, 120*, 209–234.

Magnusson, D., Klinteberg, B.A., and Stattin, H. (1992). Autonomic activity/reactivity, behavior, and crime in a longitudinal perspective. In J. McCord (Ed.), *Facts, frameworks, and forecasts: Advances in criminological theory* (Vol. 3, pp. 287–318). New Brunswick, NJ: Transaction.

Mannuzza, S., Klein, R.G., Bessler, A., Malloy, P., and LaPadula, M. (1993). Adult outcome of hyperactive boys: Educational achievement, occupational rank, and psychiatric status. *Archives of General Psychiatry, 50*, 565–576.

Matthys, W., Cuperus, J.M., and Van Engeland, H. (1999). Deficient social problem solving in boys with ODD/CD, with ADHD, and with both disorders. *Journal of the American Academy of Child and Adolescent Psychiatry, 38*, 311–321.

Milch-Reich, S., Campbell, S.B., Pelham, W.E., Connelly, L.M., and Geva, D. (1999). Developmental and individual differences in children's on-line representations of dynamic social events. *Child Development, 70*, 413–431.

Milich, R. and Dodge, K.A. (1984). Social information processing in child psychiatric populations. *Journal of Abnormal Child Psychology, 12*, 471–490.

Milich, R. and Kramer, J. (1984). Reflections on impulsivity: An empirical investigation of impulsivity as a construct. *Advances in Learning and Behavioral Disabilities, 3*, 57–94.

Milich, R. and Landau, S. (1982). Socialization and peer relations in hyperactive children. In K. Gadow and I. Bailer (Eds.), *Advances in learning and behavioral disabilities* (Vol. 1, pp. 283–339). Greenwich, CT: JAI.

Milich, R. and Landau, S. (1989). The role of social status variables in differentiating subgroups of hyperactive children. In J. Swanson and L. Bloomingdale (Eds.), *Attention deficit disorders: IV. Current concepts and emerging trends in attentional and behavioral disorders of childhood* (pp. 1–16). London: Pergamon.

Milich, R. and Lorch, E.P. (1994). Television viewing methodology to understand cognitive processing of ADHD children. In T.H. Ollendick and R.J. Prinz (Eds.), *Advances in clinical child psychology* (Vol. 16, pp. 177–201). New York: Plenum.

Milich, R., Landau, S., Kilby, G., and Whitten, P. (1982a). Preschool peer perceptions of the behavior of hyperactive and aggressive children. *Journal of Abnormal Child Psychology, 10*, 497–510.

Milich, R., Loney, J., and Landau, S. (1982b). Independent dimensions of hyperactivity and aggression: A validation with playroom observation data. *Journal of Abnormal Psychology, 91*, 183–198.

Milich, R., Wolraich, M., and Lindgren, S. (1986). Sugar and hyperactivity: A critical review of empirical findings. *Clinical Psychology Review, 6*, 493–513.

Moffitt, T.E. (1990). Juvenile delinquency and attention deficit disorder: Boys' developmental trajectories from age 3 to age 15. *Child Development, 61*, 893–910.

Moffitt, T.E. and Silva, P.A. (1988). Self-reported delinquency, neuropsychological deficit, and history of attention deficit disorder. *Journal of Abnormal Child Psychology, 16*, 553–569.

Molina, B.S.G. and Pelham, W.E. (2003). Childhood predictors of adolescent substance use in a longitudinal study of children with ADHD. *Journal of Abnormal Psychology, 112*, 497–507.

MTA Cooperative Group (1999a). A 14-month randomized clinical trial of treatment strategies for attention-deficit/hyperactivity disorder. *Archives of General Psychiatry, 56*, 1073–1086.

MTA Cooperative Group (1999b). Moderators and mediators of treatment response for children with attention-deficit/hyperactivity disorder. *Archives of General Psychiatry, 56*, 1088–1096.

MTA Cooperative Group (2004a). National Institute of Mental Health Multimodal Treatment Study of ADHD follow-up: 24-month outcomes of treatment strategies for attention-deficit/hyperactivity disorder. *Pediatrics, 113*, 754–761.

MTA Cooperative Group (2004b). National Institute of Mental Health Multimodal Treatment Study of ADHD follow-up: Changes in effectiveness and growth after the end of treatment. *Pediatrics, 113*, 762–769.

Murphy, D.A., Pelham, W.E., and Lang, A.R. (1992). Aggression in boys with attention deficit-hyperactivity disorder: Methylphenidate effects on naturalistically observed aggression, response to provocation, and social information processing. *Journal of Abnormal Child Psychology, 20*, 451–466.

Murray, L.K. and Kollins, S.H. (2000). Effects of methylphenidate on sensitivity to reinforcement in children diagnosed with attention deficit hyperactivity disorder. *Journal of Applied Behavior Analysis, 33*, 573–591.

Nagin, D. and Tremblay, R.E. (1999). Trajectories of boys' physical aggression, opposition, and hyperactivity on the path to physically violent and nonviolent juvenile delinquency. *Child Development, 70*, 1181–1196.

Nichols, S. and Waschbusch, D.A. (2004). A review of the validity of laboratory cognitive tasks used to assess symptoms of ADHD. *Child Psychiatry and Human Development, 34*, 297–315.

NIH Consensus Statement (1998). *Diagnosis and treatment of attention-deficit hyperactivity disorder.* Kensington, MD: National Institutes of Health Consensus Development Project.

Northup, J. and Gulley, V. (2001). Some contributions of functional analysis to the assessment of behaviors associated with attention deficit hyperactivity disorder and the effects of stimulant medication. *School Psychology Review, 30*, 227–238.

Offord, D.R., Boyle, M.H., Szatmari, P., Rae-Grant, N.I., Links, P.S., Cadman, D.T., et al. (1987). Ontario Child Health Study II: Six month prevalence of disorder and rates of service utilization. *Archives of General Psychiatry, 44*, 832–836.

Offord, D.R., Boyle, M.H., and Racine, Y. (1989). Ontario child health study: Correlates of disorder. *Journal of the American Academy of Child and Adolescent Psychiatry, 28*, 856–860.

Oosterlaan, J., Logan, G.D., and Sergeant, J.A. (1998). Response inhibition in AD/HD, CD, comorbid AD/HD+CD, anxious, and control children: A meta-analysis of studies with the stop task. *Journal of Child Psychology and Psychiatry, 39*, 411–425.

Palmer, E.D. and Finger, S. (2001). An early description of ADHD (inattentive subtype): Dr. Alexander Crichton and "mental restlessness" (1789). *Child Psychology and Psychiatry Review, 6*, 66–73.

Patterson, G.R., DeBaryshe, B.D., and Ramsey, E. (1989). A developmental perspective on antisocial behavior. *American Psychologist, 44*, 329–225.

Pelham, W.E. (1999a). *Attention deficit hyperactivity disorder: Diagnosis, nature, etiology, and treatment.* Buffalo, NY: State University of New York at Buffalo.

Pelham, W.E. (1999b). The NIMH multimodal treatment study for ADHD: Just say yes to drugs? *Clinical Child Psychology Newsletter, 14*, 1–6.

Pelham, W.E. and Bender, M.E. (1982). Peer relationships in hyperactive children: Description and treatment. In K. Gadow and I. Bailer (Eds.), *Advances in learning and behavioral disabilities* (Vol. 1, pp. 365–436). Greenwich, CT: JAI.

Pelham, W.E. and Lang, A.R. (1993). Parental alcohol consumption and deviant child behavior: Laboratory studies of reciprocal effects. *Clinical Psychology Review, 13*, 763–784.

Pelham, W.E. and Waschbusch, D.A. (1999). Behavioral intervention in ADHD. In H.C. Quay and A.E. Hogan (Eds.), *Handbook of disruptive behavior disorders* (pp. 255–278). New York: Plenum.

Pelham, W.E., Schnedler, R.W., Bologna, N., and Contreras, A. (1980). Behavioral and stimulant treatment of hyperactive children: A therapy study with methylphenidate probes in a within-subject design. *Journal of Applied Behavior Analysis*, *13*, 221–236.

Pelham, W.E., Schnedler, R.W., Bender, M.E., Nilsson, D.E., Miller, J., Budrow, M.S., et al. (1988). The combination of behavior therapy and methylphenidate in the treatment of attention deficit disorders: A therapy outcome study. In L. Bloomingdale (Ed.), *Attention deficit disorders III: New research in attention, treatment, and psycho-pharmacology* (pp. 29–48). London: Pergamon.

Pelham, W.E., Milich, R., Murphy, D.A., and Murphy, H.A. (1989a). Normative data on the IOWA Conners teacher rating scale. *Journal of Clinical Child Psychology*, *18*, 259–262.

Pelham, W.E., Walker, J.L., Sturges, J., and Hoza, J. (1989b). Comparative effects of methylphenidate on ADD girls and ADD boys. *Journal of the American Academy of Child and Adolescent Psychiatry*, *28*, 773–776.

Pelham, W.E., Gnagy, E.M., Greenslade, K.E., and Milich, R. (1992a). Teacher ratings of DSM-III-R symptoms for the disruptive behavior disorders. *Journal of the American Academy of Child and Adolescent Psychiatry*, *31*, 210–218.

Pelham, W.E., Schneider, W., Carlson, C.L., and Evans, S.W. (1992b). Sustained attention and ADHD: Vigilence performance and methylphenidate effects in the laboratory and the natural environment. Paper presented at the Society for Research in Child and Adolescent Psychopathology, Sarasota, FL, June.

Pelham, W.E., Carlson, C., Sams, S.E., Vallano, G., Dixon, M.J., and Hoza, B. (1993). Separate and combined effects of methylphenidate and behavior modification on boys with attention deficit-hyperactivity disorder in the classroom. *Journal of Consulting and Clinical Psychology*, *61*, 506–515.

Pelham, W.E., Hoza, B., Sams, S.E., Gnagy, E.M., Greiner, A.R., Waschbusch, D.A., et al. (1994). Rock music and video movies as distractors for ADHD boys in comparison with controls, individual differences, and medication effects. Paper presented at the International Society for Research in Child and Adolescent Psychopathology, London, July.

Pelham, W.E., Lang, A.R., Atkeson, B., Murphy, D.A., Gnagy, E.M., Greiner, A.R., et al. (1997). Effects of deviant child behavior on parental distress and alcohol consumption in laboratory interactions. *Journal of Abnormal Child Psychology*, *25*, 413–424.

Pelham, W.E., Wheeler, T., and Chronis, A.M. (1998). Empirically supported psycho-social treatment for attention deficit hyperactivity disorder. *Journal of Clinical Child Psychology*, *27*, 190–205.

Pelham, W.E., Hoza, B., Pillow, D.R., Gnagy, E.M., Kipp, H.L., Greiner, A.R., et al. (2001). Effects of methylphenidate and expectancy on children with ADHD: Behavior, academic performance, and attributions in a Summer Treatment Program and regular classroom setting. *Journal of Consulting and Clinical Psychology*, *70*, 320–335.

Pelham, W.E., Erhardt, D., Gnagy, E.M., Greiner, A.R., Arnold, L.E., Abikoff, H.B., et al. (under review). Parent and teacher evaluation of treatment in the MTA: Consumer satisfaction and perceived effectiveness.

Pliszka, S.R., Greenhill, L.L., Crimson, M.L., Sedillo, A., Carlson, C., Conners, C.K., et al. (2000). The Texas Children's Medication Algorithm Project: Report of the Texas Consensus Conference Panel on Medication Treatment of Childhood Attention-Deficit/Hyperactivity Disorder. Part I. *Journal of the American Academy of Child and Adolescent Psychiatry*, *39*, 908–919.

Pope, A.W. and Bierman, K.L. (1999). Predicting adolescent peer problems and antisocial activities: The relative roles of aggression and dysregulation. *Developmental Psychology, 35*, 335–346.

Pope, A.W., Bierman, K.L., and Mumma, G.H. (1991). Aggression, hyperactivity, and inattention-immaturity: Behavior dimensions associate with peer rejection in elementary boys. *Developmental Psychology, 27*, 663–671.

Reitman, D., Hupp, S.D.A., O'Callaghan, P.M., Gulley, V., and Northup, J. (2001). The influence of a token economy and methylphenidate on attentive and disruptive behavior during sports with ADHD-diagnosed children. *Behavior Modification, 25*, 305–323.

Rutter, M., Silberg, J., O'Connor, T., and Simonoff, E. (1999a). Genetics and child psychiatry: I. Advances in quantitative and molecular genetics. *Journal of Child Psychology and Psychiatry, 40*, 3–18.

Rutter, M., Silberg, J., O'Connor, T., and Simonoff, E. (1999b). Genetics and child psychiatry: II. Empirical research findings. *Journal of Child Psychology and Psychiatry, 40*, 19–55.

Samudra, K. and Cantwell, D.P. (1999). Risk factors for attention-deficit/hyperactivity disorder. In H.C. Quay and A.E. Hogan (Eds.), *Handbook of disruptive behavior disorders* (pp. 199–220). New York: Plenum.

Sergeant, J.A., Oosterlaan, J., and van der Meere, J. (1999). Information processing and energetic factors in attention-deficit/hyperactivity disorder. In H.C. Quay and A.E. Hogan (Eds.), *Handbook of disruptive behavior disorders* (pp. 75–104). New York: Kluwer Academic/Plenum.

Sterling-Turner, H.E., Robinson, S.L., and Wilczynski, S.M. (2001). Functional assessment of distracting and disruptive behavior in the school setting. *School Psychology Review, 30*, 211–226.

Stevens, J., Quittner, A.L., and Abikoff, H. (1998). Factors influencing elementary school teachers' ratings of ADHD and ODD behaviors. *Journal of Clinical Child Psychology, 27*, 406–414.

Stevenson, J. (1992). Evidence for genetic etiology in hyperactivity in children. *Behavior Genetics, 22*, 337–344.

Stouthamer-Loeber, M., Loeber, R., Wei, E., Farrington, D.P., and Wikström, P.O.H. (2002). Risk and promotive effects in the explanation of persistent serious delinquency in boys. *Journal of Consulting and Clinical Psychology, 70*, 111–123.

Swanson, J.M. (1996). The SNAP-IV teacher and parent rating scale: http://www.adhd.net/

Swanson, J.M., Kraemer, H.C., Hinshaw, S.P., Arnold, L.E., Conners, C.K., Abikoff, H.B., et al. (2001). Clinical relevance of the primary findings of the MTA: Success rates based on severity of ADHD and ODD symptoms at the end of treatment. *Journal of the American Academy of Child and Adolescent Psychiatry, 40*, 168–179.

Swanson, J.M., Gupta, S., Williams, L., Agler, D., Lerner, M., and Wigal, S. (2003). Efficacy of a new pattern of delivery of methylphenidate for the treatment of ADHD: Effects on activity level in the classroom and on the playground. *Journal of the American Academy of Child and Adolescent Psychiatry, 41*, 1306–1314.

Tannock, R. (1998). Attention deficit hyperactivity disorder: Advances in cognitive, neurobiological, and genetic research. *Journal of Child Psychology and Psychiatry, 39*, 65–99.

Tripp, G. and Alsop, B. (1999). Sensitivity to reward frequency in boys with attention deficit hyperactivity disorder. *Journal of Clinical Child Psychology, 28*, 366–375.

Waschbusch, D.A. (2002). A meta-analytic examination of comorbid hyperactive/impulsive/inattention problems and conduct problems. *Psychological Bulletin, 128*, 118–150.

Waschbusch, D.A. (2004). Empirically supported treatment of ADHD: Outcome data and relationship with information processing. Paper presented at the Center for Children and Families, University at Buffalo, November.

Waschbusch, D.A. and Hill, G.P. (2003). Empirically supported, promising, and unsupported treatments for attention-deficit/hyperactivity disorder. In S.O. Lilienfield, J.M. Lohr, and S.J. Lynn (Eds.), *Science and pseudoscience in contemporary clinical psychology* (pp. 333–362). New York: Guilford.

Waschbusch, D.A., King, S., and Northern Partners In Action for Children and Youth (in press). Should sex-specific norms be used to assess Attention-Deficit Hyperactivity Disorder (ADHD) or Oppositional Defiant Disorder (ODD)? *Journal of Consulting and Clinical Psychology.*

Weiss, G. and Hechtman, L.T. (1993). *Hyperactive children grown up: ADHD in children, adolescents, and adults.* New York: Guilford.

Whalen, C.K. and Henker, B. (1985). The social worlds of hyperactive (ADHD) children. *Clinical Psychology Review, 5*, 447–478.

Whalen, C.K. and Henker, B. (1999). The child with attention-deficit/hyperactivity disorder in family contexts. In H.C. Quay and A.E. Hogan (Eds.), *Handbook of disruptive behavior disorders* (pp. 139–155). New York: Kluwer Academic/Plenum.

Whalen, C.K., Henker, B., Collins, B., McAuliffe, S., and Vaux, A. (1979). Peer interaction in a structured communication task: Comparisons of normal and hyperactive boys and of methylphenidate (ritalin) and placebo effects. *Child Development, 50*, 388–401.

Willoughby, M.T. (2003). Developmental course of ADHD symptomatology during the transition from childhood to adolescence: A review with recommendations. *Journal of Child Psychology and Psychiatry, 44*, 88–106.

Wolraich, M.L., Feurer, I.D., Hannah, J.N., Baumgaertel, A., and Pinnock, T.Y. (1998). Obtaining systematic teacher reports of disruptive behavior disorders utilyzing DSM-IV. *Journal of Abnormal Child Psychology, 26*, 141–152.

Wright, K.D., Waschbusch, D.A., and Franklin, B.W. (under review). A comparison of a structured clinical interview and a behavior rating scale in the diagnosis of ADHD.

4

ANXIETY DISORDERS

Roma A. Vasa and Daniel S. Pine

Anxiety is a normal and ubiquitous emotion that enhances performance, protects against dangers, and facilitates important developmental transitions. In children, anxiety predictably occurs at different stages of development. For example, 9 month old infants experience stranger and separation anxiety, 2 to 4 year old children exhibit fears of the dark and animals, and 7 to 10 year old children have fears of bodily injury, death, and school performance.

Anxiety disorders are characterized by excessive or developmentally inappropriate anxiety that interferes with psychological, academic, and social functioning. Childhood anxiety disorders can result in school refusal, somatic complaints, social withdrawal, avoidance behavior, and low self-esteem. Despite these adverse consequences, these conditions are often neglected or misdiagnosed leaving many children untreated.

Research on childhood anxiety disorders is rapidly accumulating with current data revealing many important clinical characteristics about these conditions. Anxiety disorders are the most common psychiatric disorders afflicting children and adolescents. These disorders are often comorbid with childhood depressive and disruptive behavior disorders. Anxiety disorders are transient in many children. A subset of children will face a chronic and fluctuating course that culminates in adult anxiety, depression, substance abuse, and suicide attempts. Treatment studies show that pharmacotherapy and cognitive-behavioral therapy are effective for over 50 percent of children, which although promising, leaves a substantial number of affected children. Research on pathophysiology may reveal important insights that may help to develop more effective treatments. Developments in the fields of affective neuroscience and developmental psychopathology offer promising avenues to uncover the behavioral and neural basis of these conditions.

This chapter begins with a broad overview of the clinical characteristics of childhood anxiety disorders and highlights many important areas of future research. The next section presents data on the pathophysiology of three common disorders: separation anxiety disorder, generalized anxiety disorder, and social phobia. These disorders have recently been grouped together because they share similar clinical features and responses to treatment. The final section reviews empirically supported treatments for these three disorders.

Clinical characteristics

Phenomenology/nosology

The *Diagnostic and Statistical Manual of Mental Disorders, 4th edition* (DSM-IV; American Psychiatric Association, 1994) lists twelve different anxiety disorders that can affect children and adolescents. These disorders are classified according to symptoms and behaviors that reflect different foci of anxiety. Differentiating between normal and pathological anxiety is based on fulfillment of DSM-IV criteria for symptom count and duration, as well as clinically significant impairment or extreme distress. Although the categorical approach has facilitated communication amongst clinicians, it does not assume clinical homogeneity across individuals with the same disorder. As a result, there is significant heterogeneity within individual disorders, which poses significant dilemmas for disorder-specific research on the pathophysiology and treatment.

Descriptions of the twelve disorders are as follows: *Separation anxiety disorder* (SAD) is characterized by excessive fears about separation from a caregiver; this is the only disorder that is classified separately under the DSM-IV subheading of "Other Disorders of Infancy Childhood or Adolescence". *Social phobia* (SoP) is defined as an irrational fear of being judged in social situations. *Specific phobia* is a fear of specific objects or situations. *Generalized anxiety disorder* (GAD) is characterized by excessive and uncontrollable worry about life events. *Obsessive-compulsive disorder* (OCD) is characterized by intrusive illogical thoughts (e.g., obsessions) and repetitive behaviors often related to the obsessions (e.g., compulsions). *Panic disorder* (with and without agoraphobia) is characterized by discrete fear attacks that are associated with cognitive and physical symptoms. *Posttraumatic stress disorder* (PTSD) is a reaction to a severe trauma that is comprised of three symptom clusters: reexperiencing of the event, hyperarousal, and avoidance symptoms. *Acute stress disorder* is phenomenologically similar to PTSD, however the duration of symptoms is one month or less. *Agoraphobia* (with and without panic) is a fear of being in places that are difficult to escape. *Adjustment disorder with anxiety* and *Adjustment disorder with anxiety and depressed mood* are anxious reactions to an identifiable stressor. *Anxiety secondary to general medical condition* occurs when anxiety is the physiological result of a medical condition.

Epidemiology

Anxiety disorders are the most common psychiatric disorders affecting children and adolescents. Large scale epidemiological studies conducted in the United States, Canada, New Zealand, and Puerto Rico report that approximately 10 to 20 percent of children and adolescents will develop an anxiety disorder at some time during development (see review by Costello and Angold, 1995). Anxiety disorders occur across all age groups and in all socioeconomic and ethnic groups. Some studies show that boys and girls are equally affected, although the weight of the evidence suggests an increased prevalence in girls relative to boys and in adolescents relative to children (Bowen et al., 1990; McGee et al., 1990).

Although most of the epidemiological studies are largely similar, there are some methodological differences across studies, which may partly account for variations in prevalence. Variables such as age, race and ethnicity, assessment measures, methods to integrate parent and child reports, and differential impairment thresholds are some of the factors affecting prevalence estimates in epidemiological data. In general, only data from community samples provide information that is generalizable to the population, due to factors affecting clinically referred children that may confound the rates (e.g., adverse family factors, comorbidity). Rates of anxiety disorders are also extremely sensitive to impairment criteria. For example, in the Methods for the Epidemiology of Child and Adolescent Mental Disorders (MECA) study, Shaffer et al. (1996) demonstrated that applying more stringent impairment thresholds significantly decreased the prevalence of anxiety disorders according to both parent and child reports. This effect was particularly large for the anxiety disorders, relative to other psychiatric syndromes. Another notable point about these studies is that the samples were primarily Caucasian, African-American, or Hispanic.

Research on the prevalence of anxiety disorder in other ethnic groups, such as Asian and Middle Eastern, is needed. Knowledge of the study methods is therefore important before drawing firm conclusions about prevalence.

Despite the different methods, some general patterns of prevalence emerge from the data. Separation anxiety disorder occurs in approximately 3 to 4 percent of children (Anderson et al., 1987; Benjamin et al., 1990). Generalized anxiety disorder occurs in less than 5 percent of children although one study reported a rate of 15.4 percent in adolescents (Anderson et al., 1987; Benjamin et al., 1990). Rates of social phobia are more variable and range from 2 to 7 percent (Anderson et al., 1987; Verhulst et al., 1997). Similarly, rates of simple phobia range from 2 to 7 percent (Anderson et al., 1987; Fergusson et al., 1993; Verhulst et al., 1997). Obsessive-compulsive disorder occurs in 1 to 3 percent of children (Hollingsworth et al., 1980; Valleni-Basile et al., 1994). Rates of PTSD vary markedly across studies and on multiple factors such as the nature of the trauma, time of assessment, and the diagnostic criteria used. For example, PTSD was present in 12 percent of children who were exposed to an industrial fire (March et al., 1997), whereas the disorder manifested in 70 percent of children after the 1988 earthquake in Armenia (Pynoos et al., 1995). Panic disorder and agoraphobia are rare in children, and only case reports have been described. Even among adolescents, less than 1 percent of the population is likely to be affected with either of these disorders.

Another noteworthy point is the development differences in prevalence rates for various disorders. For example, SAD occurs in younger children and then tends to decline in adolescence (Bowen et al., 1990; Kashani and Orvaschel, 1988; Verhulst et al., 1997), whereas rates of GAD and SoP increase with age (King et al., 1994; Last et al., 1987). Developmental epidemiological studies of community and clinic-based samples are needed to examine prevalence patterns, as well as the specific risk and protective factors for disorders at each developmental stage.

Comorbidity

Anxiety disorders are highly comorbid with other anxiety disorders, depressive disorders, and disruptive behavior disorders. Comorbidity complicates the clinical management in many respects. First, symptom overlap between anxiety and depression, and symptom overshadowing by behavioral disorders, confounds the diagnostic assessment of anxiety. Second, differentiating impairment due to anxiety from impairment due to other psychiatric disorders is difficult to ascertain. Finally, treatment decisions must consider which disorder takes precedence and how treatment of comorbid disorders may affect the primary anxiety syndrome.

There is considerable data demonstrating significant coaggregation and symptom overlap amongst three particular disorders, GAD, SAD, and SoP (Gurley et al., 1996). These three disorders share similar core features of anxiety, respond to similar treatments, and distinctly differ from PTSD, OCD, and simple phobia (Bell-Dolan and Brazeal, 1993; Birmaher et al., 1994; Kendall, 2000; Kendall et al., 1997; Pine et al., 1998; RUPP Anxiety Study Group, 2001). For example, in a descriptive study of clinically referred children, Last et al. (1987) reported that 40 to 60 percent of children with an anxiety disorder had one or more comorbid anxiety disorders, usually SAD, SoP, or overanxious disorder (OAD), which is the DSM-IV equivalent of GAD. Strauss and Last (1993) found that about two-thirds of children with SoP had a comorbid anxiety disorder, mostly OAD. Pharmacological and cognitive-behavioral treatment studies show that over two-thirds of clinically anxious children presented with one or more of these three disorders (Kendall et al., 1997; RUPP Anxiety Study Group, 2001). In community samples, Kashani and Orvaschel (1990) reported similar rates of anxiety comorbidity in 8, 12 and 17 year old children; other studies of community samples however report much lower rates of comorbidity (Lewinsohn et al., 1997). These data indicate that although a single anxiety disorder is possible, coaggregation is the more likely presentation.

High rates of comorbidity amongst GAD, SAD, and SoP reflect the presence of phenotypic heterogeneity across the disorders when DSM-IV clinical criteria are used to ascertain diagnosis. Phenotypic heterogeneity is one of the major impediments to pathophysiological research. As such, there are ongoing debates about whether these three disorders should be viewed as distinct diagnoses, with disorder-specific pathophysiological mechanisms, or as one common disorder with a similar set of neural mechanisms. One approach to delineating more homogeneous anxiety phenotypes is to examine the behavioral correlates of anxiety using behaviorally based tasks and functional neuroimaging methods.

Adding to this complexity is the significant comorbidity between anxiety, depression, and disruptive behavior disorders. In a review by Brady and Kendall (1992), rates of comorbidity between anxiety and depression ranged from 15 to 60 percent depending on the study methods. Rates of comorbid disruptive behavior disorder also vary across samples but tend to range from 16 to 40 percent (Anderson et al., 1987; Last et al., 1987). The chronology of developing comorbid conditions is unknown. However, two studies support the hypothesis that anxiety may be a vulnerability factor for general psychopathology. For example, in a study of 75 children, Kovacs et al. (1984) reported that anxiety disorders heralded the onset of depressive and conduct disorders. Strauss et al. (1988) studied a clinically referred sample of 5 to 17 year old anxious children, and found that children with comorbid depression and anxiety were older and experienced more severe anxiety symptoms. Future studies on the clinical and treatment characteristics of comorbid anxiety syndromes is needed.

Course

Although anxiety disorders are transient and self-limited in many children, a subset of children exhibit a chronic and fluctuating course that progresses to adult psychopathology. Children who remain untreated and who repeatedly encounter stressful experiences and exposures to the feared stimulus are at greatest risk for chronic disturbances. At least three studies illustrate the continuity of childhood anxiety disorders for up to five years after initial onset of the disorder. Last et al. (1996) followed a cohort of one hundred 5 to 18 year old clinically referred anxious children for up to four years and found that although 82 percent of children had a remission of their original anxiety disorder, 15 percent developed a different anxiety disorder, 13 percent developed a depressive disorder, and 7 percent had an externalizing disorder. In a longitudinal study of 7 to 12 year old children, Beidel et al. (1996) found that anxiety disorders and symptoms were present in the majority of children after six months. Baker and Cantwell (1987) found that one-third of children attending a speech and hearing clinic were diagnosed with another anxiety disorder three years later. Some limitations of these studies include their small sample size and lack of control groups. Nevertheless, the data reflect the relatively high degree of persistence and stability of anxiety disorders over time.

Prospective and retrospective studies confirm the longitudinal association between child anxiety and risk for adult anxiety, depression, substance abuse, and suicide attempts (Achenbach et al., 1995; Ferdinand and Verhulst, 1995; Klein, 1995; Pine et al., 1998). For example, in a follow-up study of 776 adolescents, Pine et al. (1998) reported that adolescent anxiety or depression carried a two- to three-fold increased risk for anxiety or depression in early adulthood. Findings from retrospective studies mirror the prospective data, that is, many adults report having a significant history of childhood anxiety. Therefore, it is imperative to identify the risk and protective factors that distinguish children who develop long-term morbidity from those with a more self-limited course.

Risk factors

Some studies of risk for pediatric anxiety emphasize the role of two key empirically supported factors: behavioral inhibition and familial predisposition. Behavioral inhibition (BI) is a temperamental construct characterized by "a consistent tendency to display fear and withdrawal in unfamiliar situations" (Biederman et al., 2001).

A growing body of data demonstrates that BI is correlated with increased risk for anxiety disorders, particularly social anxiety disorder (Biederman et al., 1990, 1993, 2001). Behavioral inhibition is associated with enhanced sympathetic activity (Kagan et al., 1987) and family history of anxiety disorder (Rosenbaum et al., 1988; Battaglia et al., 1997). Furthermore, Schwartz et al. (2003) demonstrated that adults with a history of BI show increased amygdalar activity to novel versus familiar faces, a finding that raises questions about whether BI in childhood is correlated with neurophysiological hyperreactivity. A greater understanding of the developmental mechanisms that mediate the progression of BI to anxiety disorders may help to identify and treat children early in development.

Family studies using both top-down and bottom-up approaches have consistently demonstrated that childhood anxiety disorders are familial. For example, three notable top-down studies describe familial transmission of anxiety from parents to children. Weissman et al. (1984) found that parental major depressive disorder (MDD) plus panic disorder or agoraphobia conferred increased risk for childhood depression or anxiety. Similarly, Warner et al. (1995) demonstrated that parental MDD conferred risk for "any anxiety disorder" in the offspring. Another study found that parental MDD not GAD increased risk for OAD in younger children (Breslau et al., 1987). In a bottom-up study, Last et al. (1991) found increased rates of anxiety disorders in first-degree relatives of children with anxiety disorders.

Behavioral genetic studies using twin samples provide the first step towards understanding the genetic and environmental contributions of anxiety. For example, Thapar and McGuffin (1996) examined 198 same sex twin pairs, ages 8 to 16 years, and found that both genetics and non-shared environmental factors contributed to the development of neurotic symptoms. An Australian twin study in adolescents with separation anxiety symptoms found that female gender and increased age were more likely mediated by genetic influences (Feigon et al., 2001). In a twin sample of 174 monozygotic and 152 dizygotic 7 year old twin pairs, Warren et al. (1999) found that self-reported physiological and social anxiety symptoms were more likely to be genetically influenced. These data lay the groundwork for further behavioral as well as more advanced molecular genetic studies that search for genes that confer risk for anxiety-related traits or anxiety disorders.

Summary of clinical characteristics

Considerable progress has been made in advancing our knowledge of the clinical characteristics of childhood anxiety disorders. Empirical data confirm that these disorders are highly prevalent, and exhibit significant phenotypic variation both within and across diagnostic categories across development. Many children will experience an uncomplicated course of anxiety; others however will be afflicted with chronic morbidity. Behavioral inhibition and family predisposition are two well-established risk factors for these disorders.

Pathophysiology

Background

Prior research on pathophysiology has been based on the prevailing view that childhood anxiety disorders are a downward extension of adult disorders and that similar biological mechanisms mediate both child and adult disorders. As a result, the theories and methods applied to research on adult anxiety disorders have been extended to childhood anxiety. Most of these studies attempt to correlate biological markers with distinct DSM-IV anxiety disorders. Some of the pathophysiological avenues that have been explored include involvement of physiological (hypothalamic-endocrine-adrenal (HPA) axis, noradrenergic, respiratory, cardiac, autonomic), cognitive, and neural (anatomical, chemical, physiological) systems. Although these disparate lines of investigation have yielded some novel insights, no consistent biological marker has yet been identified. As a result, there is a great need to develop more complex and integrative pathophysiologic models of childhood anxiety disorders.

The conceptual and methodological framework used to study childhood anxiety has consequently shifted in three respects (Pine and Grun, 1999). First, the perspective of developmental psychopathology is now heavily incorporated into the research hypotheses and methods. This perspective asserts that growth and reorganization of cognitive and affective brain circuits throughout childhood results in different mechanisms, behavioral patterns, and expressions of anxiety across development, and between children and adults (Cicchetti and Cohen, 1995). Developmental changes in brain structure and function have now been documented and these data have significant implications for understanding the mechanisms mediating physiological and pathological emotions such as fear and anxiety (Giedd et al.,1999).

Second, instead of searching for correlates of DSM-IV disorders, there is a paradigmatic shift towards identifying discrete observable behaviors underlying anxiety disorders across development using a variety of experimental laboratory procedures. These behaviors are objectively measurable in the laboratory setting and are hypothesized to correlate with DSM-IV clinical symptoms as well as with underlying neural dysfunction (Figure 4.1). Changes in complex behaviors can be correlated with neurophysiological changes through the use of tools, such as functional magnetic resonance imaging (fMRI). This work will allow for postulating developmental behavioral and neural models of childhood anxiety disorders, which ultimately may lead to delineation of more homogeneous anxiety phenotypes.

Third, hypotheses for studying brain–behavior relationships in anxiety are derived from the field of affective neuroscience. This field is part of a larger scientific movement that integrates knowledge from cognitive psychology, basic science, and clinical psychiatry to understand the neural basis of emotion, such as anxiety. Delineating the neural basis of normal fear and anxiety may provide clues to the dysfunctional mechanisms underlying anxiety disorders. Various scientists

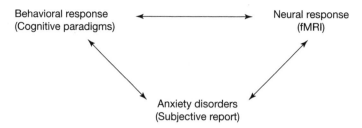

Figure 4.1 Pathophysiological model of brain–behavior relationships in child-hood anxiety disorders throughout development

(e.g., LeDoux, Rolls, Damasio) have written about different theories and definitions of fear. A common theme emerging from this body of work is that fear is a broad and complex phenomenon that is subserved by a distributed network of brain regions, rather than a single brain region or system. The study of fear therefore rests on dissecting this complex phenomenon into its constituent behavioral components and ultimately identifying their corresponding neural correlates.

Cognitive processes are an integral component of fear and anxiety (Beck et al., 1985). Cognitive theories propose that the initial processing of a threatening stimulus may contribute to the development and maintenance of anxiety disorders (Mogg and Bradley, 1998). This model embraces the strong interrelationship between cognitive and affective systems in the pathophysiology of anxiety. The nature of this cognitive-affective relationship may change across development. For example, older children demonstrate stronger cognitive and affective control and modulation of their responses to threat stimuli (Flavell, 1985; Posner and Rothbart, 1998).

The cognitive processing of a threatening stimulus is a complex multistage process that involves rapid and unconscious, as well as slow and deliberate responses (Panksepp, 1998). Cognitive processing can be decomposed into basic cognitive functions, such as attention, perception, and memory that operate on different time scales or in stages. Emotional information is hypothesized to actively and reciprocally flow within these different stages, and processing is influenced by both biological and learned factors. Chronic hypersensitivity of neural systems subserving different cognitive processes is hypothesized to activate affective circuits, thereby contributing to the origins and maintenance of anxiety disorders (Beck, 1997). Cognitive abnormalities may be universal across all anxiety disorders or disorder specific.

To test these theories, cognitive paradigms derived from the field of experimental cognitive psychology are administered to healthy and anxious subjects in the laboratory setting to examine the behavioral response to a threat stimulus. The paradigms include stimuli (e.g., words, faces) of different emotional categories (e.g., threat, happy) to probe different stages of cognitive processing. The stimulus characteristics (e.g., stimulus salience and duration) must be suitable to the child's developmental level to insure task validity and reliability. Performance on these tasks yields an objective behavioral response to threat that is a measure of cognitive function. These behavioral responses can be correlated with neural function using functional neuroimaging methods.

The clinical applications of this work are multifold. For example, behavioral tasks that probe cognitive dysfunction can help to delineate more precise anxiety phenotypes. Identifying cognitive biases can also help to understand the various sources of impairment associated with anxiety. For example, do attentional and memory biases compromise the capacity to encode and remember other types of information? Do these biases correlate with secondary sequelae such as avoidance, academic underachievement, social impairment, or self-esteem? Finally, do the cognitive abnormalities in anxious children confer risk for adult psychopathology? Understanding these relationships may lead to novel therapeutic interventions such as cognitive-behavioral therapies that remediate attentional and memory biases or novel receptor or circuit specific pharmacological therapies.

The following sections review data on the cognitive and neural correlates of anxiety disorders. The adult data are initially presented to serve as a guiding light for pursuing research in children. Consistent with the developmental perspective, the mechanisms mediating childhood anxiety may be the same or different from the findings in adults. The child behavioral data are summarized in Table 4.1.

Several important points should be noted when reading these studies. The behavioral studies typically use a case-control design to compare the behavioral response to different emotionally valent stimuli (e.g., threat, happy, sad) between subject groups. Most of these studies use single word and pictoral stimuli that are derived from normative data sets (e.g., International Affective Picture Series or IAPS) that report on the emotional salience of these stimuli in adult populations. Studies using naturalistic ecologically valid stimuli, such as facial emotional expressions, are also emerging. The neural studies examine the neurophysiological response to facial emotional expressions in healthy or clinically anxious samples. There is a preponderance of behavioral and neural adult data compared to child data, which underscores the need for much more research in children (see reviews by Daleiden and Vasey, 1997; Ehrenreich and Gross, 2002).

Behavioral studies

Attention

Attention is defined as a process by which an individual focuses on select features of the environment at the relative exclusion of others (Merriam-Webster, 1994). Selective attention to threat is an adaptive and automatic process mediated by a biologically prepared mechanism (LeDoux, 1995). Excessive attentional allocation to threat, i.e., attentional bias, is hypothesized in the etiology and maintenance of anxiety disorders (McNally, 1996).

Considerable data in adults supports the presence of an attentional bias to

Table 4.1 Information-processing studies in childhood anxiety

Study	Task	Age (years)	Diagnosis	Results
Attention studies				
Martin et al. (1992)	Stroop	6 to 13	Spider fear versus No spider fear	AB towards spider-relevant words in spider fear group
Vasey et al. (1995)	Dot probe	9 to 14	Clinically anxious versus Healthy controls	AB towards threat words in clinically anxious group
Manassis et al. (1996)	Dichotic listening task	8 to 11	Clinically anxious versus ADHD versus Healthy controls	AB towards hearing words with emotion in anxious group
Vasey et al. (1996)	Dot probe	11 to 14	High state versus Low state anxiety	AB towards threat words in high test anxious group; bias away from threat material in low test anxious group
Kindt et al. (1997a)	Stroop	8 to 12	Spider fear versus No spider fear	AB towards spider words in spider fear and control groups
Kindt et al. (1997b)	Stroop	8 to 9	High trait versus Low trait anxiety	AB towards threat in high anxious group and low anxious girls
Kindt and Brosschot (1999)	Stroop	8 to 12	Spider fear versus No spider fear	AB towards threat words in spider fear groups
Taghavi et al. (1999)	Dot probe	9 to 18	Clinically anxious versus Anxious + depressed versus Healthy controls	AB towards threat words in clinically anxious groups
Manassis et al. (2000)	Dichotic listening task	8 to 12	Clinically anxious versus ADHD versus Anxiety + ADHD versus Healthy controls	Reduced auditory recognition of emotion in control group versus controls; no bias in anxiety-only group
Dalgleish et al. (2003)	Dot probe	7 to 18	GAD versus PTSD versus Depression versus Healthy controls	AB towards threat words in GAD and PTSD
Taghavi et al. (2003)	Stroop	13.5 (mean)	GAD versus Healthy controls	AB towards negative emotional information in anxious group

continued

Table 4.1 (continued)

Study	Task	Age (years)	Diagnosis	Results
Perception studies				
Bell-Dolan (1995)	Ambiguous story	9 to 11	Clinically anxious versus Non-anxious	Enhanced misinterpretation of hostile situations in anxious group
Chorpita et al. (1996)	Ambiguous story	9 to 13	Clinically anxious versus Non-clinically anxious	Bias towards interpreting ambiguous situations as threatening in anxious group
Barrett et al. (1996)	Ambiguous story	7 to 14	Clinically anxious versus ODD versus Healthy controls	Bias towards perceiving stories as threatening in both clinical groups
Hadwin et al. (1997)	Ambiguous words	7 to 9	High trait versus Low trait anxiety	Bias towards interpreting word fragments as threatening in high anxiety group
Dalgleish et al. (1997)	Anticipation of negative events	9 to 18	Clinically anxious versus Clinically depressed versus Control	Stronger prediction of negative future events in anxious group
Bogels and Zigterman (2000)	Ambiguous story	9 to 18	Social Phobia, GAD, SAD versus Healthy controls	Enhanced perception of danger in anxious group
Muris et al. (2000a)	Ambiguous story	8 to 13	High trait versus Low trait anxiety	Enhanced threat perception in high anxiety group
Muris et al. (2000b)	Ambiguous story	8 to 13	Social phobia versus Healthy controls	Enhanced perception of threat and greater negative feelings in anxious group
Taghavi et al. (2000)	Ambiguous words	8 to 16	Clinically anxious versus Healthy controls	Bias towards interpreting word fragments as threatening in anxious group
Shortt et al. (2001)	Ambiguous story	6 to 14	Clinically anxious versus Externalizing disorders versus Control	Bias towards threatening interpretations in anxious and externalizing groups

Muris et al. (2003a)	Ambiguous and anxiety response stories	8 to 13	Non-clinically anxious	Enhanced threat perception anxious group
Muris et al. (2003b)	Ambiguous story	8 to 13	General and state anxiety versus Healthy controls	Enhanced threat perception in general and state anxiety groups
Memory studies				
Daleiden (1998)	Semantic and procedural memory	11 to 13	High trait versus Low trait anxiety	Memory bias towards threat material in high trait anxiety
Merikangas et al. (1999)	Visual and spatial memory	7 to 17	Family history of anxiety versus No family history	Memory deficit in family history group
Pine et al. (1999)	Visual and spatial memory	7 to 11	Boys at risk for disruptive behavior disorders	Memory deficit predicted anxiety at one year
Toren et al. (2000)	Verbal memory	6 to 18	Clinically anxious versus Non-clinically anxious	Lower memory scores in anxiety disorder group
Rusinek et al. (2002)	Event recall	11 to 12	High trait versus Low trait anxiety	Memory bias towards tone and intensity of a previously heard speech in high trait group
Dalgleish et al. (2003)	Verbal memory	7 to 18	GAD versus PTSD versus Depression versus Healthy	No memory bias found between any groups

Note: AB = Attentional bias

threatening stimuli in the environment across a variety of anxiety disorders. Two cognitive paradigms, the emotional Stroop task and the dot probe task, have been instrumental in capturing attentional biases. The emotional Stroop is a variant of the traditional color-word Stroop test that is commonly used in cognitive psychology to study interference processes. In the emotional Stroop test, anxious subjects are shown emotionally valent words printed in different colors, and they are asked to name the word color while ignoring the word meaning (McNally, 1996; Mathews and MacLeod, 1985). Color-naming delay occurs when the word meaning interferes with the subject's ability to attend to the word color (McNally, 1996). Increased color-naming delay in response to threatening words compared to neutral words (Mathews and MacLeod, 1985; Mogg and Bradley, 1998) reflects the presence of an attentional bias. Anxious subjects are hypothesized to demonstrate increased reaction times to naming colors of threat but not neutral words. Using this task, attentional biases have been detected for every type of anxiety disorder including simple animal phobia (Watts et al., 1986), social phobia (Hope et al., 1990; Mattia et al., 1993), obsessive-compulsive disorder (Foa et al., 1993), panic disorder (Ehlers et al., 1988; McNally et al., 1990b), posttraumatic stress disorder (McNally et al., 1990a), and generalized anxiety disorder (Mathews and MacLeod, 1985). One study of adults with spider phobia reported similar findings using pictorial stimuli (Lavy and van den Hout, 1993). These studies also report some degree of content-specificity in underlying effects, that is, longer response times are present when the word closely relates to the focus of the subject's anxiety (McNally, 1996).

The "dot probe" task is a specific measure of visual attention allocation. In this task, a pair of stimuli (e.g., words or facial expressions), one threatening and one neutral, are briefly (500ms) presented on a computer screen after which one of the stimuli immediately disappears and is replaced by a dot; subjects are required to respond (button press) as quickly as possible to the dot probe. Preferential allocation to threat is inferred when the reaction time to threat stimuli is shorter than the reaction times to other stimuli. The effects of threatening stimuli on attention are inferred from measuring reaction times to various stimuli. Adults with GAD responded more quickly to dot probes that replaced threat words compared to neutral words relative to depressed and control subjects (MacLeod et al., 1986; Mogg and Bradley, 1998; Mogg et al., 1992). Bradley et al. (1999) reported that adults with GAD selectively attended to threat faces compared to neutral faces compared to control subjects.

Although the adult data appear to consistently yield attentional biases in anxiety disorders, some inconsistent and unexplored areas should be noted. First, Martin et al. (1991) found an attentional bias to both positive and threat words in GAD, which indicates that the attentional bias is not specific to threat. Second, one study found that social anxiety was associated with an attentional bias away from threat cues, suggesting the possibility of disorder-specific patterns of attentional dysfunction (Clark and Wells, 1995). Third, no one has tested whether attentional biases predict treatment response. Finally, there is some question as to whether these biases relate to the effects of state or trait anxiety (McNally, 1996). Therefore, although the data on attentional bias in adult anxiety appear robust, more work is needed to understand the specificity and prognostic significance of these findings.

Similar to adults, preliminary data in children reveals the same pattern of attentional bias towards threat. To date, at least three studies demonstrate a relationship between childhood anxiety disorders and preferential allocation to threat using the dot probe test. Vasey and colleagues (1995) reported attentional biases in 9 to 14 year old clinically anxious children compared to healthy controls. Taghavi et al. (1999) reported similar results in 8 to 18 year children with anxiety disorders but not children with comorbid depression and anxiety. Dalgleish et al. (2003) found attentional biases in 7 to 18 year old children with GAD and PTSD. It should be noted that sample size was small and included broad age groups. Additionally, the assessment measures did not include structural diagnostic interviews and positively valenced stimuli.

Perception

Perception is a broad term that encompasses different levels of sensory awareness (Merriam-Webster, 1994). In this review, perception refers to two processes: an individual's subjective response to a threatening stimulus or an individual's ability to interpret a situation as threatening. Threat perception bias refers to an exaggerated subjective response or interpretation of a fearful stimulus. Perceptual bias is the cardinal feature of many anxiety disorders. A preponderance of functional neuro-imaging studies demonstrate perceptual abnormalities in adult anxiety disorders. Behavioral studies, although fewer in number, also capture these abnormalities in the laboratory setting using a variety of stimuli.

One set of behavioral studies examines the perceptual response to biological stimuli (e.g., carbon dioxide, yohimbine), which are considered innately threatening. In these studies, subjects are administered the biological stimulus and patterns of anxious responding are assessed (e.g., self-reported fear, panic symptoms). Many studies show that clinically anxious adults exhibit heightened anxiety when different biological stimuli are administered (Bruce et al., 1992; Charney et al., 1985, 1987, 1989; Gorman et al., 1990; Perna et al., 1999; Verburg et al., 1995). For example, when adults with agoraphobia, panic disorder, SoP, or GAD are administered a carbon dioxide challenge, there is increased anxiety across all clinical groups (Holt and Andrews, 1989).

Facial expressions have also been shown to elicit perceptual biases in anxiety. For example, Richards et al. (2002) found that high trait socially anxious adults displayed hypersensitivity to faces containing some fearful components compared to low trait anxious adults. Winton et al. (1995) report similar findings in adults with high social anxiety.

Behavioral studies in children also demonstrate threat perception biases in childhood anxiety disorders. Muris and colleagues (2000a, 2000b, 2003a, 2003b) conducted most of the studies in this field by administering stories with threat and non-threat content to children with and without anxiety, and assessing different measures of perception in response to the story. These data consistently show that high anxiety correlates with lower thresholds for experiencing fear and interpreting a situation as threatening. For example, non-referred socially anxious 8 to 13 year old children needed less information to perceive a story as threatening, and displayed more negative feelings than healthy children (Muris et al., 2000b). Similarly, non-clinical children with high anxiety showed early threat detection and increased negative cognitions on this task (Muris et al., 2003a).

Behavioral paradigms that include other types of stimuli also reveal perceptual biases in childhood anxiety. For example, Pine et al. (2005) found that adolescents with family history of anxiety reported more fear in response to angry faces compared to those without family history. Pollak and Kistler (2002) report similar findings, i.e., perceptual bias to angry faces, in children with abusive histories and/or psychopathology. Finally, similar to responses in adults, increased anxious responding is also present in children who receive biological challenges. This includes substances such as carbon dioxide or yohimbine (Pine et al., 2000; Sallee et al., 2000). Collectively, these data provide support for perceptual biases in children, although further work is needed to solidify these findings in clinical samples using ecologically valid stimuli, such as emotional facial expressions.

Memory

Memory refers to the encoding, storage, and retrieval of information. Emotional memory or emotional learning refers to memory for emotionally significant experiences (LeDoux, 1993). The phenomenon of some anxiety disorders is characterized by recurrent intrusive thoughts related to danger. Information processing theories postulate anxiety disorders may therefore be characterized by a memory bias such that threat stimuli are selectively encoded and retrieval compared to other types of emotional stimuli (McNally 1997).

Emotional memory systems can be probed implicitly or explicitly. Explicit or declarative memory is the most common type of memory studied and refers to conscious recollection of previously recalled material, either via free recall, cued recall, or recognition (McNally, 1996). Implicit memory refers to memory that is based on facilitated performance on a behavioral measure or changes in physiology without conscious recollection (McNally, 1996).

The data on explicit and implicit memory in adult anxiety disorders are equivocal, particularly when word stimuli are used in the behavioral paradigms (Mogg et al., 1987). With respect to explicit memory, some evidence supports a memory bias for threat stimuli in panic disorder (Becker et al., 1994; Cloitre and Leibowitz 1991; Cloitre et al., 1994), but these findings are not consistently present in GAD or SoP (Becker et al., 1999; Coles and Heimberg, 2002). Three studies using facial stimuli show that SoP is associated with memory bias for negative faces (e.g., critical, angry, disgust) relative to positive faces compared to controls (Foa et al., 2000; Gilboa-Schectman et al., unpublished data; Lundh and Ost, 1996), but two other studies report no group differences (D'Argembeau et al., 2003; Perez-Lopez and Woody, 2001).

Implicit memory is assessed using word-stem completion paradigms (Mathews et al., 1989) that involves studying words of varying valence (e.g., coffin, charm) and then asking subjects to complete word stems (e.g., cof) with the first word that comes to mind; a memory bias is demonstrated when subjects complete a greater proportion of stems with previously presented threat words (e.g., coffin) compared to neutral words (e.g., coffee) (McNally, 1996). Two studies report implicit memory biases in GAD (Mathews et al., 1989) and SoP (Lundh and Ost, 1997), but others have failed to replicate these findings (Mathews et al., 1995; Otto et al., 1994; Rapee et al., 1994). Some contend that these inconsistencies may be due to methodological factors, such as the nature of the encoding task, stimulus characteristics or state versus trait factors (Becker et al., 1999; Daleiden, 1998).

Preliminary behavioral data in children demonstrate different types of memory abnormalities in childhood anxiety, despite variability in the methods across studies.

Daleiden (1998) found a memory bias towards threat in 11 to 13 year old children with high trait versus low trait anxiety. Rusinek et al. (2002) found that high trait anxious children recalled more information about the tone and intensity of a previously heard speech than low trait anxious children. Pine et al. (1999) found a temporal relationship between verbal and design memory deficits and risk for future anxiety. Merikangas et al. (1999) found that a family history of anxiety predicted memory deficits, which suggests that cognitive dysfunction may confer risk for future anxiety. Only one clinical study examines the relationship between emotional memory and anxiety. Dalgleish et al. (2003) examined 93 children, ages 8 to 18 years, with GAD and PTSD and found no memory bias in either group. The age range was broad in this sample, which prevents understanding of how memory may relate to anxiety in specific age groups. Since the relationship between memory and anxiety may differ across development, additional clinical studies of more narrow groups are needed.

Summary of behavioral data

Behavioral data provide support for cognitive processing deficits in adults, and possibly children with clinical anxiety. Attentional and perceptual biases to threat are the most consistent findings implicated in both physiological and pathological anxiety, although much more work is needed to understand the specificity and prognostic significance of these findings. Data on the relationship between memory dysfunction and anxiety are equivocal in adults is tenuous, but requires further investigation in children. These data indicate that there may be some common cognitive phenotypes across child and adult disorders.

Neural studies

The neural circuits mediating cognitive and affective responses to threat are complex and include many distributed interrelated circuits involved in fear and cognition. Most of the research focuses on dysregulation of three particular regions in the threat response, the amygdala, the orbital frontal cortex (OFC), and the anterior cingulate cortex (ACC) (Charney, 2003). Provocative neuroimaging studies demonstrate that these regions are consistently activated across a variety of anxiety disorders. Lesions of the prefrontal cortex (PFC) and ACC are correlated with a reduction in intractable anxiety, as well as reduction in affect (Damasio and Van Hoesen, 1983; Weingarten, 1999).

The amygdala is a functionally diverse structure that is comprised of over ten different interconnected nuclei that can be differentiated on both cytoarchitectural and connectional grounds (Sah et al., 2003). This structure is located in the temporal lobe and possesses extensive interconnections with other cortical and subcortical brain regions (Sah et al., 2003). An abundance of animal and human data implicate the basolateral nucleus of the amygdala in the appraisal of an incoming stimulus and the central nucleus of the amygdala in the autonomic, behavioral, and emotional response to that stimulus (LeDoux, 1995, 1998).

The OFC is part of the PFC and subserves a variety of neuropsychological and neurobehavioral functions (Zald and Kim, 1996). The OFC has vast inter-connections with other brain regions; it is the only prefrontal region that has strong reciprocal connections with the amygdala (Zald and Kim, 1996). An imbalance in the OFC–amygdala connection has been implicated in the expression of anxiety (Gallagher et al., 1999; Izquierdo and Murray, 2000; Schoenbaum et al., 1998).

The anterior cingulate is a region situated between the two cerebral hemispheres and is implicated in emotional, attentional, and motivational processes (Cunningham et al., 2002). More specifically, this region is implicated in coordinating and integrating activity in multiple attentional systems (Carter et al., 2000; Peterson et al., 1999), a function which significantly affects emotional processes. Maturing connections between the anterior cingulate and the amygdala are hypothesized to contribute to better cognitive and affective control of stimulus processing (Cunningham et al., 2002; Posner and Rothbart, 1998).

Little is known about the development of the human amygdala, OFC, and anterior cingulate. Non-human primate data show that the amygdala is mature at birth and lesions of the amygydala shortly after birth affect the fear response later in development (Machado and Bachevalier, 2003). The OFC develops connections with other PFC regions towards the end of gestation and matures in early childhood (Schwartz and Goldman-Rakic, 1991). Connections between the anterior cingulate and the basolateral nucleus of the amygdala are hypothesized to develop during the postnatal period (Cunningham et al., 2002). It is possible that anxiety disorders may be considered neurodevelopmental conditions that are characterized by early developmental dysfunction of the pediatric amygdala, OFC, and anterior cingulate, which manifests behaviorally throughout development.

Many questions however remain unanswered. For example, does amygdalar or OFC dysfunction manifest before or after the onset of an anxiety disorder? Do these abnormalities correlate with particular behavioral or clinical signs? How do structural and functional abnormalities in these brain regions correlate with dysregulation in serotoninergic systems? What happens to these regions during adolescence, which is a vulnerable time for developing emotional disorders? The data presented below are a first step towards addressing these complex questions regarding the integrated network of brain regions involved in the pathogenesis of anxiety.

It is important to note that many recent neuroimaging studies document involve-ment of the amygdala and the prefrontal cortex, particularly the OFC, in the pathogenesis of adult major depressive disorder. For example, position-emission tomography (PET) (Drevets, 2003), structural (Frodl et al., 2002), and fMRI (Sheline et al., 2001) studies reveal amygdalar abnormalities in clinically depressed adults. Changes in the OFC are also present in adult depression (Ballmaier et al., 2004; Baker et al., 1997; Bremner et al., 2002; Pardo et al., 1993). Preliminary data reveal similar neural abnormalities in pediatric depression (Thomas et al., 2001b; Steingard et al., 2000). The amygdala and OFC may therefore be common substrates

94

in both anxiety and depression. More research is needed to determine the functional role of these regions towards the development of these two distinct disorders.

The following section reviews neural studies that examine the role of these brain regions in normal and pathological anxiety. Neuroimaging studies, particularly fMRI data, that examine the neurophysiological responses associated with attentional, perceptual, and mnemonic responses to threat are reported. Relevant lesion data that correlate brain damage with affective changes are also described. In summary, the majority of adult data support a role for the amygdala, the OFC and anterior cingulate in the cognitive response to threatening stimuli. Data on the neural mechanisms mediating childhood disorders is relatively lacking. The available studies however provide preliminary support for involvement of the amygdala in the fear response. Furthermore, these data highlight the utility of fMRI to examine the physiological and pathological fear responses across development.

Attention

Brain circuits implicated in attentional conflict or allocation are hypothesized to involve activity in a variety of cortical regions, particularly components of the cingulate gyrus. In situations where there are competing demands on attentional systems, the cingulate may be involved in the weighing of alternative choices for further processing. Individuals with anxiety disorders are hypothesized to display an attentional bias for potentially dangerous stimuli when faced with weighing different choices. This bias may manifest as abnormal reaction times during conflict tasks, such as the Stroop, where existing fMRI studies document the engagement of the anterior cingulate gyrus (Isenberg et al., 1999; Peterson et al., 1999). The degree to which engagement of this region varies as a function of performance however remains unclear. Additional work is needed to delineate the neural circuits mediating attentional processes in anxiety disorders.

Perception

Lesion and neuroimaging data implicate the amygdala and OFC in threat perception. In terms of lesion data, many case studies report correlations between amygdala damage and impaired fear recognition (Aggleton, 2000). For example, adults with amygdalar damage provide less intense ratings of fearful faces compared to healthy controls (Adolphs et al., 1999). Lesions to the OFC correlate with both increased and decreased anxiety. For example, right OFC lesions correlate with increased anxiety and edginess in adults with penetrating head injury (Grafman et al., 1986), whereas ventromedial PFC lesions (Damasio, 1996) and lesions that sever PFC-subcortical connections (Weingarten, 1999) decrease anxiety.

Functional neuroimaging data in healthy adults demonstrate changes in the amygdala and OFC in response to presentation of emotional faces, particularly fearful faces. For example, Morris et al. (1996, 1998) reported increased amygdalar activation in response to viewing fearful faces in healthy adults; this response was positively correlated with increasing fearfulness (Morris et al., 1996). Breiter et al. (1996) demonstrated preferential amygdalar activation in response to fearful and happy faces compared to neutral faces suggesting a nonspecific response to emotional stimuli. In contrast to a fairly consistent response to fearful faces, the response to angry faces is equivocal. For example, Whalen et al. (2001) reported amygdalar activation in response to fearful faces but not angry faces, whereas Hariri et al. (2000, 2003) reported amygdalar activation in response to both fearful and angry faces. Blair et al. (1999) reported OFC but not amygdalar activation in response to angry faces.

Interestingly, Hariri et al. (2002) found that adults with one or two copies of the short allele of the serotonin transporter promoter gene (SLC6A-4) demonstrate increased amygdalar activation in response to fearful faces compared to adults who are homozygous for the long allele. Prior work has shown that this polymorphism is linked to anxiety related personality traits, and is hypothesized to decrease 5-HTT expression and 5-HT uptake in lymphoblasts (Lesch et al., 1996). Additional studies using positive stimuli are needed to determine the specificity of this relationship.

Enhanced amygdalar activation in response to fearful stimuli or situations has been demonstrated in anxiety disorders. In a study of seven adults with social phobia and five healthy controls, Birbaumer et al. (1998) reported amygdalar activation in response to fear relevant stimuli. Similarly, Stein et al. (2002) found significant changes in the amygdala in response to angry and contemptuous but not fearful faces in fifteen adults with generalized social phobia. These data converge with the abundance of symptom provocation that implicate amydalar and across a variety of adult anxiety disorders (Bremner, 2002; Furmark et al., 2002; Fredrikson et al., 1995; Rauch et al., 1994, 1995; Tillfors et al., 2001). Symptom provocation studies also implicate the OFC in adult anxiety disorders, although the direction of activation differs across studies (Bremner et al., 2002; Rauch et al., 1994, 1995).

Neuroimaging studies of childhood anxiety disorders, particularly GAD, SAD, and SoP, are gradually accumulating. Four volumetric studies implicate the amgydala or OFC in the pathophysiology of these disorders. First, De Bellis et al. (2000) reported enlarged amygdalar volumes in twelve children with GAD compared to twenty-four controls. Furthermore, MacMillan et al. (2003) found that in children with depression and anxiety, severity of anxiety of depression was associated with amygdala-hippocampal ratios. Another study however reported reduced amygdalar volumes in children with SAD, GAD, or SoP (Milham et al., 2005). Differences in the study samples, particularly anxiety diagnosis, may partly account for the discrepant results amongst these three studies. In terms of changes in the OFC, a prospective study of posttraumatic brain injury outcomes indicated a correlation between increased OFC damage and decreased risk for anxiety disorders and symptoms at one year (Vasa et al., 2003).

Pediatric fMRI studies employ very similar study designs and stimuli that are used in adult studies. These studies aim to first examine the developmental responses to threat, which can serve as a baseline for understanding the mechanisms that go awry in clinical disorders. To date, there are at least six fMRI studies that examine the brain's response to threatening stimuli; only one of these studies includes a clinically anxious sample of children (Thomas et al., 2001a). All of these studies use some variation of a face viewing paradigm. Baird et al. (1999) conducted the first fMRI face perception study in 12 to 17 year old adolescents. Using a facial affect recognition task, the data showed amygdalar activation in response to fearful faces. Killgore et al. (2001) reported amygdalar activation to fearful faces, and changes in the amygdala and PFC during face viewing. Monk et al. (2003) found activation in the amygdala, OFC, and anterior cingulate in response to fearful faces when adolescents performed a non-emotional behavioral task during face viewing. In contrast, Thomas et al. (2001a) used a passive viewing task to document greater amygdalar responses to fearful faces relative to fixation but not compared to neutral faces in twelve children (M = 11 years, SD = 2.4 years). Pine et al. (2001) failed to engage the amygdala in adolescents or adults using a masked face task.

Thomas et al. (2001a) conducted the only fMRI study that examined the neurophysiological responses to threat in a clinically anxious sample. The methods included administering a passive face viewing task to twelve children, ages 8 to 16 years (M = 12.8, SD = 2.1), with GAD or panic disorder. The findings revealed amygdalar activation to fearful faces. The degree of amygdalar activation positively correlated with symptom severity.

Several factors limit the interpretation of these pediatric fMRI studies. Most of the studies included broad age groups, failed to include positively valenced stimuli, and selectively imaged the amydgala only, which precluded observation of other brain regions. Additionally, findings from these studies may have been influenced by whether or not subjects were performing behavioral tasks to constrain attention during face viewing. Constraining attention is critical to eliciting differential responses to emotional stimuli (Critchley et al., 2000; Hariri et al., 2000; Monk et al., 2003; Pessoa et al., 2002). Therefore, the findings of amygdalar dysfunction in the threat response are suggestive but not definitive and clearly many more developmental and clinical studies are needed to understand how the brain responds to threat in children.

Memory

Functional MRI studies document involvement of distinct brain circuits in various aspects of memory, i.e., encoding, storage, and retrieval. The neural networks mediating emotional memory are stored through both the amygdala and the hippocampus, in contrast to systems that mediate storage of experiences devoid of emotion, which draw less consistently on the amygdala.

Data in healthy adults implicate the amygdala in encoding emotional stimuli and facilitating long-term memory storage (Adolphs et al., 2000). For example, adults with amygdalar damage show impaired memory for emotional but not neutral stimuli (Adolphs et al., 1999, 2000). Neuroimaging data demonstrate a positive correlation between the degree of amygdala activation and arousal at encoding, and later recall for emotional material (Cahill, 1999; Cahill et al., 1996; Canli et al., 2000; Hamann et al., 1999). This modulatory effect of arousal may be mediated by amygdalar influences on hippocampal activity (Cahill et al., 1996).

Only one fMRI study examines emotional memory in a pediatric sample. Nelson et al. (2003) asked adolescents to provide different ratings of faces during fMRI, and then take a post-scan memory test. The data showed correlations between anterior cingulate activation at encoding and recall of angry faces, and right temporal pole activation and recall of fearful faces. These data suggest that threatening information may be more readily recalled due to chronic partial activation of fear structures, which may decrease the activation threshold at which ongoing processing is influenced (Daleiden, 1998; Foa and Kozak, 1986). Future fMRI studies are needed to examine whether neural systems underlying emotional memory processes are affected in childhood anxiety disorders.

Summary of neural data

The adult and pediatric fMRI studies are the first steps towards mapping the neural circuitry of the brain's responses threat. Converging evidence supports a role for the amygdala, OFC, and anterior cingulate in the cognitive response to threatening stimuli, particularly fearful faces, in both physiological and pathological anxiety. Although much more work is needed to unravel the neural basis of anxiety, this conceptual and methodological framework, which relies on principles of affective neuroscience and developmental psychopathology, provides a solid foundation on which to build further knowledge of brain–behavior relationships in anxiety.

Clinical implications

Pharmacotherapy and cognitive-behavioral therapies are two empirically supported treatment modalities for childhood anxiety disorders (see review by Labellarte et al., 1999). Both of these treatments are equally effective for treatment of SAD, GAD, and SoP, and combined therapy has shown to be superior to either pharmacotherapy or psychotherapy alone. In general, for many children, anxiety disorders are treatable or manageable conditions if the appropriate therapies are provided.

Multimodal treatment may offer the best possibility for maximizing successful outcomes. The goal of therapy is to treat the primary anxiety disorder, address comorbidities, and correct the various sources of impairment by building on the child and family's strengths. In addition to working with the child and family, child psychiatrists will often collaborate with psychologists, behavior therapists, school nurses and mental health counselors, and teachers to develop a multidisciplinary intervention that can be consistently generalized across the home and school settings. Components of this plan include pharmacotherapy, cognitive-behavioral therapy, strategies to target associated symptoms such as school refusal and somatic complaints, addressing family anxiety and parenting style, social skills training, and in severe cases, academic modification. Using this approach is likely to maximize chances of treating the primary and secondary sequelae associated with anxiety.

Many controlled studies indicate that cognitive-behavior therapy (CBT) is an efficacious short-term treatment for childhood anxiety disorders (Roblek and Piacentini, 2005). The central goal of CBT is to help the child find new ways of thinking and reacting to anxiety provoking situations. Key components to CBT include illness education, cognitive restructuring, and exposure to the feared stimulus or situation through gradual exposure, systematic densensitization, flooding. Therapy is usually time-limited and typically consists of approximately sixteen sessions and occasional "booster" sessions to solidify gains.

Randomized control trials and observational studies have demonstrated that selective serotonin-reuptake inhibitors (SSRI) are the first line of treatment for the treatment of GAD, SAD, SoP, and OCD. The most notable study is the NIH sponsored multi-site treatment study that demonstrated the efficacy of fluvoxamine in 128 children, ages 6 and 17 years, with SAD, GAD, and SoP (2001). Over an eight-week period, half of the children were treated with fluvoxamine while the other half received a placebo. A significant decrease in anxiety symptoms was found in 76 percent of children receiving fluvoxamine whereas only 29 percent of children demonstrated a response to placebo. Additional studies are needed to replicate these findings as well as to compare the efficacy of SSRIs, CBT, and combination therapy for childhood anxiety.

The SSRIs are usually well-tolerated and take four to six weeks to take effect. Acute adverse effects include gastrointestinal upset, sleep disturbance, and possibly behavioral activation. Additionally, in the United States, SSRIs and other anti-depressants carry a 'black box' warning of an increased risk of suicidal ideation associated with use of these medications. This warning was based on the US Food and Drug Administration Advisory (FDA) Committee's review of a meta-analysis from 24 acute placebo controlled trials involving over 4,400 children and adolescents with a diagnosis of MDD, anxiety, or other psychiatric disorders. Results of this meta-analysis revealed that the average risk of suicidal behavior was 4 percent in the medication group and 2 percent in the placebo group. The response in the United Kingdom preceded the US FDA warning and consisted of a directive contraindicating the use of paroxetine, sertraline, citalopram, escitalopram, and venlafaxine for treatment of pediatric depression. A detailed account of these events can be found in Licinio and Wong (2005).

In light of these data, concerns about the use of SSRIs are understandable. Pediatric anxiety disorders however demonstrate a robust response to SSRIs (Birmaher et al., 2003; Riddle et al., 2001; RUPP Anxiety Study Group 2001; Wagner et al., 2004a). Therefore, weighing the risk-benefit ratio for each child is necessary when making treatment decisions. Some of the factors to consider in the decision making process include illness severity and impairment, comorbidity, and family history.

Other classes of medications that may help to alleviate more severe symptoms include the benzodiazepines and neuroleptics. Benzodiazepines can be used to relieve acute anxiety so that children are more receptive to exposure therapy. These medications must be used cautiously in children due to concerns about behavioral activation, tolerance, and sedation. Benzodiazepines should initially be prescribed together with the SSRI, and then gradually discontinued as the SSRI becomes effective. Low dose neuroleptics can be used if the child is extremely agitated, or experiencing delusions, disorganized thoughts, or derealization experiences. There are no empirical data on the efficacy of other medications, such as buspar or the dual serotoninergic-norepinephrine reuptake inhibitors (e.g., mirtazapine, nefazodone, trazodone, venlafaxine) for childhood anxiety.

Treating the concomitant comorbidities associated with anxiety disorders is also critical since the presence of depression, ADHD, and substance abuse may complicate the course of anxiety as well as the response to treatment. The SSRIs are also helpful in treating comorbid disorders such as depression or mood dysregulation secondary to ADHD. Treatment of ADHD with stimulant therapy may cause exacerbated anxiety or tics. Alpha-adrenergic blockers such as clonidine may help to alleviate ADHD symptoms as well as diminish sympathetically mediated arousal secondary to anxiety. As a last resort, tricyclic antidepressants can be considered although close cardiac monitoring is warranted.

Conclusion

Anxiety disorders are the most common forms of psychopathology affecting children and adolescents. These conditions can potentially exhibit an unstable and fluctuating course and are potentially associated with acute and chronic comorbid psychopathology. It is therefore imperative that clinicians identify and treat these conditions early to prevent long-term suffering. Research on the behavioral and neural correlates of these conditions is revealing potential links between cognitive processing abnormalities in child and adult anxiety disorders. New technologies, both neuroimaging and genetics, together with methods grounded in affective, developmental, and cognitive sciences, are likely to continue to advance our understanding of the pathophysiology of these disorders.

References

Achenbach, T.M., Howell, C.T., McConaughy, S.H., and Stanger, C. (1995). Six-year predictors of problems in a national sample of children and youth: I. Cross-informant syndromes. *Journal of the American Academy of Child and Adolescent Psychiatry, 34*, 336–347.

Adolphs, R., Tranel, D., Hamann, S., Young, A.W., Calder, A.J., Phelps, E.A., et al. (1999). Recognition of facial emotion in nine individuals with bilateral amygdala damage. *Neuropsychologia, 37*, 1111–1117.

Adolphs, R., Tranel, D., and Denburg, N. (2000). Impaired emotional declarative memory following unilateral amygdala damage. *Learning and Memory, 7*, 180–186.

Aggleton, J.P. (Ed.) (2000). *The amygdala: A functional analysis.* Oxford: Oxford University Press.

American Psychiatric Association (1994). *Diagnostic and statistical manual of mental disorders*, 4th edn, (DSM-IV). Washington, DC: APA.

Anderson, J.C., Williams, S., McGee, R., and Silva, P.A. (1987). DSM-III disorders in preadolescent children: Prevalence in a large sample from a general population. *Archives of General Psychiatry, 44*, 69–76.

Baird, A.A., Gruber, S.A., Fein, D.A., Maas, L.C., Steingard, R.J., Renshaw, P.F., et al. (1999). Functional magnetic resonance imaging of facial affect recognition in children and adolescents. *Journal of the American Academy of Child and Adolescent Psychiatry, 38*, 195–199.

Baker, L. and Cantwell, D.P. (1987). A prospective psychiatric follow-up of children with speech/language disorders. *Journal of the American Academy of Child and Adolescent Psychiatry, 26*, 546–553.

Baker, S.C., Frith, C.D., and Dolan, R.J. (1997). The interaction between mood and cognitive function studied with PET. *Psychological Medicine, 27*, 565–578.

Ballmaier, M., Toga, A.W., Blanton, R.E., Sowell, E.R., Lavretsky, H., Peterson, J., et al. (2004). Anterior cingulate, gyrus rectus, and orbitofrontal abnormalitie in elderly depressed patients: an MRI-based parcellation of the prefrontal cortex. *American Journal of Psychiatry, 161*, 99–108.

Barrett, P.M., Rapee, R.M., Dadds, M.M., and Ryan, S.M. (1996). Family enhancement of cognitive style in anxious and aggressive children. *Journal of Abnormal Child Psychology, 24*, 187–203.

Battaglia, M., Bajo, S., Strambi, L.F., Brambilla, F., Castronovo, C., Vanni, G., et al. (1997). Physiological and behavioral responses to minor stressors in offspring of patients with panic disorder. *Journal of Psychiatric Research, 31*, 365–76.

Beck, A.T. (1997). The past and future of cognitive therapy. *Journal of Psychotherapy Practice and Research, 6(4)*, 276–284.

Beck, A.T., Emergy, G., and Greenberg, R.L. (1985). *Anxiety disorders and phobias: A cognitive perspective.* New York: Basic Books.

Becker, E., Rinck, M., and Margraf, J. (1994). Memory bias in panic disorder. *Journal of Abnormal Psychology, 103*, 396–399.

Becker, E.S., Roth, W.T., Andrich, M., and Margraf, J. (1999). Explicit memory in anxiety disorders. *Journal of Abnormal Psychology, 108*, 153–163

Beidel, D.C., Fink, C.M., and Turner, S.M. (1996). Stability of anxious symptomatology in children. *Journal of Abnormal Child Psychology, 24*, 257–269.

Bell-Dolan, D.J. (1995). Social cue interpretation of anxious children. *Journal of Clinical Child Psychology, 24*, 1–10.

Bell-Dolan, D.J., and Brazeal, T.J. (1993). Separation anxiety disorder, overanxious disorder, and school refusal. *Child and Adolescent Psychiatric Clinics of North America, 2*, 563–580.

Benjamin, R.S., Costello, E.J., and Warren, M. (1990). Anxiety disorders in a pediatric sample. *Journal of Anxiety Disorders, 4*, 293–316.

Biederman, J., Rosenbaum, J.F., Hirshfeld, D.R., Faraone, S.V., Bolduc, E.A., Gersten, M., et al. (1990). Psychiatric correlates of behavioral inhibition in young children of parents with and without psychiatric disorders. *Archives of General Psychiatry, 47*, 21–26.

Biederman, J., Rosenbaum, J.F., Bolduc-Murphy, E.A., Faraone, S.V., Chaloff, J.,

Hirshfeld, D.R., et al. (1993). A 3-year follow-up of children with and without behavioral inhibition. *Journal of the American Academy of Child and Adolescent Psychiatry, 32*, 814–821.

Biederman, J., Hirshfeld-Becker, D.R., Rosenbaum, J.F., Herot, C., Friedman, D., Snidman, N., et al. (2001). Further evidence of association between behavioral inhibition and social anxiety in children. *American Journal of Psychiatry, 158*, 1673–1679.

Birbaumer, N., Grodd, W., Diedrich, O., Kose, U., Erb, M., Lotze, M., et al. (1998). fMRI reveals amygdala activation to human faces in social phobia. *Neuroreport, 9*, 1223–1226.

Birmaher, B., Waterman, G.S., Ryan, N., Cully, M., Balach, L., Ingram, J., et al. (1994). Fluoxetine for childhood anxiety disorders. *Journal of the American Academy of Child and Adolescent Psychiatry, 33*, 993–999.

Blair, R.J., Morris, J.S., Frith, C.D., Perrett, D.I., and Dolan, R.J. (1999). Dissociable neural responses to facial expressions of sadness and anger. *Brain, 122*, 883–893.

Bogels, S.M. and Zigterman, D. (2000). Dysfunctional cognitions in children with social phobia, separation anxiety disorder, and generalized anxiety disorder. *Journal of Abnormal Child Psychology, 28*, 205–211.

Bowen, R.C., Offord, D.R., and Boyle, M.H. (1990). The prevalence of overanxious disorder and separation anxiety disorder: results from the Ontario Child Health Study. *Journal of the American Academy of Child and Adolescent Psychiatry, 29*, 753–758.

Bradley, B.P., Mogg, K., White, J., Groom, C., and deBono, J. (1999). Attentional bias for emotional faces in generalized anxiety disorder. *British Journal of Clinical Psychology, 38*, 267–278.

Brady, E.U. and Kendall, P.C. (1992). Comorbidity of anxiety and depression in children and adolescents. *Psychological Bulletin, 111*, 244–255.

Breiter, H.C., Etcoff, N.L., Whalen, P.J., Kennedy, W.A., Rauch, S.L., and Buckner, R.L. (1996). Response and habituation of the human amygdala during visual processing of facial expression. *Neuron, 17*, 875–887.

Bremner, J.D. (2002). Neuroimaging studies in post-traumatic stress disorder. *Current Psychiatry Reports, 4*, 254–263.

Bremner, J.D., Vythilingam, M., Vermetten, E., Nazeer, A., Adil, J., Khan, S., et al. (2002). Reduced volume of orbitofrontal cortex in major depression. *Biological Psychiatry, 51*, 273–279.

Breslau, N., Davis, G.C., and Prabucki, K. (1987). Searching for evidence on the validity of generalized anxiety disorder: psychopathology in children of anxious mothers. *Psychiatry Research, 20*, 285–297.

Bruce, M., Scott, N., Shine, P., and Lader, M. (1992). Anxiogenic effects of caffeine in patients with anxiety disorders. *Archives of General Psychiatry, 49*, 867–869.

Cahill, L. (1999). A neurobiological perspective on emotionally influenced, long-term memory. *Seminars in Clinical Neuropsychiatry, 4*, 266–273.

Cahill, L., Haier, R.J., Fallon, J., Alkire, M.T., Tang, C., Keator, D., et al. (1996). Amygdala activity at encoding correlated with long-term, free recall of emotional information. *Proceedings of the National Academy of Sciences, 93*, 8016–8021.

Canli, T., Zhao, Z., Brewer, J., Gabrieli, J.D., and Cahill, L. (2000). Event-related activation in the human amygdala associates with later memory for individual emotional experience. *Journal of Neuroscience, 20*, RC99.

Carter, C.S., MacDonald, A.M., Botvinick, M., Ross, L.L., Stenger, V.A., Noll, D., et al.

(2000). Parsing executive processes: strategic vs. evaluative functions of the anterior cingulate cortex. *Proceedings of the National Academy of Sciences*, *15*, 1944–1949.

Charney, D.S. (2003). Neuroanatomical circuits modulating fear and anxiety behaviors. *Acta Psychiatrica Scandinavica Supplement*, *417*, 38–50.

Charney, D.S., Heninger, G.R., and Jatlow, P.I. (1985). Increased anxiogenic effects of caffeine in panic disorders. *Archives of General Psychiatry*, *42*, 233–243.

Charney, D.S., Woods, S.W., Goodman, W.K., and Heninger, G.R. (1987). Neurobiological mechanisms of panic anxiety: biochemical and behavioral correlates of yohimbine-induced panic attacks. *American Journal of Psychiatry*, *144*, 1030–1036.

Charney, D.S., Woods, S.W., and Heninger, G.R. (1989). Noradrenergic function in generalized anxiety disorder: effects of yohimbine in healthy subjects and patients with generalized anxiety disorder. *Psychiatry Research*, *27*, 173–182.

Chorpita, B.F., Albano, A.M., Heimberg, R.G., and Barlow, D.H. (1996). A systematic replication of the prescriptive treatment of school refusal behavior in a single subject. *Journal of Behavior Therapy and Experimental Psychiatry*, *27*, 281–290.

Cicchetti, D. and Cohen, D. (1995). *Developmental psychopathology. Vol. 1: Theory and method; Vol. 2: Risk, disorder, and adaptation*. New York: Wiley.

Clark, D. and Wells, A. (1995). A cognitive model of social phobia. In R. Heimberg, M. Liebowitz, D.A. Hope, and F.R. Scheier (Eds.), *Social phobia: Diagnosis, assessment, and treatment* (pp. 69–93). New York: Guilford.

Cloitre, M. and Liebowitz, M.R. (1991). Memory bias in panic disorder: an investigation of the cognitive avoidance hypothesis. *Cognitive Therapy and Research*, *15*, 371–386.

Cloitre, M., Shear, M.K., Cancienne, J., and Zeitlin, S.B. (1994). Implicit and explicit memory for catastrophic associations to bodily sensation words in panic disorder. *Cognitive Therapy and Research*, *18*, 225–240.

Coles, M.E. and Heimberg, R.G. (2002). Memory biases in the anxiety disorders: Current status. *Clinical Psychology Review*, *22*, 587–627.

Costello, E.J. and Angold, A. (1995). Epidemiology. In J.S. March (Ed.). *Anxiety disorders in children and adolescents* (pp. 109–124). New York: Guilford.

Critchley, H., Daly, E., Phillips, M., Brammer, M., Bullmore, E., Williams, S., et al. (2000). Explicit and implicit neural mechanisms for processing of social information from facial expressions: a functional magnetic resonance imaging study. *Human Brain Mapping*, *9*, 93–105.

Cunningham, M.G., Bhattacharyya, S., and Benes, F.M. (2002). Amygdalo-cortical sprouting continues into early adulthood: implications for the development of normal and abnormal function during adolescence. *Journal of Comprehensive Neurology*, *453*, 116–130.

Daleiden, E.L. (1998). Childhood anxiety and memory functioning: A comparison of systemic and processing accounts. *Journal of Experimental and Child Psychology*, *68*, 216–235.

Daleiden, E.L. and Vasey, M.W. (1997). An information-processing perspective on childhood anxiety. *Clinical Psychology Review*, *17*, 407–429.

Dalgleish, T., Taghavi, R., Neshat-Doost, H., Moradi, A., Yule, W., and Canterbury, R. (1997). Information processing in clinically depressed and anxious children and adolescents. *Journal of Child Psychology and Psychiatry and Allied Disciplines*, *38*, 535–541.

Dalgleish, T., Taghavi, R., Neshat-Doost, H., Moradi, A., Canterbury, R., and Yule, W. (2003). Patterns of processing bias for emotional information across clinical disorders:

A comparison of attention, memory, and prospective cognition in children and adolescents with depression, generalized anxiety, and posttraumatic stress disorder. *Journal of Clinical Child and Adolescent Psychology*, *32*, 10–21.

Damasio, A.R. (1996). The somatic marker hypothesis and the possible function of the prefrontal cortex. *Philosophical Transactions of the Royal Society of London B*, *351*, 1413–1420.

Damasio, A.R. and Van Hoesen, G.W. (1983). Emotional disturbances associated with focal lesions of the limbic frontal lobe. In K.M. Heilman and P. Satz (Eds.). *Neuropsychology of human emotion* (pp. 85–110). New York: Guilford.

D'Argembeau, A., Van der Linden, M., Etienne, A., and Comblain, C. (2003). Identity and expression memory for happy and angry faces in social anxiety. *Acta Psychologica*, *114*, 1–15.

De Bellis, M.D., Casey, B.J., Dahl, R.E., Birmaher, B., Williamson, D.E., Thomas, K.M., et al. (2000). A pilot study of amygdala volumes in pediatric generalized anxiety disorder. *Biological Psychiatry*, *48*, 51–57.

Drevets, W.C. (2003) Neuroimaging abnormalities in the amygdala in mood disorders. *Annals of the New York Academy of Sciences*, *985*, 420–444.

Ehlers, A., Margraf, J., Davies, S.O., and Roth, W.T. (1988). Selective processing of threat cues in subjects with panic disorder. *Journal of Abnormal Psychology*, *101*, 371–382.

Ehrenreich, J.T. and Gross, A.M. (2002). Biased attentional behavior in childhood anxiety: A review of theory and current empirical investigation. *Clinical Psychology Review*, *22*, 991–1008.

Feigon, S.A., Waldman, I.D., Levy, F., and Hay, D.A. (2001). Genetic and environmental influences on separation anxiety disorder symptoms and their moderation by age and sex. *Behavior Genetics*, *31*, 403–411.

Ferdinand, R.F. and Verhulst, F.C. (1995). Psychopathology from adolescence into young adulthood: An 8-year follow-up study. *American Journal of Psychiatry*, *152*, 586–594.

Fergusson, D.M., Horwood, L.J., and Lynskey, M.T. (1993). Prevalence and comorbidity of DSM-III-R diagnoses in a birth cohort of 15 year olds. *Journal of the American Academy of Child and Adolescent Psychiatry*, *32*, 1127–1134.

Flavell, J.H. (1985). *Cognitive development*. Englewood Cliffs, NJ: Prentice-Hall.

Foa, E.B. and Kozak, M.J. (1986). Emotional memory of fear: exposure to corrective information. *Psychological Bulletin*, *99*, 20–35.

Foa, E.B., Ilai, D., McCarthy P.R., Shoyer B., and Murdock, T.B. (1993). Information-processing in obsessive-compulsive disorder. *Cognitive Therapy and Research*, *17*, 173–189.

Foa, E.B., Gilboa-Schechtman, E., Amir, N., and Freshman, M. (2000). Memory bias in generalized social phobia: remembering negative emotional expressions. *Journal of Anxiety Disorders*, *14*, 501–519.

Fredrikson, M., Wik, G., Annas, P., Ericson, K., and Stone-Elander, S. (1995). Functional neuroanatomy of visually elicited simple phobic fear: additional data and theoretical analysis. *Psychophysiology*, *32*, 43–48.

Frodl, T., Meisenzahl, E., Zetzsche, T., Bottlender, R., Born, C., Groll, C., et al. (2002). Enlargement of the amygdala in patients with a first episode of major depresson. *Biological Psychiatry*, *51*, 708–714.

Furmark, Ý., Tillfors, M., Marteinsdottir, I., Fischer, H., Pissota, A., Langstrom, B., et al. (2002). Common changes in cerebral blood flow in patients with social phobia treated with citalopram or cognitive-behavioral therapy. *Archives of General Psychiatry, 59,* 425–433.

Gallagher, M., McMahan, R.W., and Schoenbaum, G. (1999). Orbitofrontal cortex and representation of incentive value in associative learning. *Journal of Neuroscience, 19,* 6610–6614.

Giedd, J.N., Blumenthal, J., Jeffries, N.O., Castellanos, F.X., Liu, H., Zijdenbos, A., et al. (1999). Brain development during childhood and adolescence: a longitudinal MRI study. *Nature Neuroscience, 2,* 861–863.

Goenjian, A.K., Pynoos, R.S., Steinberg, A.M., Najarian, L.M., Asarnow, J.R., Karayan, I. et al. (1995). Psychiatric comorbidity in children after the 1988 earthquake in Armenia. *Journal of the American Academy Child and Adolescent Psychiatry, 34,* 1174–1184.

Gorman, J.M., Papp, L.A., Martinez, J., Goetz, R.R., Hollander, E., Liebowitz, M.R., et al. (1990). High-dose carbon dioxide challenge test in anxiety disorder patients. *Biological Psychiatry, 28,* 743–757.

Grafman, J., Vance, S., Weingartner, H., Salazer, A., and Amin, D. (1986). The effects of lateralized frontal lesions on mood regulation. *Brain, 109,* 1127–1148.

Gurley, D., Cohen, P., Pine, D.S., and Brook, J. (1996). Discriminating depression and anxiety in youth: a role for diagnostic criteria. *Journal of Affective Disorders, 39,* 191–200.

Hadwin, J., Frost, S., French, C.C., and Richards, A. (1997). Cognitive processing and trait anxiety in typically developing children: Evidence for an interpretation bias. *Journal of Abnormal Psychology, 106,* 486–490.

Hamann, S.B., Ely, T.D., Grafton, S.T., and Kilts, C.D. (1999). Amygdala activity related to enhanced memory for pleasant and aversive stimuli. *Nature Neuroscience, 2,* 289–293.

Hariri, A.R., Bookheimer, S.Y., and Mazziotta, J.C. (2000). Modulating emotional response: effects of a neocortical network on the limbic system. *Neuroreport, 11,* 43–48.

Hariri, A.R., Mattay, V.S., Tessitore, A., Kolachana, B., Fera, F., Goldman, D., et al. (2002). Serotonin transporter genetic variation and the response of the human amygdala. *Science, 297,* 400–403.

Hariri, A.R., Mattay, V.S., Tessitore, A., Fera, F., and Weinberger, D.R. (2003). Neocortical modulation of the amygdala response to fearful stimuli. *Biological Psychiatry, 53,* 494–501.

Hollingsworth, C.E., Tanquay, P.E., Grossman, L., and Pabst, P. (1980). Long-term outcome of obsessive-compulsive disorder in childhood. *Journal of the American Academy of Child Psychiatry, 19,* 134–144.

Holt, P.E. and Andrews, G. (1989). Provocation of panic: Three elements of the panic reaction in four anxiety disorders. *Behaviour Research and Therapy, 27,* 253–261.

Hope, D.A., Rapee, R.M., Heimberg, R.G., and Dombeck, M.J. (1990). Representations of the self in social phobia: Vulnerability to social threat. *Cognitive Therapy and Research, 14,* 177–189.

Isenberg, N., Silbersweig, D., Engelien, A., Emmerich, S., Malavade, K., Beattie, B., et al. (1999). Linguistic threat activates the human amygdala. *Proceedings of the National Academy of Sciences, 96,* 10456–10459.

Izquierdo, A.D. and Murray, E.A. (2000). Bilateral orbital prefrontal cortex lesions disrupt reinforcer devaluation effects in rhesus monkeys. *Society for Neuroscience Abstracts, 26,* 978.

Kagan, J., Reznick, J.S., and Snidman, N. (1987). The physiology and psychology of behavioral inhibition in children. *Child Development, 58,* 1459–1473.

Kashani, J.H. and Orvaschel, H. (1988). Anxiety disorders in mid-adolescence: A community sample. *American Journal of Psychiatry, 145*, 960–964.

Kashani, J.H. and Orvaschel, H. (1990). A community study of anxiety in children and adolescents. *American Journal of Psychiatry, 147*, 313–318.

Kendall, P.C. (2000). *Child and adolescent therapy: Cognitive-behavioral procedures*, 2nd edn. New York: Guilford.

Kendall, P.C., Flannery-Schroeder, E., Panichelli-Mindel, S.M., Southam-Gerow, M., Henin, A., and Warman, M. (1997). Therapy for youths with anxiety disorders: A second randomized clinical trial. *Journal of Consulting and Clinical Psychology, 65*, 366–380.

Killgore, W.D.S., Oki, M., and Yurgelun-Todd, D.A. (2001). Sex-specific developmental changes in amygdala response to affective faces. *Neuroreport, 12*, 427–433.

Kindt, M. and Brosschot, J.F. (1999). Cognitive bias in spider-phobic children: Comparison of a pictorial and linguistic spider stroop. *Journal of Psychopathology and Behavioral Assessment, 21*, 207–220.

Kindt, M., Bierman, D., and Brosschot, J.F. (1997a). Cognitive bias in spider fear and control children: assessment of emotional interference by a card format and a single-trial of the stroop task. *Journal of Experimental Child Psychology, 66*, 163–179.

Kindt, M., Brosschot, J.F., and Everaerd, W. (1997b). Cognitive processing bias of children in a real life stress situation and a neutral situation. *Journal of Experimental Child Psychology, 64*, 79–97.

King, N.J., Ollendick, T.H., and Mattis, S.G. (1994). Panic in children and adolescents: Normative and clinical studies. *Australian Psychologist, 29*, 89–93.

Klein, R.G. (1995) Is panic disorder associated with childhood separation anxiety disorder? *Clinical Neuropharmacology, 18(S2)*, S7–S14.

Kovacs, M., Feinberg, T.L., Crouse-Novak, M.A., Paulauskas, S.L., and Finkelstein, R. (1984). Depressive disorders in childhood. I. A longitudinal prospective study of characteristics and recovery. *Archives of General Psychiatry, 41*, 229–237.

Labellarte, M.J., Ginsburg, G.S., Walkup, J.T., and Riddle, M.A. (1999). The treatment of anxiety disorders in children and adolescents. *Biological Psychiatry, 46*, 1567–1578.

Last, C.G., Hersen, M., Kazdin, A.E., Francis, G., and Grubb, H.J. (1987). Psychiatric illness in the mothers of anxious children. *American Journal of Psychiatry, 144*, 1580–1583.

Last, C.G., Hersen, M., Kazdin, A., Orvaschel, H., and Perrin, S. (1991). Anxiety disorders in children and their families. *Archives of General Psychiatry, 48*, 928–934.

Last, C.G., Perrin, S., Hersen, M., and Kazdin, A.E. (1996). A prospective study of childhood anxiety disorders. *Journal of the American Academy of Child and Adolescent Psychiatry, 35*, 1502–1510.

Lavy, E., and van den Hout, M. (1993). Selective attention evidenced by pictorial and linguistic Stroop tasks. *Behaviour Therapy, 24*, 645–657.

LeDoux, J.E. (1993). Emotional memory systems in the brain. *Behavioural Brain Research, 58*, 69–79.

LeDoux, J.E. (1995). Emotion: Clues from the brain. *Annual Review of Psychology, 46*, 209–235.

LeDoux, J.E. (1998). Fear and the brain: Where have we been, where are we going? *Biological Psychiatry, 44*, 1229–1238.

Lesch, K.P., Bengel, D., Heils, A., Sabol, S.Z., Greenberg, B.D., Petri, S., et al. (1996). Association of anxiety-related traits with a polymorphism in the serotonin transporter gene regulatory region. *Science, 274*, 1527–1531.

Lewinsohn, P.M., Zinbarg, R., Seeley, J.R., Lewinsohn, M., and Sack, W.H. (1997). Lifetime comorbidity among anxiety disorders and between anxiety disorders and other mental disorders in adolescents. *Journal of Anxiety Disorders*, *11*, 377–394.

Licinio, J. and Wong, M. (2005). Depression, antidepressants and suicidality: a critical appraisal. *Nature Reviews*, *4*, 165–171.

Lundh, L.G. and Ost, L.G. (1996). Recognition for critical faces in social phobics. *Behaviour Research and Therapy*, *34*, 787–794.

Lundh, L.G. and Ost, L.G. (1997). Explicit and implicit memory bias in social phobia: The role of subdiagnostic type. *Behaviour Research and Therapy*, *35*, 305–317.

McGee, R., Feehan, M., Williams, S., Partridge, F., Silva, P.A., and Kelly, J. (1990). DSM-III disorders in large sample of adolescents. *Journal of the American Academy of Child and Adolescent Psychiatry*, *29*, 611–619.

MacLeod, C., Mathews, A., and Tata, P. (1986). Attentional bias in emotional disorders. *Journal of Abnormal Psychology*, *95*, 15–20

MacMillan, S., Szeszko, P.R., Moore, G.J., Madden, R., Lorch, E., Ivey, J., et al. (2003). Increased amygdala: hippocampal volume ratios associated with severity of anxiety in pediatric major depression. *Journal of Child and Adolescent Psychopharmacology*, *13*, 65–73.

McNally, R.J. (1996). Cognitive bias in the anxiety disorders. *Nebraska Symposium on Motivation*, *43*, 211–250.

McNally, R.J. (1997). Memory and anxiety disorders. *Philosophical Transactions of the Royal Society of London Biological Sciences*, *352*, 1755–1759.

McNally, R.J., Kaspi, S.P., Riemann, B.C., and Zeitlin, S. (1990a). Selective processing of threat cues in posttraumatic stress disorder. *Journal of Abnormal Psychology*, *99*, 398–402.

McNally, R.J., Riemann, B.C., and Kim, E. (1990b). Selective processing of threat cues in panic disorder. *Behaviour Research and Therapy*, *28*, 407–412.

Machado, C.J. and Bachevalier, J. (2003). Non-human primate models of childhood psychopathology: The promise and the limitations. *Journal of Child Psychology and Psychiatry*, *44*, 64–87.

Manassis, K., Tannock, R., and Masellis, M. (1996). Cognitive differences between anxious, normal, and ADHD children on a dichotic listening task. *Anxiety*, *2*, 279–285.

Manassis, K., Tannock, R., and Barbosa, J. (2000). Dichotic listening and response inhibition in children with comorbid anxiety disorders and ADHD. *Journal of the American Academy of Child and Adolescent Psychiatry*, *39*, 1152–1159.

March, J.S., Amaya-Jackson, L., Terry, R., and Costanzo, P. (1997). Post-traumatic symptomatology in children and adolescents after an industrial fire. *Journal of the American Academy of Child and Adolescent Psychiatry*, *36*, 1080–1088.

Martin, M., Williams, R., and Clark, D. (1991). Does anxiety lead to selective processing of threat-related information? *Behaviour Research and Therapy*, *29*, 147–160.

Martin, M., Horder, P., and Jones, G.V. (1992). Integral bias in naming of phobia-related words: Brief report. *Cognition and Emotion*, *6*, 479–486.

Mathews, A. and MacLeod, C. (1985). Selective processing of threat cues in anxiety states. *Behaviour Research and Therapy*, *31*, 57–62.

Mathews, A., Mogg, K., May, J., and Eysenck, M.W. (1989). Implicit and explicit memory bias in anxiety. *Journal of Abnormal Psychology*, *98*, 31–34.

Mathews, A., Mogg, K., Kentish, J., and Eysenck, M.W. (1995). Effect of psychological treatment on cognitive bias in generalized anxiety disorder. *Behaviour Research and Therapy, 33,* 293–303.

Mattia, J.I., Heinberg, R.G., and Hope, D.A. (1993). The revised Stroop color-naming task in social phobics. *Behaviour Research and Therapy, 31,* 305–314.

Merikangas, K.R., Avenevoli, S., Dierker, L., and Grillon, C. (1999). Vulnerability factors among children at risk for anxiety disorders. *Biological Psychiatry, 46,* 1523–1535.

Merriam-Webster (1994). *Merriam-Webster Dictionary.* Incorporated. Springfield, MA: Merriam-Webster.

Milham, M.P., Nugent, A.C., Drevets, W.C., Dickstein, D.P., Leibenluft, E., Ernst, M., Charney, D., Pine, D.S. (2005). Selective reduction in amygdala volume in pediatric anxiety disorders: a voxel-based morphometry investigation. *Biological Psychiatry, 57,* 961–966.

Mogg, K. and Bradley, B.P. (1998). A cognitive-motivational analysis of anxiety. *Behaviour Research and Therapy, 36,* 809–848.

Mogg, K., Mathews, A., and Weinman, J. (1987). Memory bias in clinical anxiety. *Journal of Abnormal Psychology, 96,* 94–98.

Mogg, K., Mathews A., and Eysenck, M.W. (1992). Attentional bias to threat in clinical anxiety states. *Cognition and Emotion, 6,* 149–159.

Monk, C.S., McClure, E.B., Nelson, E.E., Zarahn, E., Bilder, R.M., Leibenluft, E., et al. (2003). Adolescent immaturity in attention-related brain engagement to emotional facial expressions. *NeuroImage, 20,* 420–428.

Morris, J.S., Friston, C.D., Perrett, D.I., Rowland, D., Young, A.W., Calder, A.J., et al. (1996). A differential neural response in the human amygdala to fearful and happy facial expression. *Nature, 398,* 115–118.

Morris, J.S., Friston, K.J., Buchel, C., Frith, C.D., Young, A.W., and Calder, A.J. (1998). A neuromodulatory role for the human amygdala in processing emotional facial expressions. *Brain, 121,* 47–57.

Muris, P., Leurmans, J., Merckelbach, H., and Mayer, B. (2000a). "Danger is lurking everywhere": The relation between anxiety and threat perception abnormalties in normal children. *Journal of Behavior Therapy and Experimental Psychiatry, 31,* 123–136.

Muris, P., Merckelbach, H., and Damsma, E. (2000b). Threat perception bias in nonreferred, socially anxious children. *Journal of Clinical Child Psychology, 29,* 348–359.

Muris, P., Merckelbach, H., Schepers, S., and Meesters, C. (2003a). Anxiety, threat perception abnormalties, and emotional reasoning in nonclinical Dutch children. *Journal of Clinical Child and Adolescent Psychology, 32,* 453–459.

Muris, P., Rapee, R., Meesters, C., Schouten, E., and Geers, M. (2003b). Threat perception abnormalties in children: The role of anxiety disorders symptoms, chronic anxiety, and state anxiety. *Journal of Anxiety Disorders, 17,* 271–287.

Nelson, E.E., McClure, E.B., Monk, C.S., Zarahn, E., Leibenluft, E., Pine, D.S., et al. (2003). Developmental differences in neuronal engagement during implicit encoding of emotional faces: An event-related fMRI study. *Journal of Child Psychology and Psychiatry, 44,* 1015–1024.

Norrholm, S.D. and Ouimet, C.C. (2000). Chronic fluoxetine administration to juvenile rats prevents age-associated dendritic spine proliferation in hippocampus. *Brain Research, 883,* 205–215.

Otto, M.W., McNally, R.J., Pollack, M.H., Chen, E., and Rosenbaum, J.F. (1994). Hemispheric laterality and memory bias for threat in anxiety disorders. *Journal of Abnormal Psychology, 103,* 828–831.

Panksepp, J. (1998). *Affective neuroscience: The foundations of human and animal emotions.* New York: Oxford University Press.

Pardo, J.V., Pardo, P.J., and Raichle, M.E. (1993). Neural correlates of self-induced dysphoria. *American Journal of Psychiatry, 150,* 713–719.

Perez-Lopez, J.R., and Woody, S.R. (2001). Memory for facial expressions in social phobia. *Behaviour Research and Therapy, 39,* 967–975.

Perna, G., Bussi, R., Allevi, L., and Bellodi, L. (1999). Sensitivity to 35 percent carbon dioxide in patients with generalized anxiety disorder. *Journal of Clinical Psychiatry, 60,* 379–384.

Pessoa, L., McKenna, M., Gutierrez, E., and Ungerleider, L.G. (2002). Neural processing of emotional faces requires attention. *Proceedings of the National Academy of Sciences, 99,* 11458–11463.

Peterson, B.S., Skudlarski, P., Gatenby, J.C., Zhang, H., Anderson, A.W., and Gore, J.C. (1999). An fMRI study of Stroop word-color interference: Evidence of cingulate subregions subserving multiple distributed attentional systems. *Biological Psychiatry, 45,* 1237–1258.

Pine, D.S. (2002). Treating children and adolescents with selective serotonin reuptake inhibitors: How long is appropriate? *Journal of Child and Adolescent Psychopharmacology, 12,* 189–203.

Pine, D.S. and Grun, J. (1999). Childhood anxiety: integrating developmental psychopathology and affective neuroscience. *Journal of Child and Adolescent Psychopharmacology, 9,* 1–12.

Pine, D.S., Cohen, P., Gurley, D., Brook, J., and Ma, Y. (1998). The risk for early-adulthood anxiety and depressive disorders in adolescents with anxiety and depressive disorders. *Archives of General Psychiatry, 55,* 56–64.

Pine, D.S., Wasserman, G.A., and Workman, S.B. (1999). Memory and anxiety in prepubertal boys at risk for delinquency. *Journal of the American Academy of Child and Adolescent Psychiatry, 38,* 1024–1031.

Pine, D.S., Klein, R.G., Coplan, J.D., Papp, L.A., Hoven, C.W., Martinez, J., et al. (2000). Differential carbon dioxide sensitivity in childhood anxiety disorders and a nonill group. *Archives of General Psychiatry, 57,* 960–967.

Pine, D.S., Grun, J., Zarahn, E., Fyer, A., Koda, V., Li, W., et al. (2001). Cortical brain regions engaged by masked emotional faces in adolescents and adults: An fMRI study. *Emotion, 1,* 137–147.

Pine, D.S., Klein, R.G., Mannuzza, S., Moulton, J.L., Lissek, S., Guardino, M. et al. (2005). Face-emotion processing in offspring at risk for panic disorder. *Journal of the American Academy Child and Adolescent Psychiatry, 44,* 664–672.

Pollak, S.D. and Kistler, D.J. (2002). Early experience is associated with the development of categorical representations for facial expressions of emotion. *Proceedings of the National Academy of Sciences, 99,* 9072–9076.

Posner, M.I. and Rothbart, M.K. (1998). Attention, self-regulation and consciousness. *Philosophical Transactions of the Royal Society of London Biological Sciences, 353,* 1915–1927.

Rapee, R.M., McCallum, S.L., Melville, L.F., Ravenscroft, H., and Rodney, J.M. (1994). Memory bias in social phobia. *Behaviour Research and Therapy, 32,* 89–99.

Rauch, S.L., Jenike, M.A., and Alpert, N.A. (1994). Regional cerebral blood flow measurement during symptom provocation in obsessive-compulsive disorder using 15-O labeled CO_2 and positron emission tomography. *Archives of General Psychiatry, 52,* 20–28.

Rauch, S.L., Savage, C.R., Alpert, N.M., Miguel, E.C., Baer, L., Breiter, H.C., et al. (1995). A positron emission tomographic study of simple phobic symptom provocation. *Archives of General Psychiatry, 52*, 20–26.

Richards, A., French, C.C., Calder, A.J., Webb, B., Fox, R., and Young, A.W. (2002). Anxiety-related bias in the classification of emotionally ambiguous facial expressions. *Emotion, 2*, 273–287.

Riddle. M.A., Reeve, E.A., Yaryura-Tobias, J.A., Yang, H.M., Claghorn, J.L., Gaffney, G. (2001). Fluvoxamine for children and adolescents with obsessive-compulsive disorder: a randomized, controlled, multicenter trial. *Journal of the American Academy Child and Adolescent Psychiatry, 40*, 222–229.

Roblek, T. and Piacentini, J. (2005). Cognitive-behavior therapy for childhood anxiety disorders. *Child and Adolescent Psychiatric Clinics of North America, 14*, 863–876.

Rosenbaum, J.F., Biederman, J., Gersten, M., Hirshfeld, D.R., Meminger, S.R., Herman, J.B., et al. (1988). Behavioral inhibition in children of parents with panic disorder and agoraphobia: A controlled study. *Archives of General Psychiatry, 45*, 463–470.

Rusinek, S., Hautekèete, M., Danes, H., Deregnaucourt, I., and Lemmen, V. (2002). Biais d'interprétations d'événements scolaires chez des enfants anxieux. *Journal de Therapie Comportementale et Cognitive, 12*, 59–65.

RUPP Anxiety Study Group (2001). Fluvoxamine for the treatment of anxiety disorders in children and adolescents. *New England Journal of Medicine, 344*, 1279–1285.

Sah, P., Faber, S.L., Lopez De Armentia, M., and Power, J. (2003). The amygdaloid complex: Anatomy and physiology. *Physiological Reviews, 83*, 803–834.

Sallee, F.R., Sethuraman, G., Sine, L., and Liu, H. (2000). Yohimbine challenge in children with anxiety disorders. *American Journal of Psychiatry, 157*, 1236–1242.

Schoenbaum, G., Chiba, A.A., and Gallagher, M. (1998). Obitofrontal cortex and basolateral amygdala encode expected outcomes during learning. *Nature Neuroscience, 1*, 155–159.

Schwartz, C.E., Wright, C.I., Shin, L.M., Kagan, J., and Rauch, S.L. (2003). Inhibited and uninhibited infants "grown up": Adults' amygdalar response to novelty. *Science, 300*, 1952–1953.

Schwartz, M.L. and Goldman-Rakic, P.S. (1991). Prenatal specification of callosal in rhesus monkey. *Journal of Comparative Neurology, 307*, 144–162.

Shaffer, D., Fisher, P., Dulcan, M.K., Davies, M., Piacentini, J., Schwab-Stone, M.E., et al. (1996). The NIMH Diagnostic Interview Schedule for Children Version 2.3 (DISC-2.3): Description, acceptability, prevalence rates, and performance in the MECA Study. *Journal of the American Academy of Child and Adolescent Psychiatry, 35*, 865–877.

Sheline, Y.I., Barch, D.M., Donnelly, J.M., Ollinger, J.M., Snyder, A.Z., and Mintun, M.A. (2001) Increased amygdala response to masked emotional faces in depressed subjects resolves with antidepressant treatment: an fMRI study. *Biological Psychiatry, 50*, 651–658.

Shortt, A.L., Barrett, P.M., Dadds, M.R., and Fox, T.L. (2001). The influence of family and experimental context on cognition in anxious children. *Journal of Abnormal Child Psychology, 29*, 585–596.

Stein, M.B., Goldin, P.R., Sareen, J., Zorrilla, L.T., and Brown, G.G. (2002). Increased amygdala activation to angry and contemputous faces in generalized social phobia. *Archives of General Psychiatry, 59*, 1027–1034.

Steingard, J., Yurgelun-Todd, D.A., Hennen, J., Moore, J.C., Moore, C.M., Vakili, K., et al. (2000). Increased orbitofrontal cortex levels of choline in depressed adolescents as detected by in vivo proton magnetic resonance spectroscopy. *Biological Psychiatry*, *48*, 1053–1061.

Strauss, C.C. and Last, C.G. (1993). Social and simple phobias in children. *Journal of Anxiety Disorders*, *7*, 141–152.

Strauss, C.C., Last, C.G., Hersen, M., and Kazdin, A.E. (1988). Association between anxiety and depression in children and adolescents with anxiety disorders. *Journal of Abnormal Child Psychology*, *16*, 57–68.

Taghavi, M.R., Neshat-Doost, H.T., Moradi, A.R., Yule, W., and Dalgleish, T. (1999). Biases in visual attention in children and adolescents with clinical anxiety and mixed anxiety-depression. *Journal of Abnormal Child Psychology*, *27*, 215–223.

Taghavi, M.R., Moradi, A.R., Neshat-Doost, H.T., Yule, W., and Dalgleish, T. (2000). Interpretation of ambiguous emotional information in clinicallyanxious children and adolescents. *Cognition and Emotion*, *14*, 809–822.

Taghavi, M.R., Dalgleish, T., Moradi, A.R., Neshat-Doost, H.T., and Yule, W. (2003). Selective processing of negative emotional information in children and adolescents with Generalized Anxiety Disorder. *British Journal of Clinical Psychology*, *42*, 221–230.

Thapar, A. and McGuffin, P. (1996). A twin study of antisocial and neurotic symptoms in childhood. *Psychological Medicine*, *26*, 1111–1118.

Thomas, K.M., Drevets, W.C., Dahl, R.E., Ryan, N.D., Birmaher, B., Eccard, C.H., et al. (2001a). Amygdala response to fearful faces in anxious and depressed children. *Archives of General Psychiatry*, *58*, 1057–1063.

Thomas, K.M., Drevets, W.C., Whalen, P.J., Eccard, C.H., Dahl, R.E., Ryan, N.D., et al. (2001b). Amygdala response to facial expressions in children and adults. *Society of Biological Psychiatry*, *49*, 309–316.

Tillfors, M., Furmark, T., Marteinsdottir, I., Fischer, H., Pissiota, A., Langstrom, B., et al. (2001). Cerebral blood flow in subjects with social phobia during stressful speaking tasks: A PET study. *American Journal of Psychiatry*, *158*, 1220–1226.

Toren, P., Sadeh, M., Wolmer, L., Eldar, S., Koren, S., Weizman, R., et al. (2000). Neurocognitive correlates of anxiety disorders in children: a preliminary report. *Journal of Anxiety Disorders*, *14*, 239–247.

Valleni-Basile, L.A., Garrison, C.Z., Jackson, K.L., Waller, J.L., McKeown, R.E., Addy, C.L., et al. (1994). Frequency of obsessive-compulsive disorder in a community sample of young adolescents. *Journal of the American Academy of Child and Adolescent Psychiatry*, *33*, 782–791.

Vasa, R.A., Grados, M., Slomine, B., Herskovits, E.H., Thompson, R.E., Salorio, C., et al. (2003). Neuroimaging correlates of anxiety after pediatric traumatic brain injury. *Biological Psychiatry*, *55*, 208–216.

Vasey, M.W., Daleiden, E.L., Williams, L.L., and Brown, L.M. (1995). Biased attention in childhood anxiety disorders: A preliminary study. *Journal of Abnormal Child Psychology*, *23*, 267–279.

Vasey, M.W., El-Hag, N., and Daleiden, E.L. (1996). Anxiety and the processing of emotionally threatening stimuli: Distinctive patterns of selective attention among high-and-low-test-anxious children. *Child Development*, *67*, 1173–1185.

Verburg, K., Griez, E., Meijer, J., and Pols, H. (1995). Discrimination between panic disorder and generalized anxiety disorder by 35 percent carbon dioxide challenge. *American Journal of Psychiatry*, *152*, 1081–1083.

Verhulst, F.C., van der Ende, J., Ferdinand, R.F., and Kasius, M.C. (1997). The prevalence of DSM-III-R diagnoses in a national sample of Dutch adolescents. *Archives of General Psychiatry*, *54*, 329–336.

Warner, V., Mufson, L., and Weissman, M.M. (1995). Offspring at high and low risk for depression and anxiety: Mechanisms of psychiatric disorder. *Journal of the American Academy of Child and Adolescent Psychiatry*, *34*, 786–797.

Warren, S.L., Schmitz, S., and Emde, R.N. (1999). Behavioral genetic analyses of self-reported anxiety at 7 years of age. *Journal of the American Academy of Child and Adolescent Psychiatry*, *38*, 1403–1408.

Watts, F., McKenna, F.P., Sharrock, R., and Trezise, L. (1986). Color naming of phobia-related words. *British Journal of Psychology*, *77*, 97–108.

Weingarten, S.M. (1999). Psychosurgery. In B.L. Miller and J.L. Cummings (Eds.), *The human frontal lobes: Functions and disorders*. New York: Guilford.

Weissman, M.M., Leckman, J.F., Merikangas, K.R., Gammon, G.D., and Prusoff, B.A. (1984). Depression and anxiety disorders in parents and children: Results from the Yale family study. *Archives of General Psychiatry*, *41*, 845–852.

Whalen, P.J., Shin, L.M., McInerney, S.C., Fischer, H., Wright, C.I., and Rauch, S.L. (2001). A functional MRI study of human amygdala responses to facial expressions of fear versus anger. *Emotion*, *1*, 70–83.

Winton, E.C., Clark, D.M., and Edelmann, R.J. (1995). Social anxiety, fear of negative evaluation and the detection of negative emotion in others. *Behaviour Research and Therapy*, *33*, 193–196.

Zald, D.H. and Kim, S.W. (1996). Anatomy and function of the orbital frontal cortex II: Anatomy, neurocircuitry and obsessive-compulsive disorder. *Journal of Neuropsychiatry*, *8*, 249–261.

5

DEPRESSIVE DISORDERS

Helen Z. Reinherz, Jennifer L. Tanner, Angela D. Paradis,
William R. Beardslee, Eva M. Szigethy,
and Abigail E. Bond

Consequences of childhood and adolescent depression are far-reaching. Depressive disorder during these formative years not only impairs well-being, but also undermines normal development resulting in threats to developmentally salient achievements. Findings from longitudinal studies that have followed depressed youth into adulthood have documented a substantial degree of continuity and severely impaired functioning across multiple domains well into adulthood (Fergusson and Woodward, 2002; Lewinsohn et al., 1999; Pine et al., 1998; Rao et al., 1995; Reinherz et al., 2000; Weissman et al., 1999).

Since the mid 1980s increasing attention has been given to these disabling disorders as evidenced by the volume of literature on child and adolescent depression. However, there remains a need to delineate specific and multiple developmental pathways tracing the onset and course of depression in youth. Given that most individuals experience their first depressive episode in childhood or adolescence (Hankin et al., 1998), accurate understanding of depression in youth is vitally important for the development of effective intervention, prevention, and treatment programs that may curtail the development of a chronic course of illness.

The purpose of this chapter is to review the current state of the literature on childhood and adolescent depressive disorders, which includes major depressive disorder and dysthymic disorder. As an overview, we report on issues concerning definition and classification, risk factors and correlates, course, associated outcomes and available treatments, as well as identify areas for future research. Most studies highlighted in this review are based on community samples (rather than clinical or referred samples) as they provide insight into the natural history of depressive disorders in the general population of youth.

Classification of child and adolescent depression

There is wide variation in meaning when the term depression is used to describe youth who exhibit a core set of depressive symptoms (see Merikangas and

Avenevoli, 2002, for a discussion). It was not until 1980 that the American Psychiatric Association provided diagnostic criteria for major depressive disorder and dysthymia in children and adolescents (DSM-III; APA, 1980). Current criteria, operationalized in the DSM-IV (APA, 1994), share a high degree of similarity with those for adult major depressive disorder and dysthymia (APA, 1994) and those outlined in the tenth revision of the International Statistical Classification of Diseases and Mental Health Problems (ICD-10; World Health Organization, 1992).

Children and adolescents who meet DSM-IV criteria for major depressive disorder (MDD) must exhibit at least one core symptom, in addition to four more of nine symptoms:

- Depressed or irritable mood (core symptom)
- Diminished interest or pleasure in previously preferred activities (core symptom)
- Significant weight loss or gain
- Insomnia or hypersomnia
- Psychomotor agitation or retardation
- Fatigue or loss of energy
- Feelings of worthlessness or inappropriate guilt
- Diminished ability to think or concentrate
- Recurrent thoughts of death.

The occurrence of these symptoms must result in a change from previous functioning, may not be due to a medical condition, and must interfere with daily functioning of the affected youth.

Dysthymic disorder (DD) is a mild, chronic form of depression. In children and adolescents, depressed mood for most of the day more days than not (by subjective account or observation by others) must be present. Two or more of the following must also be present:

- Poor appetite or overeating
- Insomnia or hypersomnia
- Low energy or fatigue
- Low self-esteem
- Poor concentration or difficulty making decisions
- Feelings of hopelessness.

Cases in which, between episodes of MDD, the youth never returns to a state of previous functioning, but rather, to a state of dysthymia are referred to as "double-depression." Double-depression has been associated with severe impairments in functioning beyond those found for cases of MDD or DD (Goodman et al., 2000).

Despite the widespread use of the DSM classification system to trace the natural history of depressive disorders in children and adolescents, three arguments speak to the controversy concerning the validity of the current system. First, the developing status of children and adolescents gives rise to the question of whether criteria created for adults is appropriate for use with children and adolescents. As an illustration of this point, Luby et al. (2002) found that DSM-IV criteria failed to capture 76 percent of preschoolers (ages 3 to 5.6 years) who met MDD when criteria were age-appropriately modified. Additionally, there is increasing evidence that a single set of criteria may not accurately describe the phenomenon of childhood and adolescent depression. Weiss and Garber (2003) reviewed evidence suggestive of developmental differences in depressive symptoms in youth under age 18, indicating that even a global set of criteria for those under age 18 may be inadequate.

Second, some studies have shown that rates of subthreshold depression in adolescents are as high, if not higher, than rates of MDD (e.g., Kessler, 2002). Various investigations indicate that youth with subthreshold levels of the disorder may experience deficits in psychosocial functioning similar to youth who meet full diagnostic criteria (Lewinsohn et al., 2000b), and that adolescents with subthreshold symptoms are at increased risk for future psychiatric diagnoses (Angold et al., 1999c). Given the importance of subthreshold depressive symptomatology, it has been suggested that depression may be best conceptualized as a continuum (Lewinsohn et al., 2000b; see Santor and Coyne, 2001, for contrasting findings).

Third, the co-occurrence of depressive disorders with other psychiatric problems in children and adolescents suggests that there are relatively few pure cases of depression. In recent years, research on psychiatric comorbidity has increased due to recognition by clinicians and researchers of its importance in diagnosis, prognosis, and treatment (Kessler et al., 1994). Researchers have found that 40–70 percent of depressed adolescents meet criteria for comorbid conditions (Angold et al., 1999a; Ford et al., 2003). Although comorbidity is common, there appears to be systematic co-occurrence of specific disorders with MDD. A meta-analysis (Angold et al., 1999a) of psychiatric comorbidity found that anxiety disorders were eight times as common in depressed as compared to non-depressed youth; moreover, conduct and oppositional defiant disorders were over six times as common, and attention deficit/hyperactivity disorder was over five times as common. These three areas of research draw attention to the validity of the current taxonomy. Developmentally sensitive diagnostic strategies should be a primary focus of future inquiry.

Epidemiology of depressive disorders

Prevalence and incidence of depressive disorders in children and adolescents

Prevalence studies of childhood depression are limited in number. Thus, knowledge about the occurrence of depressive disorders in youth is largely based on the adolescent period. The available research suggests that MDD is relatively rare in the first decade of life and increases dramatically in mid to late adolescence (Kessler et al., 1993). While this may reflect a truly limited number of cases during early childhood, it may be partially attributable to the lack of valid assessment tools available for use with this younger age group.

Point prevalence estimates of MDD among pre-pubertal youth range from 1.8 to 2.0 percent (Cohen et al., 1993) and from 0.7 to 2.6 percent in adolescents (Fergusson et al., 1993; Lewinsohn et al., 1993). Lifetime prevalence of depression in adolescents is comparable to what is found for adults, ranging from 4.0 to 24.0 percent (Angst and Merikangas, 1997; Essau et al., 2000; Kessler and Walters, 1998; Lewinsohn et al., 1993; Reinherz et al., 1999).

Although there are far fewer studies of DD prevalence among children and adolescents, it appears to follow a developmental pattern similar to MDD, with higher prevalence among adolescents than children. Point prevalence ranges between 0.6 and 1.7 percent in preschool age children (Kashani and Carlson, 1987) and from 1.6 to 8.0 percent in adolescents (Fergusson et al., 1993; Lewinsohn et al., 1993). Lifetime prevalence of dysthymia among adolescents ranges from 1.8 to 5.6 percent (Angst and Merikangas, 1997; Essau et al., 2000).

While prevalence estimates provide important information about the occurrence of depressive disorders among youth, incidence rates, referring to the emergence of new cases of disorder over a specified time interval, are critical for estimating age of onset and the appropriate timing of interventions (Newman et al., 1996). Incidence rates, however, are rarely reported because they require frequent assessment points in a longitudinal study design. Studies reporting incidence rates generally find the highest rates in mid to late adolescence. Lewinsohn et al. (1993) reported one-year incidence rates for MDD and DD in a high school sample (ages 14 to 18) of 5.7 percent and 0.07 percent, respectively. In another community study of high school students, Garrison and colleagues (1997) found a one-year incidence of MDD of 3.4 percent. It is also important to note that there has been a reported increase of depression in more recent generations of youth (Fombonne, 1994; Klein et al., 1995).

Due to the pervasive nature of depressive disorders in youth and the impact of its occurrence on development, it is critical to study risk factors and correlates of childhood and adolescent depression along with its comorbid concomitants (Kessler et al., 1996). The next section of this review surveys theoretically and empirically important correlates and risk factors from many domains affecting the onset and course of depressive disorders.

Correlates and risk factors for childhood and adolescent depression

The emergence of developmental epidemiology (Costello and Angold, 2000) and developmental psychopathology (Cicchetti and Toth, 1998) paradigms has underscored the necessity of considering the role of risk exposure on the course and outcomes associated with psychopathology. Moving beyond single risk factor models, findings from prospective, longitudinal studies of depressive disorders have begun to test developmental pathways that integrate multiple levels of risk from neurobiological to societal level factors. Due largely to emerging analytic

116

techniques that aid in furthering our understanding of the complex etiology of psychopathology across the life span (Susser et al., 2002), the most recent approaches have attempted to cast light on the interactions of risk factors and developmental status as they affect the onset and continuity of depression (Cicchetti and Toth, 1991; Costello and Angold, 2000).

Researchers and clinicians have stressed the need to identify malleable risk factors that can be targeted for preventive intervention (Beardslee, 1998; Carbonell et al., 2002). However, identification of risk profiles that describe not only the etiology, but also the course and outcome of depressive disorders in childhood and adolescence, is a complex endeavor. This research is complicated by the fact that there are clear developmental differences in children's responses to specific risks (Rutter, 2002) and it is not always possible to determine the temporal sequence of risk factors and disorder (Kraemer et al., 1997). Indeed, emerging theoretical models suggest bidirectional influences between risk and disorder (Cicchetti and Toth, 1998; Costello and Angold, 2000). Thus, this overview of correlates and risks surveys a broad array of factors that interact in complex ways across different developmental stages.

Age

Both prospective, longitudinal studies of youth and retrospective studies of adults have identified mid to late adolescence as a particularly vulnerable time for the development of major depression (Giaconia et al., 1994; Hammen and Rudolph, 1996; Lewinsohn et al., 1993), as well as a crucial time for delineating factors protecting at-risk youth (Carbonell et al., 2002). Most index episodes of dysthymia also occur during this pivotal age period. Identifying the age at which depressed youth experience their first episode is critical as it may be related to course of disorder. Early onset depressive disorders have been associated with a protracted course of illness and increased risk for the later development of other mental disorders. For instance, Klein and Santiago (2003) found that 70 percent of children with DD in their study went on to develop MDD before adulthood. MDD has also been found to confer substantial risk for later substance disorders (Costello et al., 1999; Lewinsohn et al., 1999; Kessler and Walters, 1998). A greater understanding about age of onset is important for the timing of prevention efforts.

Gender

Most studies find no gender differences in the prevalence of major depression in pre-pubertal children (Nolen-Hoeksema, 2002). However, beginning in early adolescence, rates of depressive symptoms (Nolen-Hoeksema and Girgus, 1994; Leadbeater et al., 1995) and major depressive disorder (Lewinsohn et al., 1993; Reinherz et al., 1999) between male and female populations diverge, revealing a greater risk for disorder in females. It appears that gender differences in depressive symptoms are moderate and consistent among referred youth (Compas et al., 1997)

117

and approach a 2:1 female to male ratio for MDD by age 15 in epidemiologic studies (Kessler et al., 1993; Weissman et al., 1991).

Mechanisms underlying this shift in prevalence are not fully understood, but may reflect the interplay of gender socialization, social and hormonal mechanisms, and stressful events associated with adolescence (Cyranowski et al., 2000). Although most research has found that gender-based differences in prevalence continue throughout the life span, several studies (Cohen et al., 1993; Reinherz et al., 1999) have noted a temporary decrease in these differences during early adulthood. One hypothesis suggested to explain this shift is that entrance into college may empower young women, making them less vulnerable to depression (Nolen-Hoeksema, 1990).

Gender differences exist both in pathways to depression as well as in course of disorder (Cicchetti and Toth, 1998; Compton et al., 2003). Most studies have found that females experience greater severity of symptoms (McCauley et al., 1993; Reinherz et al., 1993), are more likely to have recurrent episodes (Lewinsohn and Essau, 2002), have a higher likelihood of continuity of depression into adulthood, and higher rates of comorbidity with anxiety and other affective disorders (Breslau et al., 2000; Kovacs et al., 2003).

Socioeconomic status and race/ethnicity

Findings concerning the impact of socioeconomic status (SES) on the development of childhood and adolescent depression are inconsistent. McLeod and Shanahan (1996) reported that children with histories of persistent poverty had a higher occurrence of childhood depression. However, other researchers have not found SES to be significantly related to child and adolescent depression (Miech et al., 1999; Poulton et al., 2002). Since low SES frequently co-occurs with many other risk factors, such as parental psychopathology and stressful home environment, these factors may confound the relationship between SES and depression (Goodman and Gotlib, 1999; Kraemer et al., 2001). Additional methodological problems, such as restricted ranges of SES in study samples, may also erode the ability to find differences among groups.

Most epidemiologic studies do not have sufficiently large minority samples to provide statistical power to test for differences across racial and ethnic groups after controlling for sociodemographic factors. The research to date has been inconclusive. While some studies report no differences in rates of disorder between African American and Caucasian youth (Costello et al., 1996), others suggest that there is increased depressive symptomatology in African American early adolescents (Garrison et al., 1989). There is also some evidence that Mexican American and Latino youth may experience more depression than Caucasian youth independent of age, gender, and SES (Roberts et al., 1997; Siegel et al., 1998). Additional research is needed to elucidate how ethnicity, culture, and race may function as risk or protective factors for childhood and adolescent depression.

118

Family and genetic factors

In childhood and adolescence, the family provides the most important environment for development. Parents also endow children with specific biological and genetic predispositions, vulnerabilities, and strengths. The influence of powerful environmental and genetic family influences has been studied and debated by numerous scholars (e.g., Lewinsohn et al., 2000a; Wallace et al., 2002). There is general agreement that untangling the contributions of family genetic endowment and environment remains an important challenge for scientists (Kendler, 1995).

Parental history of depression, particularly maternal depression, has been identified as a major risk factor for depressive disorders in children and adolescents. Beardslee et al. (1993) reported that children of depressed parents have a 60 percent chance of developing major depression by age 25. Other authors (Hammen and Brennan, 2003; Lewinsohn and Essau, 2002) have noted that the offspring of depressed parents have a 3- to 6-fold increase in the odds of experiencing depression themselves.

The mode and specificity of familial transmission of depression has also been examined (Klein et al., 2001). For example, there may be a greater possibility of transmission of MDD from same sex parents, particularly from mothers to daughters (Davies and Windle, 1997). Reinherz and colleagues (2000) have found that having a sibling with depression or a substance disorder places an individual at risk for depression. Similarly, Luthar et al. (1992) found that siblings of individuals with drug disorders were at increased risk for depression. To explain such findings, it has been suggested that depression and substance disorder may be an alternate expression of the same underlying vulnerability (Reinherz et al., 2000). The heritability of DD has also been supported. Klein et al. (1995) noted that patients (over 18) with DD had significantly higher rates of DD in first-degree relatives than patients with MDD and controls.

In reviewing possible mechanisms, Goodman and Gotlib (1999) noted that the pathways of transmission of MDD from parent to child are likely to be complex and include aspects of dysfunctional parent–child interactions, marital conflict, emotional distance of parents, as well as genetic factors. In fact, there is likely to be substantial interaction between genes and environment (Rutter, 2005). Specific evidence regarding such interactions comes from a study by Caspi et al. (2003), who investigated the relationship between functional polymorphisms of the serotonin transporter (5-HTT) gene and stressful life events. In this study, young adults with one or two short alleles of the 5-HTT promoter polymorphism were more likely to experience depression when facing life stress than those with two copies of the long allele. This influential article was one of the first to provide specific evidence suggesting both that genetic susceptibility has little effect in the absence of environmental stressors and that adverse life events have a larger impact in the face of genetic susceptibility. Gene–environment interactions associated with child and adolescent onset of depressive disorders represents the frontier of research into the etiology of these disorders.

Brain and neurochemistry

To date, no specific physiological risk markers for childhood and adolescent depression have been identified. However, physiological processes, especially those associated with stress and pubertal development, have been associated with childhood and adolescent depression. Replicating findings from studies of depressed adults, many find a link between hyperactive functioning of the hypothalamic-endocrine-adrenal (HPA) axis, the endocrine axis responsible for stress regulation, and depression in youth (Ryan et al., 1992).

Dysregulation of other hypothalamic-endocrine axes (e.g., thyroid, gonadol, and somatotropic) has been explored as a risk factor for childhood and adolescent depression (Brooks-Gunn et al., 2001). Findings indicate that dysregulated levels of growth hormone, secreted mostly nocturnally by the pituitary gland as a growth-stimulating agent during adolescence, are found in depressed youth (see De Bellis et al., 1996, for contrary results; Kutcher et al., 1991; Meyer et al., 1991).

Across such studies, there is a convergence of findings indicating that reaching puberty early is a risk factor for depressive symptoms (Graber et al., 1997; Hayward et al., 1997; Kaltiala-Heino et al., 2003). Work by Angold et al. (1999b) indicates that pubertal stage has stronger effects on depression than age and further, that changes in androgen and oestrogen levels are stronger contributors to the risk for depression than associated morphological changes.

Health

Health has emerged both as a predictor and correlate of childhood and adolescent depression (Lewinsohn et al., 1996; Reinherz et al., 1999). Several studies have found an association between reports of neonatal, postnatal, and early childhood illness and late adolescent major depression (Cohen et al., 1989; Gizynski and Shapiro, 1990). For example, Reinherz et al. (1999) found that as early as the neonatal period, serious illness in boys was predictive of MDD in late adolescence (age 18) and early adulthood (age 21). In trying to account for the long-term effects of early health problems, it has been suggested that parent–child interactions may be compromised by these illnesses, increasing the child's vulnerability to depression (Cohen et al., 1989).

Life events and stressors

Since the 1970s, studies have noted the influence of negative life events and stressors on the onset of depression for people of all ages, and research has shown that stress is specifically predictive of depressive symptoms in children and adolescents (Goodyer et al., 2000; Nolen-Hoeksema, 1992). Lewinsohn and colleagues have extensively examined the etiologic role of negative events, as well as minor hassles, on MDD during adolescence (Lewinsohn et al., 1994b; Monroe et al., 1999). Several studies have found that patients with DD report childhood adversities to a greater extent than those with MDD (Riso and Klein, 2003).

Specific sources of stress linked to depression in children and adolescents include disappointments, loss, separation, and interpersonal conflict (Cuffe et al., 2005; Monroe et al., 1999; Reinherz et al., 1989). Although some studies have not found separation/divorce to be a significant risk factor for the later development of depression (e.g., Reinherz et al., 1999), others have reported that parental divorce in childhood is associated with an increased risk for depression (Short, 2002). In the past, the primary focus of research was on the harmful effects of divorce on children's mental health, but researchers are now recognizing that marital *conflict* (which frequently co-occurs with divorce) is a more important predictor of child adjustment (see Kelly 2000, for a review).

Merikangas and Angst (1995) have noted that negative life events most frequently lead to depression when they are disruptive, chronic, and have a severe impact on the individual. Important gender differences in response to specific stressors have also been found (Little and Garber, 2000; Reinherz et al., 1993).

To explain the complex relationship between stressors and depression, Hammen et al. (1999) proposed a diathesis-stress model describing the interaction between individual vulnerability and external stressors. Some studies have also investigated the contributions of genes that may influence both the development of depressive symptoms and negative life events (Caspi et al., 2003). Although this is an emerging line of research, the clarification of these relationships offers promise.

Along with new efforts to understand mechanisms that lead from negative events to depression there is continuing need to identify modifiable stressors, such as violent and chaotic households, abusive behaviors, and peer rejection, that can be targeted by prevention and intervention programs.

Psychosocial factors

Many psychosocial factors that are both characteristic of youth with depression and predictive of later disorder reflect negative self-perceptions, including low self-esteem, peer rejection, and lack of secure familial relationships (Beardslee and Gladstone, 2001; Lewinsohn et al., 1994b; Reinherz et al., 1999). Problematic childhood behaviors, such as anxious-depressed and withdrawn behavior, have also been associated with the onset of depression by young adulthood (Caspi et al., 1996; Goodwin et al., 2004).

Among the adolescents studied by Lewinsohn et al. (1994b), those with current MDD were characterized by low self-esteem, emotional dependence, less self-reported social support, and ineffective coping. Reinherz et al. (1989, 1999) reported similar findings; study participants with depression at ages 18 and 21 were described by teachers as early as kindergarten as being more hostile to peers. Adolescents with depression also self-reported more anxiety, unpopularity, and familial rejection at age 9. Caspi et al. (1996) found that 3 year olds who were inhibited were more likely to meet criteria for MDD at age 21 than other children. Conversely, Essau and Dobson (1999) point out the protective effect of social competence and good peer relationships in later adolescence.

Several important psychosocial constructs have been identified as salient links to both current and future depression in children and adolescents. In discussing adolescent predictors of MDD in young adulthood, Lewinsohn described the construct "emotional reliance" (Lewinsohn and Seeley, 2003). This term characterizes an extreme need for support and approval which is closely linked with depression. His findings echo those of Reinherz et al. (1999), who reported that depressed 21 year olds indicated a greater need for extensive social support than their non-depressed counterparts. Other authors have also underscored the important link between insecure parental attachment and depression in youth (Cicchetti and Toth, 1998). Adolescents with a history of DD also report having less social support from peers than adolescents with past histories of MDD and other psychopathology (Klein et al., 1997). As with many predictors of MDD and DD, identification of these early warning signs may augur well for early identification and intervention altering the course of these disorders and their chronicity.

Course of disorder

Episode duration

In clinical and community studies the mean length of a major depressive episode in children and adolescents has been found to be approximately 28–36 weeks (Kovacs et al., 1984; Lewinsohn et al., 1994a; Rao et al., 1995). For dysthymia, Lewinsohn et al. (1993) reported an average duration of 134 weeks in an adolescent cohort. Factors associated with a longer index depressive episode include being female (both MDD and DD), greater episode severity, early onset (before age 15), and having received treatment for the disorder (Lewinsohn et al., 1994a). Under-standing factors contributing to protracted length of disorder is critical because prior research has shown that the longer an episode persists the greater the risk for negative effects on healthy developmental processes (Goodyer et al., 1997).

Relapse and persistence

There is considerable evidence indicating that childhood and adolescent depressive episodes often mark the onset of a recurrent or chronic course of disorder (Bardone et al., 1996; Birmaher et al., 2002; Fombonne et al., 2001; Lewinsohn et al., 1999, 2000a; Pine et al., 1998; Rao et al., 1995, 1999). Although most adolescents (nearly 90 percent) recover from their index episode of MDD within 1.5–2 years of onset, a substantial minority, 6–10 percent, develop a protracted course of illness (Kovacs, 1996; McCauley et al., 1993; Sanford et al., 1995). Findings from epidemiologic studies (Fleming et al., 1993; Lewinsohn et al., 1994a) have also documented a recurrence rate of up to 70 percent by five years after the index episode. Moreover, Pine et al. (1998) found that adolescents with major depression face a two- to four-fold greater risk for depression as young adults.

Studies investigating factors contributing to the recurrence of depressive disorders have consistently found that youth with early onset MDD have substantially increased risk for recurrence in adulthood (Bardone et al., 1996; Lewinsohn et al., 1999; Rao et al., 1995). Yet adolescent onset depression, as compared to pre-pubertal onset, is more closely associated with mood disorders in adulthood. The continuity of childhood depression with adult disorder appears to be more heterotypic, i.e., it increases the risk for multiple types of psychopathology in adulthood but not necessarily for mood disorders (Weissman et al., 1999).

Depressed youth experiencing recurrent episodes in adulthood have been found to have higher rates of recurrent MDD in first-degree relatives (Birmaher et al., 2002; Lewinsohn et al., 2000a; Wickramaratne et al., 2000). Lewinsohn et al. (2000a) also found female gender, experiencing multiple depressive episodes in adolescence, and family conflict (females only) to be predictive of recurrent depression. Both youth and adults suffering from comorbid disorders have also been found to have chronic and complicated courses of disorder (Fombonne et al., 2001; Clarke et al., 1995; Lewinsohn et al., 2000a; Merikangas et al., 2003).

Despite substantial levels of continuity, it is important to note that many individuals with MDD and DD in adolescence do not manifest clinically significant symptoms in adulthood. The identification of factors differentiating these youth from those who continue to experience depressive disorders may provide information relevant to prevention and intervention efforts. In one of the few studies to identify psychosocial predictors of recurrent MDD, Lewinsohn et al. (2000a) found that formerly depressed adolescents with low levels of emotional reliance and positive attributional style (males only) were more likely to remain disorder free in young adulthood. Programs fostering these adaptive qualities in youth may help curtail recurrent depressive episodes.

Outcome

Psychosocial impairment

Depressive disorders occurring during childhood and adolescence have been linked to psychosocial impairment across multiple domains. Youth experiencing MDD and DD have compromised social functioning and family relations, decreased self-esteem, and lower academic achievement (Geller et al., 2001; Giaconia et al., 2001; Rao et al., 1995; Reinherz et al., 1999). The extent to which depression impacts one's ability to meet normative developmental tasks during these important age periods may have long-range implications for functioning.

The growing body of literature on the long-term impact of childhood and adolescent depression on adult functioning indicates substantial morbidity. Adolescent MDD, for example, has been linked to aspects of problematic social adjustment, including interpersonal difficulties with friends and family (Leader and Klein, 1996; Lewinsohn et al., 1995). Depression during adolescence has also been found to predict early marriage and marital distress in young adulthood (Gotlib et al., 1998). Additional evidence suggests that depressed adolescents have an earlier transition to parenthood (Bardone et al., 1996). This is particularly concerning as previous studies have clearly documented an association between parental and offspring depression (Beardslee et al., 1998; Hammen and Brennan, 2003). Other research has established a relationship between adolescent depression and school drop-out as well as occupational difficulties in young adulthood (Bardone et al., 1996; Fergusson and Woodward, 2002; Kessler et al., 1997).

Psychosocial impairment tends to be more severe in depressed individuals with comorbid disorder than in people with major depression only (Fombonne et al., 2001; Kessler et al., 1994; Lewinsohn et al., 1995; Rao et al., 1999). Other factors linked to increased dysfunction from depression are early onset and greater severity of disorder, and increased number of recurrent episodes. In contrast, youth with depressive episodes limited to their pre-pubertal years tend to experience less functional impairment than do youth who experience depression during later adolescence (Geller et al., 2001; Rao et al., 1995).

Mental health and suicidal behaviors

While adolescents with MDD and DD often have concurrent comorbid psycho-pathology, they are also more likely than their non-disordered peers to later develop an array of mental health problems. Of particular note is the risk DD poses for the later development of major depression. At five years' follow-up Kovacs and colleagues (1997) found that approximately 70 percent of children with dysthymia had developed MDD. Youth with major depression are more likely than adults with the same illness to convert to bipolar disorder, with 20–40 percent developing bipolar I (periods of MDD and mania) within several years of their first depressive episode (Geller et al., 1994; Rao et al., 1995).

Youth with depressive disorders are also likely to develop alcohol and drug problems (Costello et al., 1999; Lewinsohn et al., 1999; Kessler and Walters, 1998). This increased risk for substance abuse has been found to extend into adulthood. Risk for anxiety disorders also remains elevated (Bardone et al., 1996). Additionally, Kasen et al. (2001) found that childhood depression predicts the onset of personality disorders in later adolescence and adulthood.

The serious nature of depressive disorders is most clearly underscored in the substantial levels of suicidal ideation and attempts that occur in children and adolescents with depression (Reinherz et al., 1995), especially in those who have another comorbid psychiatric condition (Angst, 1996; Beautrais et al., 1996; Giaconia et al., 2001; Harrington et al., 1994; Newman et al., 1996). For example, Weissman et al. (1999) found that youth with pre-pubertal onset MDD were three times as likely as normal controls to attempt suicide by adulthood. The life-threatening nature of depressive illness is perhaps one of the most compelling reasons given in support of the need for effective prevention and treatment programs for depressive disorders.

The lingering nature of depression

Functional impairments associated with major depression are not limited to those who are currently depressed. Prior research has demonstrated that individuals with a history of depression, who do not currently meet clinical levels of the disorder, continue to exhibit significant deficits in crucial areas of psychosocial functioning. Formerly depressed adolescents are less likely to complete college, to be more recently unemployed, have a lower income level, lower life satisfaction, and poorer physical health (Birmaher et al., 2002; Lewinsohn et al., 1999; Reinherz et al., 1999).

There is also evidence to suggest that depressive episodes leave "scars," or residual effects, on an individual that are not present prior to the onset of depression (Rohde et al., 1994). These impairments in functioning may serve to increase the likelihood of future depressive episodes. Such findings highlight the continued vulnerability of individuals with a history of depressive illness and speak to the need for continued monitoring and follow-up services with formerly depressed youth to reduce the risk of recurrence.

Treatment

This section will present an overview of available treatments with an emphasis on those that have been empirically validated. Despite increasing recognition of childhood and adolescent depressive disorders and their serious consequences, these disorders frequently remain under-diagnosed and inadequately treated (Beasley and Beardslee, 1998).

Pharmacotherapy

Although psychopharmacologic studies using tricyclic antidepressants to treat childhood and adolescent depression have generally been disappointing (e.g., Puig-Antich et al., 1987; Hughes et al., 1990), the use of selective serotonin reuptake inhibitors (SSRIs) shows greater promise (Greenberg et al., 1994). Studies of adolescents have reported a 70–90 percent response rate to fluoxetine or sertraline (DeVane and Sallee, 1996; Leonard, 1997). Moreover, an eight-week double blind study showed that both children and adolescents responded significantly better to fluoxetine than to placebo (56 percent versus 33 percent) (Emslie et al., 1997). A multicenter study examining the efficacy of paroxetine and imipramine in 275 depressed adolescents also found that youth treated with paroxetine experienced greater improvement than those receiving placebo (Keller et al., 1998).

Despite these promising results, there are several important considerations for treating children and adolescents with antidepressant medication: (1) the long-term developmental impact and effectiveness are not known; (2) rates of SSRI-induced manic episodes may be as high as 20 percent, the rate found in adult samples (Altshuler et al., 1995) which may be similar in youth populations; and (3) recent studies have linked paroxetine and venlafaxine to increasing suicidal thoughts and agitation in children and adolescents, although causality has not been demonstrated. There is much the field must learn about how psychopharmacological agents designed to alleviate depressive symptoms interact with the development of the brain and nervous system in children and adolescents. For these reasons, psychotherapy should be considered a first-line approach for treating mild to moderate depression in youth.

Psychotherapy

Most empirically supported studies of children and adolescents have utilized cognitive behavioral treatment. CBT has been shown to both decrease depressive symptoms and increase functioning across multiple domains (see Compton et al., 2004; Kaslow and Thompson, 1998, for reviews). CBT has also been used to help prevent depressive symptoms (Clarke et al., 1995). These studies, although often grouped together in meta-analytic reviews, have several important differences that may affect results: (1) a range in depression severity, (2) a range of CBT modalities (e.g., relaxation training, social skills training, and cognitive restructuring), and (3) a diversity of outcome measurements (see Michael and Crowley, 2002; Sherrill and Kovacs, 2002, for reviews).

Interpersonal therapy (IPT) has also been shown to reduce depressive symptoms and improve social functioning in adolescents (Mufson et al., 1999). IPT and CBT share many common components; both treat depressive symptoms in a problem-focused, time-limited manner with attention to engagement in activities, problem solving, cognitive reframing, and improvement of interpersonal relationships. Unlike CBT, however, IPT focuses primarily on addressing interpersonal conflicts and deficits rather than on changing cognitive patterns. Findings from a study comparing IPT, CBT, and wait-list control conditions in Puerto Rican adolescents, showed that while both treatment groups experienced improvement in depressive symptoms, social adaptation and self-esteem, IPT was more useful for adolescents with interpersonal problems or impaired social functioning (Rossello and Bernal, 1999).

Treatments incorporating family involvement have produced mixed results. While supplementation of individual CBT with monthly family meetings did not enhance outcomes for depressed adolescents in some studies (Lewinsohn and Clarke, 1999; Lewinsohn et al., 1999), others yielded more promising results. For example, the Multi-Family Psychoeducational Groups (MFPG), aimed at improving family functioning by reducing caregiver burden in a manner that is sensitive to normal developmental issues, has had positive impact on adolescent depression (Fristad et al., 2002). Beardslee et al. (1997) demonstrated that a family psycho-educational approach linked to families' life experiences, contrasted with parental group lectures, was more effective in the short- and long-term prevention of depression in adolescents with depressed parents (Beardslee et al., 2003). Another study, evaluating a family treatment protocol designed for African American girls with depression and a history of abuse, illustrates the importance of cultural and gender-sensitive considerations (Kaslow et al., 2000).

Overall, approximately 50–87 percent of depressed youth treated with psycho-therapy recover, compared to 21–75 percent of those receiving supportive therapy, and 5–48 percent of wait-list controls (Sherrill and Kovacs, 2002). However, many treated participants continue to experience depressive symptoms and high relapse rates during the year following treatment. Several reasons for these shortcomings of psychotherapy may include brevity of treatment, comorbidity, and negative familial interactions.

Even with these caveats, studies of CBT, IPT and treatments involving families show promise. Each confers a slightly different set of benefits to recipients. Research matching treatment choices with participant characteristics is an important next step in evaluating treatment efficacy. For example, IPT may be the better treatment for adolescents whose depression is associated with disrupted relation-ships. MFPG may be preferable when the family environment contributes to the development of depression or when multiple family members are depressed.

Several important limitations of these existing studies should be noted. Many clinical trials have been conducted with relatively small samples and without adequate control groups. In addition, three issues regarding treatment outcome have not been convincingly resolved: (1) specificity (whether deficits in functioning are linked to depression in particular or psychopathology in general), (2) state-dependence (whether deficits are evident only during a depressive episode or occur even when a youth is not depressed), and (3) comorbidity (whether low levels of social competence in depressed youth are accounted for by subgroups who also meet criteria for other psychiatric diagnoses). Given that depression often co-occurs with other disorders, it is critical that researchers explore strategies that effectively address problems extending beyond depression. For example, Connor-Smith and Weisz (2002) described how CBT can be adapted to accommodate a variety of comorbid disorders and problems facing adolescents with depression. In addressing these issues, the field will be better positioned to transition from demonstrating efficacy in research settings to real-world application in the treatment of childhood and adolescent depression.

Conclusions and future directions

Since the mid 1980s, volumes of research on the etiology, course, and treatment of childhood and adolescent depression have led to a better understanding of this prevalent and often disabling disorder. Researchers have delineated individual risk factors in the genetic, biological, and psychosocial domains and have begun to examine how these factors interact to increase vulnerability for depression. Studies have noted not only that adolescent depression is a lifelong condition for many youth, but also that experiencing depression places these youth at risk for the development of additional disorders. There are, however, some encouraging findings suggesting that depression in children and adolescents can be effectively treated. Despite these advances, there remains much to be learned about the pathways to childhood and adolescent depressive disorders and the most effective means of furthering their prevention and treatment.

While it is gratifying to see that the serious nature of childhood and adolescent depressive disorders is increasingly acknowledged, questions have arisen regarding the appropriateness of using a diagnostic system developed for adults with children (Weiss and Garber, 2003). Due largely to the serious nature of subthreshold depression, there also is a continuing controversy as to whether depression would be better characterized as a continuum (Angst and Merikangas, 1997; Hankin et al., 2005; Lewinsohn et al., 2000b).

An important feature of depressive disorders in childhood and adolescence is the high occurrence of comorbid disorders that may cloud both assessment and treatment (Angold et al., 1999a; Ford et al., 2003). Future research is needed to clarify the most common types of co-occurring disorders, their most frequent temporal order (i.e., do they commonly precede or come after the depressive disorder), and factors that may lead to experiencing multiple disorders.

Much progress has been made in understanding the complex, multiple pathways leading to depressive disorders in childhood and adolescence and beyond into adulthood. New knowledge from the fields of neurobiology, physiology, and genetics has been added to our existing understanding of developmental and psychosocial influences. Such models are more reflective of real life processes and their further development will aid in unraveling the development of disorders over time (Susser et al., 2002).

Although much of the work in identifying correlates of and risk factors for depressive disorders has shed light on the potency of factors such as the family (Lewinsohn et al., 2000a; Goodman and Gotlib, 1999; Reinherz et al., 2003), the field needs to acknowledge risks denoting marked vulnerabilities, such as being born to depressed parents (Beardslee et al., 1993) or experiencing early health problems (Reinherz et al., 1991; Lewinsohn et al., 1994b). These findings are useful in pinpointing vulnerable groups who are in need of intervention. Yet, an equal or greater challenge is the identification of risk factors that may be amenable to change and/or areas of specific vulnerability that may require supportive interventions. Equally essential is the identification of areas of strength (protective factors) that can be identified in children and adolescents who are at risk for developing depressive disorders. Beardslee (2002) has noted that positive relationships and interpersonal communication skills are protective factors for youth raised in households with a depressed parent. Carbonell et al. (2002) also found that strong family cohesion and social support were protective.

There also remains much to be learned about the continuity of depressive disorders, and how the course of these disorders may differ between child and adolescent onset cases (Weissman et al., 1999). Findings from long-term, prospective studies since the mid 1990s have brought appropriate attention to the extensive impairment associated with depressive disorders that is evident even after they are no longer active (Lewinsohn et al., 1999; Reinherz et al., 1999). It is apparent that substantial impairment and poor mental health are legacies of depressive disorders. Findings such as these speak to the need for instituting treatment and prevention programs as early as possible.

Our review of current treatment efforts indicates that efficacious therapeutic approaches are being developed and evaluated (Emslie et al., 1997). Additionally CBT, IPT, and family treatment methods show promise provided that treatment approaches are chosen according to participant needs. However, in spite of the serious consequences of child and adolescent depression, it remains under-diagnosed and under-treated (Beasley and Beardslee, 1998).

Finally, after surveying the accomplishments and gaps in the field, what are the proposed directions for the field of childhood and adolescent depressive disorders? Areas needing further research include gaining a greater understanding of depression in different cultural, ethnic, and racial groups, clearer elucidation of the role of gender, and the specific multifaceted pathways to depressive disorders utilizing factors from many domains. It will also be important to further examine the risk posed by early depressive symptoms and subthreshold depression. Yet most importantly, we need to further identify the developmental periods of greatest vulnerability as well as the periods presenting the greatest window of opportunity for intervention. There is hope that in the next decade many of these issues will be clarified due to advancements in the sciences of neurobiology, physiology, and genetics along with increasingly sophisticated methods in psychiatric epidemiology and developmental psychopathology.

References

Altshuler, L.L., Post, R.M., Leverich, G.S., Mikalauskas, K., Rosoff, A., and Ackerman, L. (1995). Antidepressant-induced mania and cycle acceleration: A controversy revisited. *American Journal of Psychiatry, 152*, 1130–1138.

American Psychiatric Association (1980). *Diagnostic and statistical manual of mental disorders*, 3rd edn (DSM-III). Washington, DC: APA.

American Psychiatric Association (1994). *Diagnostic and statistical manual of mental disorders*, 4th edn (DSM-IV). Washington, DC: APA.

Angold, A., Costello, E.J., and Erkanli, A. (1999a). Comorbidity. *Journal of Child Psychology and Psychiatry, 40*, 57–87.

Angold, A., Costello, E.J., Erkanli, A., and Worthman, C.M. (1999b). Pubertal changes in hormone levels and depression in girls. *Psychological Medicine, 29*, 1043–1053.

Angold, A., Costello, E.J., Farmer, E.M., Burns, B.J., and Erkanli, A. (1999c). Impaired but undiagnosed. *Journal of the American Academy of Child and Adolescent Psychiatry, 38*, 129–137.

Angst, J. (1996). Comorbidity of mood disorders: A longitudinal prospective study. *British Journal of Psychiatry, 168* (Suppl. 30), 31–37.

Angst, J. and Merikangas, K. (1997). The depressive spectrum: Diagnostic classification and course. *Journal of Affective Disorders, 45*, 31–40.

Bardone, A.M., Moffitt, T.E., Caspi, A., Dickson, N., and Silva, P.A. (1996). Adult mental health and social outcomes of adolescent girls with depression and conduct disorder. *Development and Psychopathology, 8*, 811–829.

Beardslee, W.R. (1998). Prevention and the clinical encounter. *American Journal of Orthopsychiatry*, *68*, 521–533.

Beardslee, W.R. (2002). *Out of the darkened room.* Boston, MA: Little, Brown.

Beardslee, W.R. and Gladstone, T.R.G. (2001). Prevention of childhood depression: Recent findings and future prospects. *Biological Psychiatry*, *49*, 1101–1110.

Beardslee, W.R., Keller, M.B., Lavori, P.W., Staley, J., and Sacks, N. (1993). The impact of parental affective disorder on depression in offspring: A longitudinal follow-up in a nonreferred sample. *Journal of the American Academy of Child and Adolescent Psychiatry*, *32*, 723–730.

Beardslee, W.R., Salt, P., Versage, E.M., Gladstone, T.R.G., Wright, E.J., and Rothberg, P.C. (1997). Sustained change in parents receiving preventive interventions for families with depression. *American Journal of Psychiatry*, *154*, 510–515.

Beardslee, W.R., Versage, E.M., and Gladstone, T.R.G. (1998). Children of affectively ill parents: A review of the past 10 years. *Journal of the American Academy of Child and Adolescent Psychiatry*, *37*, 1134–1141.

Beardslee, W.R., Gladstone, T.R.G., Wright, E.J., and Cooper, A.B. (2003). A family-based approach to the prevention of depressive symptoms in children at risk: Evidence of parental and child change. *Pediatrics*, *112*, e119–e131.

Beasley, P.J. and Beardslee, W.R. (1998). Depression in the adolescent patient. *Adolescent Medicine*, *9*, 351–362.

Beautrais, A.L., Joyce, P.R., and Mulder, R.T. (1996). Risk factors for serious suicide attempts among youth aged 13 through 24 years. *Journal of the American Academy of Child and Adolescent Psychiatry*, *35*, 1174–1182.

Birmaher, B., Arbelaez, C., and Brent, D. (2002). Course and outcome of child and adolescent major depressive disorder. *Child and Adolescent Psychiatric Clinics of North America*, *11*, 619–637.

Breslau, N., Chilcoat, H.D., Peterson, E.L., and Schultz, L.R. (2000). Gender differences in major depression. In E. Frank (Ed.), *Gender and its effects on psychopathology* (pp. 131–150). Washington, DC: American Psychiatric Press.

Brooks-Gunn, J., Auth, J.J., Petersen, A.C., and Compas, B.E. (2001). Physiological processes and the development of childhood and adolescent depression. In I.M. Goodyer (Ed.), *The depressed child and adolescent*, 2nd edn (pp. 79–118). New York: Cambridge University Press.

Carbonell, D.M., Reinherz, H.Z., Giaconia, R.M., Stashwick, C.K., Paradis, A.D., and Beardslee, W.R. (2002). Adolescent protective factors promoting resilience in young adults at risk for depression. *Child and Adolescent Social Work Journal*, *19*, 393–412.

Caspi, A., Moffitt, T.E., Newman, D.L., and Silva, P.A. (1996). Behavioral observations at age 3 years predict adult psychiatric disorders. *Archives of General Psychiatry*, *53*, 1033–1039.

Caspi, A., Sugden, K., Moffitt, T.E., Taylor, A., Craig, I.W., Harrington, H., et al. (2003). Influence of life stress on depression: Moderation by a polymorphism in the 5-HTT gene. *Science*, *301*, 386–389.

Cicchetti, D. and Toth, S.L. (1991). A developmental perspective on internalizing and externalizing disorders. In D. Cicchetti and S.L. Toth (Eds.), *Internalizing and externalizing expressions of dysfunction: Rochester symposium on developmental psychopathology* (pp. 1–19). Hillsdale, NJ: Lawerence Erlbaum Associates.

Cicchetti, D. and Toth, S.L. (1998). The development of depression in children and adolescents. *American Psychologist*, *53*, 221–241.

Clarke, G.N., Hawkins, W., Murphy, M., Sheeber, L.B., Lewinsohn, P.M., and Seeley, J.R. (1995). Targeted prevention of unipolar depressive disorder in an at-risk sample of high school adolescents: A randomized trial of a group cognitive intervention. *Journal of the American Academy of Child and Adolescent Psychiatry, 34,* 312–321.

Cohen, P., Velez, C.N., Brook, J.S., and Smith, J. (1989). Mechanisms of the relation between perinatal problems, early childhood illness, and psychopathology in late childhood and adolescence. *Child Development, 60,* 701–709.

Cohen, P., Cohen, J., Kasen, S., Velez, C.N., Hartmark, C., Johnson, J., et al. (1993). An epidemiologic study of disorders in late childhood and adolescence: I. Age- and gender-specific prevalence. *Journal of Child Psychology and Psychiatry, 34,* 851–867.

Compas, B.E., Oppedisano, G., Connor, J.K., Gerhardt, C.A., Hinden, B.R., Achenbach, T.M., et al. (1997). Gender differences in depressive symptoms in adolescence: Comparison of national samples of clinically referred and nonreferred youths. *Journal of Consulting and Clinical Psychology, 65,* 617–626.

Compton, K., Snyder, J., Schrepferman, L., Bank, L., and Short, J.W. (2003). The contribution of parents and siblings to antisocial and depressive behavior in adolescents: A double jeopardy coercion model. *Developmental Psychopathology, 15,* 163–182.

Compton, S.N., March, J.S., Brent, D., Albano, A.M., Weersing, V.R., and Curry J. (2004). Cognitive-behavioral psychotherapy for anxiety and depressive disorders in children and adolescents: An evidence-based medicine review. *Journal of the American Academy of Child and Adolescent Psychiatry, 43,* 930–959.

Connor-Smith, J.K. and Weisz, J.R. (2003). Applying treatment outcome research in clinical practice: Techniques for adapting interventions to the real world. *Child and Adolescent Mental Health, 8,* 3–10.

Costello, E.J. and Angold, A. (2000). Developmental psychopathology and public health: Past, present, and future. *Development and Psychopathology, 12,* 599–618.

Costello, E.J., Angold, A., Burns, B.J., Stangl, D.K., Tweed, D.L., Erkanli, A., et al. (1996). The Great Smoky Mountains Study of Youth: Goals, design, methods, and the prevalence of DSM-III-R disorders. *Archives of General Psychiatry, 53,* 1129–1136.

Costello, E.J., Erkanli, A., Federman, E., and Angold, A. (1999). Development of psychiatric comorbidity with substance abuse in adolescents: Effects of timing and sex. *Journal of Clinical Child Psychology, 28,* 298–311.

Cuffe, S.P., McKeown, R.E., Addy, C.L., and Garrison, C.Z. (2005). Family and psychosocial risk factors in a longitudinal epidemiological study of adolescents. *Journal of the American Academy of Child and Adolescent Psychiatry, 44,* 121–129.

Cyranowski, J.M., Frank, E., Young, E., and Shear, M.K. (2000). Adolescent onset of the gender difference in lifetime rates of major depression: A theoretical model. *Archives of General Psychiatry, 57,* 21–27.

Davies, P.T. and Windle, M. (1997). Gender-specific pathways between maternal depressive symptoms, family discord, and adolescent adjustment. *Developmental Psychology, 33,* 657–668.

De Bellis, M.D., Dahl, R.E., Perel, J., Birmaher, B., Al-Shabbout, M., Williamson, D.E., et al. (1996). Nocturnal ACTH, cortisol, growth hormone, and prolactin secretion in prepubertal adolescence. *Journal of the American Academy of Child and Adolescent Psychiatry, 35,* 1130–1138.

DeVane, C.L. and Sallee, F.R. (1996). Serotonin selective reuptake inhibitors in child and adolescent psychopharmacology: A review of published experience. *Journal of Clinical Psychiatry, 57,* 55–66.

Emslie, G.J., Rush, A.J., Weinberg, W.A., Kowatch, R.A., Hughes, C.W., Carmody, T., et al. (1997). A double-blind, randomized, placebo-controlled trial of fluoxetine in children and adolescents with depression. *Archives of General Psychiatry, 54*, 1031–1037.

Essau, C.A. and Dobson, K.S. (1999). Epidemiology of depressive disorders. In C.A. Essau and F. Petermann (Eds.), *Depressive disorders in children and adolescents: Epidemiology, risk factors, and treatment* (pp. 69–103). Northvale, NJ: Jason Aronson.

Essau, C.A., Conradt, J., and Petermann, F. (2000). Frequency, comorbidity, and psychosocial impairment of depressive disorders in adolescents. *Journal of Adolescent Research, 15*, 470–481.

Fergusson, D.M. and Woodward, L.J. (2002). Mental health, educational, and social role outcomes of adolescents with depression. *Archives of General Psychiatry, 59*, 225–231.

Fergusson, D.M., Horwood, L.J., and Lynskey, M.T. (1993). Prevalence and comorbidity of DSM-III-R diagnoses in a birth cohort of 15 year olds. *Journal of the Academy of Child and Adolescent Psychiatry, 32*, 1127–1134.

Fleming, J.E., Boyle, M.H., and Offord, D.R. (1993). The outcome of adolescent depression in the Ontario child health study follow-up. *Journal of the American Academy of Child and Adolescent Psychiatry, 32*, 28–33.

Fombonne, E. (1994). Increased rates of depression: Update of epidemiological findings and analytical problems. *Acta Psychiatrica Scandinavica, 90*, 145–156.

Fombonne, E., Wostear, G., Cooper, V., Harrington, R., and Rutter, M. (2001). The Maudsley long-term follow-up of child and adolescent depression: 2. Suicidality, criminality and social dysfunction in adulthood. *British Journal of Psychiatry, 179*, 218–223.

Ford, T., Goodman, R., and Meltzer, H. (2003). The British child and adolescent mental health survey 1999: The prevalence of DSM-IV disorders. *Journal of the American Academy of Child and Adolescent Psychiatry, 42*, 1203–1211.

Fristad, M.A., Goldberg-Arnold, J.S., and Gavazzi, S.M. (2002). Multi-family psychoeducation groups (MFPG) for families of children with bipolar disorder. *Bipolar Disorders, 4*, 254–262.

Garrison, C.Z., Schluchter, M.D., Schoenbach, V.J., and Kaplan, B.K. (1989). Epidemiology of depressive symptoms in young adolescents. *Journal of the American Academy of Child and Adolescent Psychiatry, 28*, 343–351.

Garrison, C.Z., Waller, J.L., Cuffe, S.P., McKeown, R.E., Addy, C.L., and Jackson, K.L. (1997). Incidence of major depressive disorder and dysthymia in young adolescents. *Journal of the American Academy of Child and Adolescent Psychiatry, 36*, 458–465.

Geller, B., Fox., L.W., and Clark, K.A. (1994). Rate and predictors of prepubertal bipolarity during follow-up of 6- to 12-year-old depressed children. *Journal of the American Academy of Child and Adolescent Psychiatry, 33*, 461–468.

Geller, B., Zimmerman, B., Williams, M., Bolhofner, K., and Craney, J.L. (2001). Adult psychosocial outcome of prepubertal major depressive disorder. *Journal of the American Academy of Child and Adolescent Psychiatry, 40*, 673–677.

Giaconia, R.M., Reinherz, H.Z., Silverman, A.B., Pakiz, B., Frost, A.K., and Cohen, E. (1994). Age of onset of psychiatric disorders in a community population of older adolescents. *Journal of the American Academy of Child and Adolescent Psychiatry, 33*, 706–717.

Giaconia, R.M., Reinherz, H.Z., Paradis, A.D., Hauf, A.M.C., and Stashwick, C.K. (2001). Major depression and drug disorders in adolescence: General and specific impairments in early adulthood. *Journal of the American Academy of Child and Adolescent Psychiatry, 40*, 1426–1433.

Gizynski, M. and Shapiro, V.B. (1990). Depression and childhood illness. *Child and Adolescent Social Work, 7*, 179–197.

Goodman, S.H. and Gotlib, I.H. (1999). Risk for psychopathology in the children of depressed parents: A developmental approach to the understanding of mechanisms. *Psychological Review, 106*, 458–490.

Goodman, S.H., Schwab-Stone, M., Lahey, B.B., Shaffer, D., and Jensen, P.S. (2000). Major depression and dysthymia in children and adolescents: Discriminant validity and differential consequences in a community sample. *Journal of the American Academy of Child and Adolescent Psychiatry, 39*, 761–770.

Goodwin, R.D., Fergusson, D.M., and Horwood, L.J. (2004). Early anxious/withdrawn behaviours predict later internalising disorders. *Journal of Child Psychology and Psychiatry, 45*, 874–883.

Goodyer, I.M., Herbert, J., Secher, S.M., and Pearson, J. (1997). Short-term outcome of major depression: I. Comorbidity and severity at presentation as predictors of persistent disorder. *Journal of the American Academy of Child and Adolescent Psychiatry, 36*, 179–187.

Goodyer, I.M., Herbert, J., Tamplin, A., and Altham, P.M. (2000). Recent live events, cortisols, dehydroepiandrosterone and the onset of major depression in high-risk adolescents. *British Journal of Psychiatry, 177*, 499–504.

Gotlib, I.H., Lewinsohn, P.M., and Seeley, J.R. (1998). Consequences of depression during adolescence: Marital status and marital functioning in early adulthood. *Journal of Abnormal Psychology, 107*, 686–690.

Graber, J.A., Lewinsohn, P.M., Seeley, J.R., and Brooks-Gunn, J. (1997). Is psychopathology associated with timing of pubertal development? *Journal of the American Academy of Child and Adolescent Psychiatry, 36*, 1768–1776.

Greenberg, R.P., Bornstein, R.F., Zborowski, M.J., Fisher, S., and Greenberg, M.D. (1994). A meta-analysis of fluoxetine outcome in the treatment of depression. *Journal of Nervous and Mental Disease, 182*, 547–551.

Hammen, C. and Brennan, P.A. (2003). Severity, chronicity, and timing of maternal depression and risk for adolescent offspring diagnoses in a community sample. *Archives of General Psychiatry, 60*, 253–258.

Hammen, C. and Rudolph, K. (1996). Childhood depression. In E.J. Mash and R.A. Barkley (Eds.), *Child psychopathology* (pp. 153–195). New York: Guilford.

Hammen, C., Rudolph, K., Weisz, J., Rao, U., and Burge, D. (1999). The context of depression in clinic-referred youth: Neglected areas in treatment. *Journal of the American Academy of Child and Adolescent Psychiatry, 38*, 64–71.

Hankin, B.L., Abramson, L.Y., Moffit, T.E., Silva, P.A., and McGee, R. (1998). Development of depression from preadolescence to young adulthood: Emerging gender differences in a 10-year longitudinal study. *Journal of Abnormal Psychology, 107*, 128–140.

Hankin, B.L., Fraley, C., Lahey, B.B., and Waldman, I.D. (2005). Is depression best viewed as a continuum or discrete category? A taxometric analysis of childhood and adolescent depression in a population-based sample. *Journal of Abnormal Psychology, 114*, 96–110.

Harrington, R., Bredenkamp, D., Groothues, C., Rutter, M., Fudge, H., and Pickles, A. (1994). Adult outcomes of childhood and adolescent depression: III. Links with suicidal behaviours. *Journal of Child Psychology and Psychiatry, 35*, 1309–1319.

Hayward, C., Killen, J.D., Wilson, D.M., Hammer, L.D., Litt, I.F., Kraemer, H.C., et al. (1997). Psychiatric risk associated with early puberty in adolescent girls. *Journal of the American Academy of Child and Adolescent Psychiatry, 36*, 255–262.

Hughes, C.W., Preskorn, S.H., Weller, E., Hassanein, R., and Tucker, S. (1990). The effect of concomitant disorders in childhood depression on predicting treatment response. *Psychopharmacology Bulletin, 26*, 235–238.

Kaltiala-Heino, R., Kosunen, E., and Rimpela, M. (2003). Pubertal timing, sexual behavior and self-reported depression in middle adolescence. *Journal of Adolescence, 26*, 531–545.

Kasen, S., Cohen, P., Skodol, A.E., Johnson, J.G., Smailes, E., and Brook, J.S. (2001). Childhood depression and adult personality disorder: Alternative pathways of continuity. *Archives of General Psychiatry, 58*, 231–236.

Kashani, J.H. and Carlson, G.A. (1987). Seriously depressed preschoolers. *American Journal of Psychiatry, 144*, 348–350.

Kaslow, N.J. and Thompson, M.P. (1998). Applying the criteria for empirically supported treatments to studies of psychosocial interventions for child and adolescent depression. *Journal of Clinical Child Psychology, 27*, 146–155.

Kaslow, N.J., Adamson, L.B., and Collins, M.H. (2000). A developmental psychopathology perspective on the cognitive components of child and adolescent depression. In A.J. Sameroff, M. Lewis, and S.M. Miller (Eds.), *Handbook of developmental psychopathology*, 2nd edn (pp. 491–510). New York: Kluwer Academic/Plenum.

Keller, M.B., Kocsis, J.H., Thase, M.E., Gelenberg, A.J., Rush, A.J., Koran, L., et al. (1998). Maintenance phase efficacy of sertraline for chronic depression: A randomized controlled trial. *Journal of the American Medical Association, 280*, 1665–1672.

Kelly, J.B. (2000). Children's adjustment in conflicted marriage and divorce: A decade review of research. *Journal of the American Academy of Child and Adolescent Psychiatry, 39*, 963–973.

Kendler, K.S. (1995). Genetic epidemiology on psychiatry. *Archives of General Psychiatry, 52*, 895–899.

Kessler, R.C. (2002). Epidemiology of depression. In I.H. Gotlib and C.L. Hammen (Eds.), *Handbook of depression* (pp. 23–42). New York: Guilford.

Kessler, R.C. and Walters, E.E. (1998). Epidemiology of DSM-III major depression and minor depression among adolescents and young adults in the National Comorbidity Survey. *Depression and Anxiety, 7*, 3–14.

Kessler, R.C., McGonagle, K.A., Swartz, M., Blazer, D.G., and Nelson, C.B. (1993). Sex and depression in the National Comorbidity Survey: I. Lifetime prevalence, chronicity, and recurrence. *Journal of Affective Disorders, 29*, 85–96.

Kessler, R.C., McGonagle, K.A., Zhao, S., Nelson, C.B., Hughes, M., Eshleman, S., et al. (1994). Lifetime and 12-month prevalence of DSM-III-R Psychiatric Disorders in the United States. *Archives of General Psychiatry, 51*, 8–19.

Kessler, R.C., Nelson, C.B., McGonagle, K.A., Edlund, M.J., Frank, R.G., and Leaf, P.J. (1996). The epidemiology of co-occurring addictive and mental disorders: Implications for prevention and service utilization. *Journal of Orthopsychiatry, 66*, 17–31.

Kessler, R.C., Berglund, P.A., Foster, C.L., Saunders, W.B., Stang, P.E., and Walters, E.E. (1997). Social consequences of psychiatric disorders: II. Teenage parenthood. *American Journal of Psychiatry, 154*, 1405–1411.

Klein, D.N. and Santiago, N.J. (2003). Dysthymia and chronic depression: Introduction, classification, risk factors, and course. *Journal of Clinical Psychology, 59*, 807–816.

Klein, D.N., Riso, L.P., Donaldson, S.K., Schwartz, J.E., Anderson, R.L., Ouimette, P.C., et al. (1995). Family study of early-onset dysthymia: Mood and personality disorders in relatives of outpatients with dysthymia and episodic major depression and normal controls. *Archives of General Psychiatry, 52,* 487–496.

Klein, D.N., Lewinsohn, P.M., and Seeley, J.R. (1997). Psychosocial characteristics of adolescents with a past history of dysthymic disorder: Comparison with adolescents with past histories of major depressive and non-affective disorders, and never mentally ill controls. *Journal of Affective Disorders, 42,* 127–135.

Klein, D.N., Lewinsohn, P.M., Seeley, J.R., and Rohde, P. (2001). A family study of major depressive disorder in a community sample of adolescents. *Archives of General Psychiatry, 58,* 13–20.

Kovacs, M. (1996). The course of childhood-onset depressive disorders. *Psychiatric Annals, 26,* 326–330.

Kovacs, M., Feinberg, T.L., Crouse-Novak, M., Paulauskas, S.L., Pollock, M., and Finkelstein, R.F. (1984). Depressive disorder in childhood: II. A longitudinal study of the risk for a subsequent major depression. *Archives of General Psychiatry, 41,* 643–649.

Kovacs, M., Devlin, B., Pollock, M., Richards, C., and Mukerji, P. (1997) A controlled family history study of childhood-onset depressive disorder. *Archives of General Psychiatry, 54,* 613–623.

Kovacs, M., Obrosky, D.S., and Sherrill, J. (2003). Developmental changes in the phenomenology of depression in girls compared to boys from childhood onward. *Journal of Affective Disorders, 74,* 33–48.

Kraemer, H.C., Kazdin, A.E., Offord, D.R., Kessler, R.C., Jensen, P.S., and Kupfer, D.J. (1997). Coming to terms with the terms of risk. *Archives of General Psychiatry, 54,* 337–343.

Kraemer, H.C., Stice, E., Kazdin, A., Offord, D., and Kupfer, D. (2001). How do risk factors work together? Mediators, moderators, and independent, overlapping, and proxy risk factors. *American Journal of Psychiatry, 158,* 848–856.

Kutcher, S., Malkin, D., Silverberg, J., Marton, P., Williamson, P., Malkin, A., et al. (1991). Nocturnal cortisol, thyroid stimulating hormone, and growth hormone secretory profiles in depressed adolescents. *Journal of the American Academy of Child and Adolescent Psychiatry, 30,* 407–413.

Leadbeater, B.J., Blatt, S.J., and Quinlan, D.M. (1995). Gender-linked vulnerabilities to depressive symptoms, stress, and problem behaviors in adolescents. *Journal of Research on Adolescence, 5,* 1–29.

Leader, J.B. and Klein, D.N. (1996). Social adjustment in dysthymia, double depression and episodic major depression. *Journal of Affective Disorders, 37,* 91–101.

Leonard, B.E. (1997). Noradrenaline in basic models of depression. *European Neuro-psychopharmacology, 7*(suppl. 1), S11–S16.

Lewinsohn, P.M. and Clarke, G.N. (1999). Psychosocial treatment for adolescent depression. *Clinical Psychology Review, 19,* 329–342.

Lewinsohn, P.M. and Essau, C.A. (2002). Depression in adolescents. In I.H Gotlib and C.L. Hammen (Eds.), *Handbook of depression* (pp. 541–559). New York: Guilford.

Lewinsohn, P.M. and Seeley, J.R. (2003). Early adult life. In I.M. Goodyer (Ed.), *Unipolar depression: A lifespan perspective* (pp. 95–122). New York: Oxford University Press.

Lewinsohn, P.M., Hops, H., Roberts, R.E., Seeley, J.R., and Andrews, J.A. (1993). Adolescent psychopathology: I. Prevalence and incidence of depression and other DSM-III-R disorders in high school students. *Journal of Abnormal Psychology, 102,* 133–144.

Lewinsohn, P.M., Clarke, G.N., Seeley, J.R., and Rohde, P. (1994a). Major depression in community adolescents: Age at onset, episode duration, and time to recurrence. *Journal of the American Academy of Child and Adolescent Psychiatry, 33*, 809–818.

Lewinsohn, P.M., Roberts, R.E., Seeley, J.R., Rohde, P., Gotlib, I.H., and Hops, H. (1994b). Adolescent psychopathology: II. Psychosocial risk factors for depression. *Journal of Abnormal Psychology, 103*, 302–315.

Lewinsohn, P.M., Rohde, P., and Seeley, J.R. (1995). Adolescent psychopathology: III. The clinical consequences of comorbidity. *Journal of the American Academy of Child and Adolescent Psychiatry, 34*, 510–519.

Lewinsohn, P.M., Seeley, J.R., Hibbard, J.S., Rohde, P., and Sack, W.H. (1996). Cross-sectional and prospective relationships between physical morbidity and depression in older adolescents. *Journal of the American Academy of Child and Adolescent Psychiatry, 35*, 1120–1129.

Lewinsohn, P.M., Rohde, P., Klein, D.N., and Seeley, J.R. (1999). Natural course of adolescent major depressive disorder: I. Continuity into young adulthood. *Journal of the American Academy of Child and Adolescent Psychiatry, 38*, 56–63.

Lewinsohn, P.M., Rohde, P., Seeley, J.R., Klein, D.N., and Gotlib, I.H. (2000a). Natural course of adolescent major depressive disorder in a community sample: Predictors of recurrence in young adults. *American Journal of Psychiatry, 157*, 1584–1591.

Lewinsohn, P.M., Solomon, A., Seeley, J.R., and Zeiss, A. (2000b). Clinical implications of 'subthreshold' depressive symptoms. *Journal of Abnormal Psychology, 109*, 345–351.

Little, S.A. and Garber, J. (2000). Interpersonal and achievement orientations and specific hassels predicting depressive and aggressive symptom in children. *Cognitive Therapy and Research, 24*, 651–671.

Luby, J.L., Heffelfinger, A.K., Mrakotsky, C., Hessler, M.J., Brown, K., and Hildebrand, T. (2002). Preschool major depressive disorder: Preliminary validation for developmentally modified DSM-IV criteria. *Journal of the American Academy of Child and Adolescent Psychiatry, 41*, 928–937.

Luthar, S.S., Anton, S.F., Merikangas, K.R., and Rounsaville, B.J. (1992). Vulnerability to substance abuse and psychopathology among siblings of opiod users. *Journal of Nervous and Mental Disease, 180*, 153–161.

McCauley, E., Myers, K., Mitchell, J., Caleron, R., Schloredt, K., and Treder, R. (1993). Depression in young people: Initial presentation and clinical course. *Journal of the American Academy of Child and Adolescent Psychiatry, 32*, 714–722.

McLeod, J.D. and Shanahan, M.J. (1996). Trajectories of poverty and children's mental health. *Journal of Health and Social Behavior, 37*, 207–220.

Merikangas, K.R. and Angst, J. (1995). The challenge of depressive disorders in adolescence. In M. Rutter (Ed.), *Psychosocial disturbances in young people* (pp. 131–165). Cambridge: Cambridge University Press.

Merikangas, K.R. and Avenevoli, S. (2002). Epidemiology of mood and anxiety disorders in children and adolescents. In M.T. Tsuang and M. Tohen (Eds.), *Textbook in psychiatric epidemiology* (pp. 657–704). New York: Wiley.

Merikangas, K.R., Zhang, H., Avenevoli, S., Acharyya, S., Neuenschwander, M., and Angst, J. (2003). Longitudinal trajectories of depression and anxiety in a prospective community study: The Zurich Cohort Study. *Archives of General Psychiatry, 60*, 993–1000.

Meyer, W.J., Richards, G.E., Cavallo, A., Holt, K.G., Hejazi, M.S., Wigg, C., et al. (1991). Depression and growth hormone. *Journal of the American Academy of Child and Adolescent Psychiatry, 30,* 335.

Michael, K.D. and Crowley, S.L. (2002). How effective are treatments for child and adolescent depression? A meta-analytic review. *Clinical Psychology Review, 22,* 247–269.

Miech, R.A., Caspi, A., Moffitt, T.E., Wright, B.E., and Silva, P.A. (1999). Low socio-economic status and mental disorders: A longitudinal study of selection and causation during young adulthood. *American Journal of Sociology, 104,* 1096–1131.

Monroe, S.M., Rohde, P., Seeley, J.R., and Lewinsohn, P.M. (1999). Life events and depression in adolescence: Relationship loss as a prospective risk factor for first onset of major depressive disorder. *Journal of Abnormal Psychology, 108,* 606–614.

Mufson, L., Weissman, M.M., Moreau, D., and Garfinkel, R. (1999). Efficacy of inter-personal psychotherapy for depressed adolescents. *Archives of General Psychiatry, 56,* 573–579.

Newman, D.L., Moffitt, T.E., Caspi, A., and Magdol, L. (1996). Psychiatric disorder in a birth cohort of young adults: Prevalence, comorbidity, clinical significance, and new case incidence from ages 11 to 21. *Journal of Consulting and Clinical Psychology, 64,* 552–562.

Nolen-Hoeksema, S. (1990). *Sex differences in depression.* Stanford, CA: Stanford University Press.

Nolen-Hoeksema, S. (1992). Children coping with uncontrollable events. *Applied and Preventive Psychology: Current Scientific Perspectives, 1,* 183–189.

Nolen-Hoeksema, S. (2002). Gender differences in depression. In I.H. Gotlib and C.L. Hammen (Eds.), *Handbook of depression* (pp. 492–509). New York: Guilford.

Nolen-Hoeksema, S. and Girgus, J.S. (1994). The emergence of gender differences in depression among adolescence. *Psychological Bulletin, 115,* 424–443.

Pine, D.S., Cohen, P., Gurley, D., Brook, J., and Ma, Y. (1998). The risk for early-adulthood anxiety and depressive disorders in adolescents with anxiety and depressive disorders. *Archives of General Psychiatry, 55,* 56–64.

Poulton, R., Caspi, A., Milne, B.J., Thomson, W.M., Taylor, A., Sears, M.R., et al. (2002). Association between children's experience of socioeconomic disadvantage and adult health: A life-course study. *Lancet, 360,* 1640–1645.

Puig-Antich, J., Perel, J.M., Lupatkin, W., Chambers, W.J., Tabrizi, M.A., King, J., et al. (1987). Imipramine in prepubertal major depressive disorders. *Archives of General Psychiatry, 44,* 81–89.

Rao, U., Ryan, N.D., Birmaher, B., Dahl, R.E., Williamson, D.E., Kaufman, J., et al. (1995). Unipolar depression in adolescents: Clinical outcome in adulthood. *Journal of the American Academy of Child and Adolescent Psychiatry, 34,* 566–578.

Rao, U., Hammen, C., and Daley, S.E. (1999). Continuity of depression during the transition to adulthood: A 5-year longitudinal study of young women. *Journal of the American Academy of Child and Adolescent Psychiatry, 38,* 908–915.

Reinherz, H.Z., Stewart-Berghauer, G., Pakiz, B., Frost, A.K., Moeykens, B.A. and Holmes, W.M. (1989). The relationship of early risk and current mediators to depressive symptomatology in adolescence. *Journal of the American Academy of Child and Adolescent Psychiatry, 28,* 942–947.

Reinherz, H.Z., Frost, A.K., and Pakiz, B. (1991). Changing faces: Correlates of depressive symptoms in late adolescence. *Family and Community Health, 14,* 52–63.

Reinherz, H.Z., Giaconia, R.M., Pakiz, B., Silverman, A.B., Frost, A.K., and Lefkowitz, E. S. (1993). Psychosocial risks for major depression in late adolescence: A longitudinal study. *Journal of the American Academy of Child and Adolescent Psychiatry*, *36*, 1155–1163.

Reinherz, H.Z., Giaconia, R.M., Silverman, A.B., Friedman, A., Pakiz, B., Frost, A.K., et al. (1995). Early psychosocial risks for adolescent suicidal ideation and attempts. *Journal of the American Academy of Child and Adolescent Psychiatry*, *34*, 599–611.

Reinherz, H.Z., Giaconia, R.M., Hauf, A.M.C., Wasserman, M.S., and Silverman, A.B. (1999). Major depression in the transition to adulthood: Risks and impairments. *Journal of Abnormal Psychology*, *108*, 500–510.

Reinherz, H.Z., Giaconia, R.M., Hauf, A.M.C., Wasserman, M.S., and Paradis, A.D. (2000). General and specific childhood risk factors for depression and drug disorders by early adulthood. *Journal of the American Academy of Child and Adolescent Psychiatry*, *39*, 223–231.

Reinherz, H.Z., Paradis, A.D., Giaconia, R.M., Stashwick, C.K., and Fitzmaurice, G. (2003). Childhood and adolescent predictors of major depression in the transition to adulthood. *American Journal of Psychiatry*, *160*, 2141–2147 .

Riso, L.P. and Klein, D.N. (2003). Risk for chronic depression: A review and preliminary model. In J. Alpert and M. Fava (Eds.), *Handbook of chronic depression*. New York: Marcel Dekker.

Roberts, R.E., Roberts, C.R., and Chen, Y.R. (1997). Ethnocultural differences in prevalence of adolescent depression. *American Journal of Community Psychology*, *25*, 95–110.

Rohde, P., Lewinsohn, P.M., and Seeley, J.R. (1994). Are adolescents changed by an episode of major depression? *Journal of the American Academy of Child and Adolescent Psychiatry*, *33*, 1289–1298.

Rossello, J. and Bernal, G. (1999). The efficacy of cognitive-behavioral and interpersonal treatments for depression in Puerto Rican adolescents. *Journal of Consulting and Clinical Psychology*, *67*, 734–745.

Rutter, M. (2002). The interplay of nature, nurture, and developmental influences: The challenge ahead for mental health. *Archives of General Psychiatry*, *59*, 996–1000.

Rutter, M. (2005). Environmentally mediated risks for psychopathology: Research strategies and findings. *Journal of the American Academy of Child and Adolescent Psychiatry*, *44*, 3–18.

Ryan, N.D., Birmaher, B., Perel, J.M., Dahl, R.E., Meyer, V., Al-Shabbout, M., et al. (1992). Neuroendocrine response to L-5 hydroxytrytophan challenge in prepubertal major depression: Depressed vs. normal children. *Archives of General Psychiatry*, *49*, 843–851.

Sanford, M., Szatmari, P., Spinner, M., Muroe-Blum, H., Jamieson, E., Walsh, C., et al. (1995). Predicting the one-year course of adolescent major depression. *Journal of the American Academy of Child and Adolescent Psychiatry*, *34*, 1618–1628.

Santor, D.A. and Coyne, J.C. (2001). Evaluating the continuity of symptomatology between depressed and nondepressed individuals. *Journal of Abnormal Psychology*, *110*, 216–225.

Sherrill, J.T. and Kovacs, M. (2002). Nonsomatic treatment of depression. *Child and Adolescent Psychiatric Clinics of North America*, *11*, 579–593.

Short, J.L. (2002). The effects of parental divorce during childhood on college students. *Journal of Divorce and Remarriage*, *38*, 143–155.

Siegel, J.M., Aneshensel, C.S., Taub, B., Cantwell, D.P., and Driscoll, A.K. (1998). Adolescent depressed mood in a multiethnic sample. *Journal of Youth and Adolescence, 27,* 413–428.

Susser, E., Bresnahan, M., and Link, B. (2002). Peering into the future of psychiatric epidemiology. In M.T. Tsuang and M. Tohen (Eds.), *Textbook in psychiatric epidemiology* (pp. 195–211). New York: Wiley-Liss.

Wallace, J., Schneider, T., and McGuffin, P. (2002). Genetics of depression. In I.H. Gotlib and C.L. Hammen (Eds.), *Handbook of depression* (pp. 169–191). New York: Guilford.

Weiss, B. and Garber, J. (2003). Developmental differences in the phenomenology of depression. *Development and Psychopathology, 15,* 403–430.

Weissman, M.M., Bruce, M.L., Leaf, P.J., and Florio, L.P. (1991). Affective disorders. In L.N. Robins and D.A. Reiger (Eds.), *Psychiatric disorders in America.* New York: The Free Press.

Weissman, M.M., Wolk, S., Goldstein, R.B., Moreau, D., Adams, P., Greenwald, S., et al. (1999). Depressed adolescents grown up. *Journal of the American Medical Academy, 281,* 1707–1713.

Wickramaratne, P., Greenwald, S., and Weissman, M.M. (2000). Psychiatric disorders in the relatives of probands with prepubertal-onset or adolescent-onset major depression. *Journal of the American Academy of Child and Adolescent Psychiatry, 39,* 1396–1405.

World Health Organization (1992). *The ICD-10 classification of mental and behavioural disorders: Diagnostic criteria for research.* Geneva: WHO.

6

THE THEORETICAL IMPLICATIONS OF RESEARCH FINDINGS ON ADOLESCENT DEPRESSION

Implications for Lewinsohn's Integrative
Model of Depression and for a lifespan
developmental theory of depression

Antonette M. Zeiss

This chapter reviews issues in a theoretical understanding of depression in adolescence into early adulthood. Although this chapter will be restricted primarily to exploration of psychosocial influences on depression, it is evident that further progress will depend on integration of an enhanced psychosocial understanding of depression with current genetic and pathophysiologic theories regarding the mergence of depression, its persistence, and its recurrence. Toward that end, the intent here is to work toward the enhanced psychosocial theoretical integration of the phenomenology and epidemiology of depression.

It is well established that major depressive disorder is a condition that can occur in early adolescence, and that the greater likelihood of depression in females emerges by late adolescence or even earlier (e.g., Kashani et al., 1987; Lewinsohn et al., 1993; McGee et al., 1990). Depressive episodes occurring in adolescence have been shown to be heterogeneous in terms of onset and course, with a greater proportion of adolescent MDD episodes apparently due to developmental challenges and stressors common in this age period (Arnett, 1999). It has even been argued that depression during adolescence is more heterogeneous than child or adult depression (Wickramaratne and Weissman, 1998). There also is diversity in the course of depression for adolescents. For most, the depression experience may be fairly transient, and most depressed adolescents recover from the initial episode of depression. However, for others, it indicates the beginning of a more chronic and debilitating condition and there is substantial risk among young adults, as with older adults, of recurrence and psychiatric comorbidity (e.g., Lewinsohn et al., 1999b; Weissman et al., 2000).

Researchers have worked to identify psychosocial factors associated with depression, and many have been identified in at least one study, including the experience of major and minor stressful life events, negative or dysfunctional cognitions and attributional styles, low self-esteem, reduced engagement in pleasant activities and problematic interpersonal relationships, often characterized by excessive interpersonal dependence (summarized in Gotlib and Hammen, 1992). However, almost all of this research has simply demonstrated correlations of these variables with concurrent depression. Thus, whether each of the variables is an antecedent, a consequence, or merely a concomitant of depression has continued to be in question.

Given the apparent heterogeneity of depression and the unclear associations of psychosocial variables with onset and continuation of depression, longitudinal data are essential for understanding the disorder. The primary question addressed in this chapter is how such longitudinal work can inform the psychosocial understanding of depression in adolescents, young adulthood, and by extension, the broader understanding of depressive disorder.

Lewinsohn's integrative theory of depression

Given the goal of examining the theoretical implications of Lewinsohn's extensive work with depression in adolescents and young adults, it is important to review the integrative theory published in 1985 (Lewinsohn et al., 1985). This model, shown in Figure 6.1, posits that risk for depressive onset occurs when a complex set of interrelated environmental and intrapersonal factors co-occur. The model begins with environmental changes, points A and B in the model, that disrupt automatic functioning in important areas of behavior for an individual. These changes are particularly likely to create increased vulnerability for depression when they increase negative experience and/or decrease positive events associated with reinforcing outcomes (point C). These events might be such things as loss of important relationships that have been part of daily behavior patterns, loss of physical function that impairs activities of daily living or ability to engage in valued activities, a move to a new area where prior activities are not possible, or hosts of other life experiences that increase unpleasant events or limit access to positive outcomes.

These experiences are hypothesized to have particularly negative impact if the individual has any of a large set of vulnerabilities to depression or lacks factors that may protect against depression (point G in the model). The theory does not state the exact variables that might be personal vulnerability or immunity factors; these were expected to emerge in research over time, and this element of the theory was expected to be one that would evolve as knowledge developed. However, some personal vulnerability factors are well known, such as female gender or a family history of depression, and others are very likely factors, such as dysfunctional cognitive patterns and lack of a strong social support system. Thus, this theory was designed to be able to incorporate important emerging knowledge both about possible biological contributants to depression and about

141

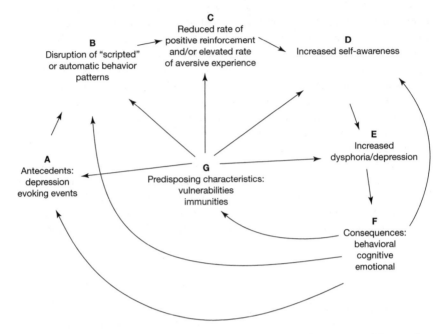

Figure 6.1 An integrative model of the etiology and maintenance of depression (Adapted from Lewinsohn et al., 1985)

cognitive processing styles that increase the likelihood of depression or protect against it.

When life events and personal vulnerabilities co-occur, the model emphasizes that a mediating step toward depression is increased self-awareness: the tendency to focus on one's internal experience and to self-monitor and self-analyze in an internally focused way (point D). Thus, the individual at risk for depression starts over-attending to mood, personal failings, and the impact of negative experiences, and this contributes to development of dysphoria and other symptoms of depression.

Unless this process is disrupted, the development of these symptoms becomes a downward spiral in which the full array of depressive symptoms emerges (point E), and the development of a depressive episode in turn becomes a feedback element that sustains the whole cycle just described (point F). For example, once depressed, people lose energy and stop initiating pleasant activities, thus further disrupting the balance of positive and negative life events. At each of these steps, personal vulnerability factors continue to play a role: some people may be more likely to become self-aware in problematic ways, some develop depression symptoms more readily, some have fewer resources to interrupt the negative impact of decreased mood on other, formerly positive areas of life experience.

In addition, the theory leaves open the possibility that some consequences of depression could become long term sequelae, even after resolution of a current episode of depression. These would become additional vulnerability factors for a future episode of depression (point G again).

Considering the theory as a whole, it makes some very specific predictions. These seem to be the most clear:

1   The theory predicts that for the first onset of depression, some set of events should be identifiable that leads to disruption of behavior patterns resulting in reduced positive experiences and/or increased negative experiences.

2   The experience of increased self-awareness is essential to the emergence of a full-blown depressive episode. While this is a specific prediction, measuring self-awareness is not a simple process, so some of the evidence for this component of the theory by necessity will be inferential.

3   Recurrence of depression could be predicted by the same pattern, or it could be triggered by lingering depressive symptoms that in themselves disrupt daily experience, leading to the same cycle of decreased reinforcement and increased self-awareness but without specific, identifiable, initial disruptive life events. Such lingering symptoms could be considered to become predisposing characteristics that obviate the necessity for readily identifiable external events as triggers for recurrent depression.

In addition, the theory suggests fruitful areas for research that would neither confirm nor disconfirm the theory, but could expand its specificity. Such research would particularly focus on the nature of predisposing characteristics that are in themselves not adequate to create depression but which greatly increase or decrease the likelihood of becoming depressed given particular life circumstances.

Factors that predict initial episodes and recurrence of depression in adolescents and young adults: how well do they fit the theory?

Lewinsohn has published several studies exploring the specific predictors of initial and recurring episodes of depression. The factors shown to be implicated appear in Tables 6.1 through 6.4; these tables show the variables identified, the study in which they were identified, and an indication of how that variable fits with Lewinsohn's integrative model of depression. In the last column, the letters refer to the point in Lewinsohn's model where this variable could best be understood to occur. In addition, Tables 6.2 and 6.4, which show the longstanding variables that represent point G in the model, also include whether the variable shows a vulnerability or protective influence. This column does not appear in other tables, since logically in the model, all other points present experiences that are innately vulnerability factors for development of depression.

Initial episodes of depression

Table 6.1 presents the variables that represent points A through F of the integrative model; these are all points in the development of a depressive episode that represent immediate influences. These are not the long-lasting vulnerability or protective factors, but rather environmental events or internal reactions to them that increase the likelihood of developing an episode of depression.

Examining Table 6.1, it seems clear that there is considerable evidence to support the hypothesis that depression is associated with important life experiences and immediate internal reactions to them. Four general experiences and three specific events corresponding to A, "Antecedents: Depression evoking events", have been

Table 6.1 Predictors of first episode of depression in adolescence or young adulthood: variable capturing immediate events and reactions to them

Study	Vulnerability factor	Relevant theory element
Lewinsohn et al., 1994*	Daily hassles	A
	Major life events	A
	Lifetime number of physical symptoms	A
	Physical health	A
	Conflict with parents	A
Lewinsohn et al., 1999a	Major life stress	A
Monroe et al., 1999	Romantic break-up	A
Lewinsohn et al., 2001	Depression onset associated with negative attributional style at low levels of stress, but not at high levels of stress **	A and G
Joiner et al., 2002	Lack of pleasurable social engagement	C
Lewinsohn et al., 1994*	Failure to complete homework	B
	Externalizing behavior problems (conduct disorder, oppositional behavior, ADHD, substance use disorder, eating disorder)	B
	Dissatisfaction with grades	C (possibly G)
	Self-consciousness	D
	Internalizing behavior problems (worry, behavioral fluctuations, state anxiety, sleep problems, hypochondriasis)	D

Notes: * Various other factors were associated with a future onset of depression in this study, but they seemed logically to suggest recurrence rather than a first episode, e.g., prior suicide attempt, prior depression, so they are not shown in this table. They do appear in Table 6.2.
    ** This pattern also was associated with recurrence of depression.

identified. In general, daily hassles, major negative life events, and physical health issues all have been shown to increase vulnerability for a first episode of depression in adolescents or young adults. Three specific kinds of stressful life experiences have been identified. One is a common event for adolescents, but it represents an important potential trigger for depression: the break-up of a romantic relationship. In addition, physical health issues can be more specifically identified as the lifetime number of physical symptoms experienced by the adolescent – the more symptoms, the more vulnerability to depression. Finally, conflict with parents is a specific life experience that often occurs in adolescence, but also represents a potential antecedent of depression, if the other steps on the model occur as a consequence of such conflict.

Each of these variables represents the A point in the model, because they are life events that now have been shown to be potential antecedents to depression. In addition, they well represent A because it is intuitively clear how each could set the stage for B, "Disruption of important behavior patterns." For example, a romantic break-up likely changes access to a variety of social situations that were formerly part of everyday life. Presence of physical symptoms clearly disrupts behavior, by making valued behaviors impossible, painful, or difficult. Conflict with parents could disrupt spending time together as a family as well as creating disruptive experiences when conflict is overtly expressed.

One study (Lewinsohn et al., 2001) also demonstrates an important verification of the theorized relationship between point A, immediate antecedents, and point G, longstanding vulnerability factors. This study reported that depression onset in adolescents was associated with negative attributional style at low levels of stress, but not at high levels of stress. At high levels of stress, attributional style became unimportant as a predictor, but as shown in other studies, the presence of high stress was itself an important predictor. Thus, if antecedent events are powerful enough, any adolescent (and perhaps adult) could be vulnerable to depression, regardless of attributional style. When stressors are less powerful, cognitive vulnerabilities in point G of the model become very important in predicting who will be most likely to become depressed, however.

Turning to B, two factors have been reported in Lewinsohn's research that could be construed to demonstrate directly the disruption of behavior patterns. Failure to complete homework is a direct measure of disrupted behavior, and certainly sets the stage for a change in reinforcement patterns (point C). In addition, "Externalizing behavior problems", which were defined in this study as conduct disorder, oppositional behavior, attentional problems, substance use disorder, and/or eating disorder, also can be construed as direct indices of behavioral disruption. With further research, these might be demonstrated to be better construed as longstanding vulnerabilities (G), rather than as patterns that emerge after an initial antecedent event. However, in this study, they were initially measured in the context of such antecedents, and such behavioral disruptions would all be associated with decreased positive reinforcement and greater likelihood of negative reactions or other experiences (C), so they are included here.

145

Direct measures of factor C are surprisingly few in the body of adolescent research reviewed here. Only two such variables were identified in the published findings. First, lack of pleasurable social engagement has been shown to predict likelihood of adolescent depression. This follows directly from the model and is the clearest demonstration to date of reduced positive reinforcement creating vulnerability for depression. Second, dissatisfaction with grades is associated with development of a first depressive episode. This variable also could be construed differently, in that "dissatisfaction" may represent a self-evaluative pattern that could better be considered a cognitive vulnerability factor. However, dissatisfaction with grades was reported in the study which also demonstrated disruption of homework, and both variables were shown to be related. Thus, it seems reasonable to expect that grades were objectively poorer for some adolescents, that they cared about grades, that they experienced reduced positive reinforcement, and thus that dissatisfaction with grades represents a point in a chain of events exactly predicted by the model.

Future research to help validate this model of depression and/or to further refine it could fruitfully focus on generating additional direct evidence regarding the role of reduced positive reinforcement or elevated aversive experience. To date, there is clear evidence that some variables are predictors of first depressive episodes that could reasonably be predicted to lead to reduced reinforcement and/or elevated negative experiences; as noted above, these include major negative life events, romantic break-ups, and physical symptoms. Still, it would be helpful to have direct evidence of their impact on the overall level of positive versus negative life experiences of adolescents (and those in other age groups) to directly and unequivocally validate the hypothesized sequence of events.

Measurement of point D, "Increased self-awareness," is difficult, particularly in longitudinal research rather than immediate laboratory situations, but two variables have been reported that may capture this aspect of the model. The clearest is "Self-consciousness", measured by self-report, which was found to be a predictor of increased likelihood for depression. In addition, internalizing behavior problems (defined in this study as worry, behavioral fluctuations, state anxiety, sleep problems, and hypochondriasis) could all be thought of as problems that involve heightened self-awareness. Thus, they can be considered to represent the tendency to respond to stressful events in ways that involve a tendency to focus on one's internal experience (e.g., mood state, physical sensations) and to self-monitor and self-analyze in an internally focused way.

Points E and F are not represented in Tables 6.1 or 6.2, since they are the end points to which the predictions allude. In the studies reviewed, extensive measures of depression status were used to identify the level of symptoms and diagnostic status. For all variables reported above, the variables shown to be predictive were associated with the presence of increased dysphoria (point E) and the host of consequences of depressed mood that lead to a diagnosis of major depressive disorder (point F).

Many variables have been reported in Lewinsohn's work on predictors of initial depressive episodes that lead to an expanded understanding of the vulnerability

Table 6.2   Predictors of first episode of depression in adolescence or young adulthood:
variables representing long-lasting vulnerability or protective factors (point G
in the integrative theory)

Study	Vulnerability factor	Protective factor	Relevant theory element
Rohde et al., 2001	Alcohol use disorder or problematic use in adolescence predicts depression in young adults		G
Lewinsohn et al., 1994	Past anxiety disorder		G
	Female gender		G
	Pessimism		G
	Attributions		G
	Other disorders (unspecified)		G
	Emotional reliance		G
		Self-esteem	G
		Self-rated social competence	G
		Coping skills	G
		Family social support	G

factors and protective factors for depression in adolescents (point G); Table 6.2
presents these variables. These are the long-lasting variables that make some
individuals more vulnerable to episodes of depression, given an equal experience
of immediate challenges. Some of these may be biological; others represent living
in long-standing stressful environments with fewer resources; others may be
developed early in life (such as particular cognitive attributional styles); and some
may accrue after an incident of depression (e.g., defining oneself as someone likely
to become depressed).

Although biological factors certainly could be included here, Lewinsohn's
research largely has not included immediate biological processes, such as cortisol
levels or other endocrine influences. Their absence in these tables does not reflect
a lack of appreciation for the potential of such variables to have major influence,
but rather the interest in building up a strong body of literature on psychosocial
influences on depression. Such psychosocial influences are relatively neglected in
many threads of current research on depression, so Lewinsohn's work represents
an important source of knowledge about which of these variables play important
roles.

Looking first at vulnerability factors, eight have been identified. In young adults,
alcohol use disorder or problematic use during adolescence predicts emergence of
an initial episode of depression in young adults. Other variables were identified in
adolescence, in relation to a first episode at that time. These include some general

experiences, such as history of a past anxiety disorder or other psychological disorder (other than depression, anxiety, or substance abuse). Some variables represent cognitive styles that are broadly understood as risk factors for depression, such as pessimism and negative attributions. Excessive emotional reliance also emerged as a personal risk factor; when adolescents depend for their sense of well-being on direct demonstrations of the approval and caring of others, they may be more vulnerable when relationships are disrupted, whether by the variables mentioned above (conflict with parents, romantic break-up) or in other situations such as changing schools or having important friends move away. Finally, female gender appeared as a risk factor for first episode, as it has in almost all other studies of depression in European and American sites. Whether its power is due to related biological variables, to cultural variables influencing women and girls, or to cognitive processing differences for each gender cannot be concluded from this research, and likely is attributable to a complex interaction of all of these influences.

Four protective variables have been identified in this body of research, and these address both personal abilities and environmental influences. Self-esteem, self-rated social competence, and coping skills each play a crucial role. These variables make sense within the model of depression, since each suggests an ability to deal with antecedent events and their potential to disrupt important behavior in effective, problem-solving ways. In addition, social support from the adolescent's family was protective. This may help in various ways: parents or siblings may step in to solve problems if the adolescent seems unable to cope; a supportive family may provide strong sources of positive reinforcement that counter-balance negative life experiences, etc. They also may be able to divert the adolescent, through planned activities or other means, in order to prevent increased self-awareness from developing to a destructive level.

Recurrence of depression

As noted above, the integrative theory of depression leads to some different predictions for recurrence of depression than for first episodes. Certainly the model would argue that subsequent episodes could be triggered by the same kinds of events that trigger initial episodes: if antecedent events are powerful enough, and personal resources sparse enough, a depressive episode would be expected to occur at any time. However, the model also emphasizes ways in which the consequences of a first depression may heighten vulnerability to subsequent episodes.

Table 6.3 first examines the variables associated with prediction of recurrence of depression that provide evidence relevant to points A through D of the model. As expected, the role of specific antecedent events is less prominent in predicting subsequent episodes. Indeed, Lewinsohn and colleagues have specifically reported that major life stress is a stronger predictor of a first episode of Major Depressive Disorder than recurrence of depression. However, just as with first episode, depression onset is associated with negative attributional style at low levels of stress, but not at high levels of stress. Even for subsequent episodes, if life stress is severe

148

Table 6.3 Predictors of recurrence of depression

Study	Vulnerability factor	Relevant theory element
Lewinsohn et al., 1999a	Major life stress stronger predictor of first MDD than recurrence	A and G
Lewinsohn et al., 2001	Depression onset associated with negative attributional style at low levels of stress, but not at high levels of stress *	A and G
Lewinsohn et al., 2000	Conflict with parents (for women only)	B

Note: * This pattern was also associated with onset of first episode of depression.

enough, the additional impact of the personal vulnerability factor and factors in point G of the model is mitigated. Finally, one specific life stressor – conflict with parents – continues to be predictive of subsequent depressive episodes, but only for women. No explanation of this is clearly supported. It may be that girls have more emotional reliance on parental relationships than boys do, or that conflict between girls and parents is more virulent than conflict between adolescent boys and parents, or some other factor may be explanatory.

Most of the variables that have been reported to be predictive of a second or further recurring episode of depression fit better with the category of long-lasting variables that make some individuals more vulnerable to episodes of depression, given an equal experience of immediate challenges, point G in the model. These appear in Table 6.4.

However, although multiple such variables have been reported in various studies by Lewinsohn and his colleagues, most of them can best be understood as some variant of the same theme: prior depression is a risk factor for future depression. These variables include, in various studies shown in Table 6.4, a prior suicide attempt, a prior episode of depression, prior adjustment disorder with depressed mood during adolescence (for young adults), and multiple episodes of depression in adolescence. While these findings fit well with a larger body of prior work demonstrating greater risk for depression in those with a prior episode (e.g., Lewinsohn et al., 1989), these particular findings shed no light on the specific vulnerability created by a prior episode.

Most of the other identified variables fit the same pattern: intriguing but not ultimately explanatory. For example, the finding that dysphoric mood or symptoms predict recurrence of depression more strongly than they do first episodes of depression is intriguing and potentially vital to understanding recurrence. It may be that self-awareness is heightened in individuals who have been depressed previously, so that increased self-monitoring of depressed mood is more prevalent. This certainly is reported clinically by individuals who have been previously

Table 6.4   Predictors of recurrence of depression

Study	Vulnerability factor	Protective factor	Relevant theory element
Lewinsohn et al., 1994*	Prior suicide attempt		G
	Prior episode of depression		G
Lewinsohn et al., 1999a	Dysphoric mood/symptoms stronger predictors of recurrence than first MDD		G
	Dysfunctional thinking stronger predictor of recurrence than first MDD		G
Lewinsohn et al., 1999b	Similar MDD in young adults for those with MDD versus Adjustment disorder with depressed mood during adolescence		G
Lewinsohn et al., 2000	Female gender		G
	Multiple episodes in adolescence predict depression in young adults		G
	Higher borderline symptoms		G
		Low levels of excessive emotional reliance	G
		For young adults, history of only single adolescent episode	G
		Low proportion of family with recurrent MDD	G
		Low antisocial and borderline symptoms	G
		Positive attributional style (for men only)	G

* *Note*: These factors were associated with a future onset of depression in this study, not specified as first onset or recurrence; they seem logically to suggest recurrence rather than a first episode.

depressed. Alternatively, attempts at problem-solving in the face of life challenges may be curtailed by those who have been previously depressed. Additionally, higher borderline symptoms have been associated with recurrence of depression, but without clarifying exploration. It seems likely that the mood problems associated with borderline disorder are as relevant to heightening recurrent depressive vulnerability as are dysphoric moods due to other causes. Future research to tease out the chain of events between events leading to dysphoria, the initial dysphoria itself, and how that escalates into depression in those who have no prior episode versus those who do would be a fruitful area for theory development.

Similarly, Lewinsohn's research group also has found that dysfunctional thinking is a stronger predictor of recurrence of depression than of first episode. However, it is hard to say why that would be. Perhaps dysfunctional thoughts are simply another aspect of heightened self-awareness, as discussed regarding the impact of dysphoric mood. Perhaps the link between dysphoric symptoms and accelerated dysfunctional thoughts is exacerbated by prior episodes of depression, in the sense that the mental pathways connecting negative experience to dysfunctional approaches of understanding them are strengthened. Further research to explore this finding also is indicated.

Finally, female gender is associated with recurrence of depression; in fact, it is even more predictive of recurrence than of first episode. As discussed above, female gender is shorthand for a wide array of possible physiological, cognitive, environmental, and cultural variables that may be the real risk factors. Why these factors would coalesce into prediction of even greater vulnerability for recurrence is not known.

The factors that protect against recurrence of depression are not generally more instructive. Adolescents and young adults with a low proportion of family members who have experienced recurrent episodes of depression are less likely to have recurrence. It is unclear whether that is due to biological mechanisms; it also could be an indication of family coping skills and modeling of such skills, of the stressfulness of the environment faced by such families, or other environmental variables. Finally, low levels of antisocial behaviors and borderline symptoms are associated with less recurrence of depression. This could reflect underlying valuable information, for example that those whose behavior is less easily disrupted by life events are less vulnerable to repeated depressive episodes, but that explanation is speculative.

Two variables are perhaps most instructive. First, low levels of excessive emotional reliance are protective against recurrence, just as excessive emotional reliance was predictive of first episodes. This seems more directly linked to the theory, as noted above: when adolescents depend for their sense of well-being on direct demonstrations of the approval and caring of others, they may be more vulnerable when relationships change and conversely, when they are more self-reliant or have broader social support, they will be less vulnerable to repeated depression. Second, positive attributional style was a protective factor for recurrence of depression, but only for men.

Looking overall at the predictors of recurrence of depression, it is striking that few specific predictors emerge. The primary finding is that for those with a history of depression, some factor associated with dysphoria is more likely to trigger a recurrence, particularly for women, for men who do not have positive attributional styles, and for those who do not have an excessive level of emotional reliance on others. In a broad sense this supports the model of depression presented by Lewinsohn, and at a clinical level it provides considerable useful information for predicting when formerly depressed individuals might be at risk of recurrence. However, it would be extremely valuable to have additional research to elucidate the internal psychological processes that set the stage for this vulnerability and that represent the steps in its emergence.

The most interesting finding regarding recurrence is not related directly to the specific predictors of depression. It could be easy to assume that when depression "recurs" it is a mirror image of a prior episode – the same person is depressed again, in presumably much the same ways. However, Lewinsohn and colleagues (2003) have found that the specific pattern of depressive symptoms is not replicated across episodes for adolescents and young adults. All of the participants included as having recurrent episodes met criteria for major depressive disorder at each episode, but which symptoms they displayed to meet criteria were not repeated. Further, the severity of episodes was not replicated, nor did episodes simply increase in severity (Lewinsohn et al., 2003). Each episode of depression had unique features and its own level of severity; duration was not reported, but these results raise the question of whether different episodes may be of quite different duration as well. The integrative model of depression does not directly explain or predict this finding. However, it is not inconsistent with the model, and at a meta-level, these results may be reminding us that, even if antecedent events play a less clear role in triggering recurrence, there may be environmental elements that play an important role in shaping the phenomenology of each episode.

Theoretical implications of research findings: are modifications of the theory suggested? What future research is most needed?

Lewinsohn and his colleagues (1998a) have previously explored the question of whether their research findings up to that point suggested modifications of the integrative theory of depression. Their main conclusions were minimal. They articulated the understanding that the model needs to attend to how recurrences of depression may be predicted differently than initial episodes, as I have sought to explore. They listed the variables that had been demonstrated to be predictive up to that point, but did not link them to specific elements of the model. The listing of predictions in this chapter incorporates additional studies and does make more explicit linkages to theory elements. Lewinsohn et al. (1998a) also indicate that a complete model of depression should include a theoretical explication of duration of episodes, as well as their development, and it should contain elements to differentiate when depression would be the primary disorder as opposed to a comorbid and secondary disorder. While the latter tasks seem invaluable ultimately, they are beyond the scope of this chapter and await further exploration.

The task that seems possible now is to consider the integrative theory of depression to see how it fits findings to date. Overall, the set of results from the research guided by Lewinsohn and performed by him and research collaborators provides consistent evidence of the strength of the integrative model of depression.

Initial episodes of depression

In particular, there is considerable evidence for the first argument presented in this chapter, i.e., that the theory predicts that for the first onset of depression, some set of events (A) should be identifiable that leads to disruption of behavior patterns (B) resulting in reduced positive experiences and/or increased negative experiences (C). Table 6.1 shows support for eight such types of events, ranging across a wide spectrum of severity, from daily hassles thorough physical problems, conflict with parents, and romantic problems, to events that could be considered major life stresses.

Other research groups studying depression in children and adults also have reported findings (e.g., Kessing et al., 2003; Patton et al., 2003) that major stressful life events are a risk factor for depression across the life span. However, no other research group, to my knowledge, has accumulated the same amount of data over a longitudinal period as Lewinsohn. While the support from other research groups is validating, the evidence flowing from the ongoing intensive study of a large, community-based sample of adolescents (now into early adulthood) is our current best source of evidence against which to compare the theoretical predictions of the integrative model of depression.

While the chain of events in points A, B, and C of the integrative model of depression is largely confirmed by the data reported thus far, the variables that would most directly affect point C, "Reduced positive reinforcement and/or elevated aversive experience," has few direct tests. There have been no contradictory findings and some support has been found; most clearly, reduced social and academic reinforcement have been shown to be predictive of depression. Factor C has been a key element in Lewinsohn's theorizing about depression since his earliest work (e.g., Lewinsohn, 1974), and it has a key role in the integrative theory in what could be considered "the tipping point" – events are external, and it is the internal experience of loss of pleasure or increase of aversive experience that creates the internal responses that develop into depression. Because point C does refer to such a subjective internal experience, it is not surprising that it is more difficult to assess and enter into predictive regression equations. However, future efforts to capture more of this internal experience and show its links to the origin of the emotional events we think of as the essence of dysphoria would be very useful.

Findings with regard to point D in the model, "Increased self-awareness," are almost identical to those with point C: there are no contradictory findings; some support has been demonstrated, but few direct tests have been reported. The model argues that depression occurs when someone facing a deteriorating pattern of positive and negative life experiences begins to focus inwardly on negative emotional experience (point D), rather than trying to deal effectively with the external life disruptions. The model argues that at this tipping point, dysphoria occurs and can develop into depression. As stated earlier in this chapter,

The experience of increased self-awareness is essential to the emergence of a full-blown depressive episode. While this is a specific prediction, measuring self-awareness is not a simple process, so some of the evidence for this component of the theory by necessity will be inferential.

This part of the model has been less emphasized in much writing about Lewinsohn's work, and often his theory is characterized as emphasizing only the external life events without attention to internal emotional processing. It may, in fact, be true that depression could be predicted without relying on this internal step. Certainly the power of simply measuring the kinds of events in point A of the model suggests that the process described in point D may be an epiphenomenon rather than an integral step in the causal chain. One challenge to this argument is the early finding (Lewinsohn et al., 1994) that increased scores on a self-report measure of self-consciousness were predictive of depression, but it would be helpful to have a more rich and complex assessment of "increased self-awareness" as an unfolding process that, when it occurs leads to depression and when it can be disrupted averts development of depression. Creating the capacity to assess this process and its timing will be a challenge for a next generation of research. Again, to date there is no reason to discard it from the integrative model of depression, but there is not yet definitive support for its essential role.

Certainly research to date has helped to flesh out many elements of the predisposing characteristics that heighten vulnerability or resistance to depression (point G). Further, high levels of stressful life events predict depression onset even in the absence of a negative attributional style, a potential predisposing characteristic (G in the model). Of particular theoretical value is the finding that, at low levels of stress, predisposing factors are important for predicting onset of depression (Lewinsohn et al., 2001), just as the integrative model would predict. Stated differently, the data reported by Lewinsohn and colleagues and reviewed above show that any of us could become depressed given severe enough antecedents; any of us are vulnerable, when personal storms are severe. Further, some individuals will be more vulnerable than others when circumstances are less stressful. One such vulnerability factor is negative attributional style, a style that other research groups also have shown to increase the likelihood of depression. The integrative model of depression captures this relationship well: negative cognitive style is a predisposing variable, serving to heighten the likelihood of depression in negative life circumstances that would not be strong enough to trigger depression in most individuals. Some will be vulnerable, even when hit by brief showers instead of major storms.

Other predisposing variables include use of alcohol, anxiety, and general pessimism, all of which seem likely to be incompatible with effective problem-solving in stressful circumstances. These factors also could help to generate life events that might set off a depressive cycle. For example, anxiety in adolescents might lead to avoidance of school or social activities, triggering the failure to complete homework or lack of pleasurable social engagement that have been shown to be trigger events for depression.

The integrative model of depression also invites us to consider protective factors, and many have been reported, including positive evaluations of oneself, effective coping abilities, and support from family members. These factors might be valuable to consider in light of attempts to develop a greater research base for point D in the model, as discussed above. For example, a supportive family may be particularly powerful at keeping an adolescent from retreating to his or her room and ruminating on personal failings during stressful times. Having effective coping skills may function just as described above in relation to the hypothesized "tipping point": adolescents who feel more self-efficacy may take action and stay focused on external events rather than turning attention inward. To date, these process links of how protective variables actually function to avert a depressive cycle have not been studied; such efforts would be an excellent next step in providing information to enrich the theoretical perspective.

Recurrence of depression

Recurrence of depression remains a compelling issue both clinically and theoretically. Clinically, a large minority of individuals who have been depressed once will become depressed again at some point in their lifetime (e.g., Lewinsohn et al., 1989). Some have argued that depression should be considered a chronic illness (e.g., Joiner, 2000), and for many individuals it is, although this is not the most likely outcome. There are more individuals who become depressed once, recover, and never have another depressive episode than there are individuals who have recurring episodes. A theoretical framework that can clarify the important differences in lifetime pattern, with some individuals having at least two and often more episodes of depression and others never having a recurrence, is essential. Certainly arguments have been voiced concerning biological vulnerability for those who have repeated episodes, and as discussed above, that certainly may play a role. The emphasis in this chapter, however, is to examine psychosocial variables in the integrative model of depression that may have theoretical relevance to the issue of recurrence.

Earlier in the chapter, I argued that the integrative model of depression predicts that recurrence of depression could be predicted by the same pattern of events that lead to an initial episode of depression, or that it could be triggered by lingering depressive symptoms that in themselves disrupt daily experience, leading to the same cycle of decreased reinforcement and increased self-awareness but without specific, identifiable, initial disruptive life events. Such lingering symptoms could be considered to become predisposing characteristics that obviate the necessity for readily identifiable external events as triggers for recurrent depression.

The idea that recurrence of depression is more independent of points A and B in the integrative model is supported by the body of research reported by Lewinsohn and colleagues. Most specifically, they have found that major life stress is a stronger predictor of a first major depressive disorder diagnosis than of recurrence

(Lewinsohn et al., 1999a). Conversely, a larger host of predisposing variables was found to predict recurrence of depression than initial episode. Most of these predisposing characteristics are related to depressive experience itself: dysphoric mood or symptoms, dysfunctional thinking, adjustment disorder with depressed mood, borderline symptoms. Thus the expectation that lingering depressive qualities set the stage for a recurrence of full-blown major depression is powerful. In addition, many variables have been reported that provide some protective influence, reducing the likelihood of a recurrent depressive episode. These include low emotional reliance on others, low antisocial and borderline symptoms, and a positive attributional style (but only for men in the latter case).

But what is the process of development of a recurrent episode? As with initial episodes, examination of how vulnerability and protective factors exert their influence at particular moments that generate or avert a depressive cycle would be invaluable. Do individuals who have dysfunctional thinking interpret neutral or ambiguous events as more disruptive and internally experience decreased positive reinforcement or increased aversive experience, even when direct evidence is not compelling? Do individuals who have lingering depressive symptoms create a negative interpersonal climate, as Coyne's (1976) early research suggested, such that they have an ongoing low level of reinforcement, and even minor disruptions tip them into a depressogenic ratio of positive to negative experience? Does the experience of a prior depression, with lingering impact, increase the likelihood of self-awareness during difficult events? Are there individuals who have been depressed once but learn in the process of recovering how to escape from heightened self-awareness and turn instead to effective problem-solving rather than emotional self-involvement? All of these patterns would be consistent with the personal characteristics reported in various studies by Lewinsohn and colleagues. Future work designed to delve into the specific processes of coping actively with distress versus turning inward to depressive rumination would help us develop a more complete theory of depressive recurrence. It also could help, as all good theories do, in understanding what interventions, with what timing, might be most effective for preventing recurrence of depression.

Summary

While much of Lewinsohn's work has focused on development of effective treatments for adolescent depression, this chapter has focused on research that elucidates variables that are predictive of depression. Findings from this body of research have been compared against Lewinsohn's integrative theoretical model of depression. The findings provide an interrelated, comprehensive pattern of support for important elements of that theory, and having a theoretical model that organizes these empirically supported psychosocial variables is enormously valuable. What can be an overwhelming listing of variables can be organized into theoretical components, as this chapter has attempted to do. Review of these relationships supports the hypotheses that:

1   For the first onset of depression, events can be identified that can lead to disruption of behavior patterns, resulting in likely reduced positive experiences and/or increased negative experiences. These events are shown to predict onset of depression in adolescents.

2   Recurrence of depression could be predicted by the same pattern, although the relationship is less strong. In addition, recurrence can be triggered by lingering depressive symptoms that likely disrupt daily experience, leading to the same cycle of decreased reinforcement and increased self-awareness but without specific, identifiable, initial disruptive life events. Such lingering symptoms could be considered to become predisposing characteristics that obviate the necessity for readily identifiable external events as triggers for recurrent depression, and further research to explore such relationships is suggested.

The experience of increased self-awareness has not yet been shown to be essential to the emergence of a full-blown depressive episode, but some supportive evidence has been obtained. Research strategies for developing additional evidence for this component of the theory were also suggested.

Lewinsohn's integrative model of depression has been well supported by research to date, and the ongoing nature of his research with this cohort will allow further research examining depression across early adulthood and perhaps ultimately across the life span. The time is ripe for a next generation of research designed explicitly to facilitate theory development.

References

Arnett, J.J. (1999). Adolescent storm and stress, reconsidered. *American Psychologist, 54*, 317–326.

Coyne, J.C. (1976). Depression and the response of others. *Journal of Abnormal Psychology, 85*, 186–193.

Gotlib, I.H. and Hammen, C. (1992). *Psychological aspects of depression: Toward an interpersonal integration*. New York: Wiley.

Joiner, T.E. (2000). Depression's vicious scree: Self-propagating and erosive process in depression chronicity. *Clinical Psychology: Science and Practice, 7*, 203–218.

Joiner, T.E., Lewinsohn, P.M., and Seeley, J.R. (2002). The core of loneliness: Lack of pleasurable engagement – more so than painful disconnection – predicts social impairment, depression onset, and recovery from depressive disorder among adolescents. *Journal of Personality Assessment, 79*, 472–491.

Kashani, J.H., Carlson, G.A., Beck, N.C., Hoeper, E.W., Corcoran, C.M., McAllister, J.A., et al. (1987). Depression, depressive symptoms, and depressed mood among a community sample of adolescents. *American Journal of Psychiatry, 144*, 931–934.

Kessing, L.V., Agerbo, E., and Mortensen, P.B. (2003). Does the impact of major stressful life events on the risk of developing depression change throughout life? *Psychological Medicine, 33*, 1177–1184.

Lewinsohn, P.M. (1974). A behavioral approach to depression. In R.J. Friedman and M.M. Katz (Eds.), *The psychology of depression: Contemporary theory and research* (pp. 157–185). New York: Wiley.

Lewinsohn, P.M., Hoberman, H., Teri, L., and Hautzinger, M. (1985) An integrative theory of depression. In S. Reiss and R.R. Bootzin (Eds.), *Theoretical issues in behavior therapy* (pp. 331–359). New York: Academic Press.

Lewinsohn, P.M., Zeiss, A.M., and Duncan, E.M. (1989). Probability of relapse after recovery from an episode of depression. *Journal of Abnormal Psychology*, *98*, 107–116.

Lewinsohn, P.M., Hops, H., Roberts, R.E., Seeley, J.R., and Andrews, J.A. (1993). Adolescent psychopathology: I. Prevalence and incidence of depression and other DSM-III-R disorders in high school students. *Journal of Abnormal Psychology*, *102*, 135–144.

Lewinsohn, P.M., Roberts, R.E., Seeley, J.R., Rohde, P., Gotlib, J.H. and Hops, H. (1994). Adolescent psychopathology: II. Psychosocial risk factors for depression. *Journal of Abnormal Psychology*, *103*, 302–315.

Lewinsohn, P.M., Gotlib, I.H., and Hautzinger, M. (1998a). Behavioral treatment of unipolar depression. In V.E. Caballo (Ed.), *International Handbook of Cognitive and Behavioral Therapies for Psychological Disorders*. Oxford: Pergamon.

Lewinsohn, P.M., Rohde, P., and Seeley, J.R. (1998b). Major Depressive Disorder in older adolescents: Prevalence, risk factors, and clinical implications. *Clinical Psychology Review*, *18*, 765–794.

Lewinsohn, P.M., Allen, N.B., Gotlib, I.H., and Seeley, J.R. (1999a). First onset versus recurrence of depression: Differential processes of psychosocial risk. *Journal of Abnormal Psychology*, *108*, 483–489.

Lewinsohn, P.M., Rohde, P., Klein, D.N., and Seeley, J.R. (1999b). Natural course of adolescent Major Depressive Disorder: I. Continuity into young adulthood. *Journal of the American Academy of Child and Adolescent Psychiatry*, *38*, 56–63.

Lewinsohn, P.M., Rohde, P., Seeley, J.R., Klein, D.N., and Gotlib, I.H. (2000). Natural course of adolescent Major Depressive Disorder in a community sample: Predictors of recurrence in young adults. *American Journal of Psychiatry*, *157*, 1584–1591.

Lewinsohn, P.M., Joiner, T.E., and Rohde, P. (2001). Evaluation of cognitive diathesis-stress models in predicting Major Depressive Disorder in adolescents. *Journal of Abnormal Psychology*, 110, 203–215.

Lewinsohn, P.M., Petit, J.W., Joiner, T.E., and Seeley, J.R. (2003). The symptomatic expression of Major Depressive Disorder in adolescents and young adults. *Journal of Abnormal Psychology*, *112*, 244–252.

McGee, R., Feehan, M., Williams, S., Partridge, F., Silva, P.A., and Kelly, J. (1990). DSM-III disorders in a large sample of adolescents. *Journal of the American Academy of Child and Adolescent Psychiatry*, *29*, 611–619.

Monroe, S.M., Rohde, P., Seeley, J.R., and Lewinsohn, P.M. (1999). Life events and depression in adolescence: Relationship loss as a prospective risk factor for first onset of Major Depressive Disorder. *Journal of Abnormal Psychology*, *108*, 606–614.

Patton, G.C., Coffey, C., Posterino, M., Carlin, J.B., and Bowes, G. (2003). Life events and early onset depression: cause or consequence? *Psychological Medicine*, *33*, 1203–1210.

Rohde, P., Lewinsohn, P.M., Kahler, C.W., Seeley, J.R., and Brown, R.A. (2001). Natural course of alcohol use disorders from adolescence to young adulthood. *Journal of the American Academy of Child and Adolescent Psychiatry*, *40*, 83–90.

Weissman, M.M., Warner, V., Wickramaratne, P., Moreau, D., and Olfson, M. (2000). Offspring at risk: Early-onset major depression and anxiety disorders over a decade. In J.L. Rapoport (Ed.), *Childhood onset of "adult" psychopathology: Clinical and research advances* (pp. 245–258). Washington, DC: American Psychopathological Association.

Wickramaratne, P.J. and Weissman, M.M. (1998). Onset of psychopathology in offspring by developmental phase and parental depression. *Journal of the American Academy of Child and Adolescent Psychiatry, 37*, 933–942.

7

ADOLESCENT EATING DISORDERS

Ruth H. Striegel-Moore and Debra L. Franko

Adolescent eating disorders, specifically anorexia nervosa and bulimia nervosa, represent an understudied area in developmental psychopathology. These disorders typically originate in adolescence and are associated with significant physical and psychosocial morbidity (Rome et al., 2003). Indeed, anorexia nervosa (AN) has the highest mortality rate of any psychiatric disorder (Sullivan, 1995). Given the clinical significance of eating disorders, advancing the scientific knowledge is a high priority. This chapter will summarize what is known about the clinical presentation, course, risk factors, and empirically proven treatments for adolescent eating disorders. Eating disorders affect primarily girls or women and few studies have included male samples. Therefore, except when describing studies of the prevalence of eating disorders (where on occasion males have been included), by necessity this chapter focuses on females.

The chapter begins with a description of the diagnostic criteria, clinical presentation, and prevalence of eating disorders. Next, research documenting the course and outcome of anorexia nervosa and bulimia nervosa (BN) is described. Finally, risk factor, prevention, and treatment outcome studies are summarized.

Defining the eating disorders

Despite multiple revisions since the introduction of anorexia nervosa (in the late nineteenth century) and bulimia nervosa (in 1980) in the medical nomenclature, the diagnostic criteria for eating disorders remain a topic of considerable discussion. Experts agree that the challenge in defining these eating disorders lies in the fact that the core symptoms occur along a severity continuum with no apparent "natural" cut-point and that the currently agreed upon thresholds as articulated in the fourth edition of the *Diagnostic and statistical manual for mental disorders* (DSM-IV; American Psychiatric Association (APA) 1994) are arbitrary (Striegel-Moore and Marcus, 1995). Specifically, anorexia nervosa is defined by the refusal to maintain a minimum normal body weight (e.g., weight loss or failure to make developmentally expected weight gain, leading to body weight less than 85 percent of that expected), presence of intense fear of becoming overweight even though under-weight, body image disturbance (e.g., denial of the seriousness of being underweight, feeling fat even though underweight, or placing undue importance on weight or shape in evaluating self-worth), and, in postmenarcheal females, absence of at least three menstrual cycles. Depending on the presence or absence of additional behavioral symptoms, two subtypes are recognized: binge-eating/purging type and restricting type, respectively. Bulimia nervosa is defined by the presence of recurrent episodes of binge eating (eating objectively large amounts of food and experiencing loss of control over these eating episodes) and recurrent inappropriate compensatory behaviors (e.g., purging, excessive exercise), and experiencing undue influence of body weight and shape on self-evaluation. The behavioral symptoms of binge eating and compensatory behaviors have to co-occur, on average, at a minimum frequency of twice a week for three months to meet the severity threshold required for a full-syndrome diagnosis. The DSM-IV includes two subtypes, characterized by vomiting, laxatives, or diuretic use (purging type) and dieting, fasting and exercise (non-purging type).

Experts have noted that these criteria are fairly restrictive, resulting in a large number of individuals presenting for eating disorder treatment that do not meet full-syndrome criteria for anorexia nervosa or bulimia nervosa, but rather fit the diagnostic criteria for Eating Disorder Not Otherwise Specified (EDNOS) (Striegel-Moore and Marcus, 1995). Studies of adult populations have shown that EDNOS is far more common than anorexia nervosa and bulimia nervosa both in treatment-seeking samples and community samples (Garfinkel et al., 1995; Kendler et al., 1991; Walters and Kendler, 1995). There is some indication that among adolescents, the rates of EDNOS relative to anorexia nervosa and bulimia nervosa are even higher than in adults (Fisher et al., 2001). This relatively higher rate of EDNOS in adolescents compared to adults may reflect that (1) some adolescents may be "on their way" to developing anorexia nervosa or bulimia nervosa i.e., the EDNOS diagnosis captures the early stage of anorexia nervosa or bulimia nervosa, (2) in adolescents, the clinical picture is somewhat different from that of adults, i.e., despite the absence of all required symptoms the adolescent does, essentially, experience anorexia nervosa or bulimia nervosa, or (3) for some individuals EDNOS may be a transient disturbance associated particularly with adolescence, that improves with maturation to the point where the person no longer meets diagnostic criteria in adulthood.

The category of EDNOS is highly problematic for several reasons. First, it encompasses several distinct clinically significant syndromes and thus represents a fairly heterogeneous diagnostic category of questionable clinical or predictive utility. Second, by definition, a diagnosis of EDNOS requires that the disturbance is associated with distress or impairment, yet the fact that the category includes syndromes that are "subthreshold variants" of full syndrome disorders such as anorexia nervosa and bulimia nervosa begs the question of whether EDNOS syndromes are less severe types of eating disturbances than the "named" eating disorders. Third, in empirical studies, operational definitions of EDNOS vary so much that comparisons across studies are difficult. Finally, in treatment research and clinical practice, individuals with EDNOS have a secondary status over other eating disorders as reflected by the fact that most studies specify strict inclusion criteria and insurance companies often fail to support treatment unless the insured meets narrowly defined diagnostic criteria.

The American Academy of Pediatrics (AAP) has developed the *Diagnostic and statistical manual for primary care (DSM-PC) child and adolescent version* (Wolraich et al., 1996) that features a diagnostic scheme where it is possible to note mental health concerns that do not reach full-syndrome levels, but nonetheless warrant clinical attention. Specifically, "variations" represent minor symptoms and "problems" indicate the more serious disturbances currently captured as EDNOS in the DSM-IV. Research has not yet examined the predictive utility of the DSM-PC distinctions of "variations" and "problems" regarding the progression from these lesser disturbances to full syndrome eating disorders. Although there is a fair amount of research illustrating that eating disorder symptoms (e.g., body image disturbance, binge eating) are widely prevalent among adolescent girls (Rodin et al., 1984) (and to a lesser extent also boys, see Muise et al., 2003) and are risk factors for subsequent full syndrome anorexia nervosa or bulimia nervosa (e.g., Attie and Brooks-Gunn, 1992; Killen et al., 1994; Patton et al., 1999; Stice et al., 2001), the question of where to best draw the line in capturing adolescent eating disorders remains unanswered.

Large, prospective studies are needed to examine the developmental progression of these symptoms and investigate their clinical significance in terms of concurrent and prospective adverse effects on health and psychosocial functioning.

Prevalence of adolescent eating disorders

Although an extensive literature exists that offers data regarding the prevalence of eating disorder symptoms, surprisingly few studies have focused on prevalence of full syndrome eating disorders in adolescent samples. Even fewer studies have employed rigorous methods to ensure representativeness of the sample or validity of the diagnostic assessment. Striegel-Moore reviewed the extant literature on prevalence of eating disorders in adolescents for the Annenberg Eating Disorder Commission and identified only fifteen studies that satisfied the rather minimal methodological criterion that diagnostic criteria be specified and diagnoses based on a research interview (rather than the far less accurate use of self-report surveys). A full discussion is beyond the scope of this chapter and the interested reader is referred to the Commission's report (Evans et al., 2005) for a critical appraisal of these studies. Numerous methodological differences make a comparison across studies difficult and a summary of this literature runs the risk of oversimplification. In brief, eight studies used a two-stage sampling approach (Graber et al., 2003; Rathner and Messner, 1993; Rosenvinge et al., 1999; Santonastaso et al., 1996; Steinhausen et al., 1997; Verhulst et al., 1997; Whitaker et al., 1990; Wlodarczyk-

Bisaga and Dolan, 1996) and six studies assessed the entire study sample for presence or history of an eating disorder (Emerson, 2003; Johnson et al., 2002a; Lewinsohn et al., 1993; McKnight Investigators, 2003; Newman et al., 1996; Wittchen et al., 1998). Only two studies used the same research interview (Johnson et al., 2002b; Verhulst et al., 1997), diagnostic criteria varied over time (from DSM-III in the earliest study, to DSM-IV in the most recent studies, and only four studies (Lewinsohn et al., 1993; Newman et al., 1996; Santonastaso et al., 1996; Wittchen et al., 1998) report both current and "lifetime" rates of eating disorders (given that many participants in these studies were not yet old enough to have gone through the peak age period where onset of eating disorders is likely, the term "lifetime rates" is a misnomer). Only eight studies recruited both females and males, whereby six reported gender specific rates (Lewinsohn et al., 1993; Newman et al., 1996; Rosenvinge et al., 1999; Steinhausen et al., 1997; Wittchen et al., 1998; Whitaker et al., 1990), and two studies reported combined rates for boys and girls (Emerson, 2003; Verhulst et al., 1997). Finally, the age ranges vary considerably, with some studies including prepubertal children (in one study as young as 5 years of age: Emerson, 2003), some studies restricting the sample to teenagers (e.g., Lewinsohn et al., 1993), and yet other studies including participants in their early twenties (e.g. as old as 24 years: Wittchen et al., 1998).

Bearing in mind that these methodological differences render any broad statement somewhat simplistic, three major findings are of note. One, as in adult samples, rates of eating disorders are far higher among females than males. Indeed, there is some indication that the gender difference may be even more pronounced in adolescent populations compared to adults, possibly due to the later age of onset of eating disorders in males compared to females (Carlat et al., 1997).

Two, not surprisingly, there is a correlation between age and prevalence rates in that studies with relatively young samples report lower rates (current or lifetime) than studies with older participants, although, surprisingly, this relationship is far from perfect. For example, the McKnight investigators (2003) reported 0 cases of anorexia nervosa and only 0.37 percent for bulimia nervosa in their sample (N = 1103) of 11 to 14 year old girls. Consequently, rates in these adolescent studies tend to be lower than rates reported in adult studies. For current anorexia nervosa or bulimia nervosa, in girls they range from a low of 0 to high of 0.9 percent (anorexia nervosa) or 1.5 percent (bulimia nervosa). In boys, current anorexia nervosa appears to be "epidemiologically undetectable," (i.e., none of the studies reported even a single case) and bulimia nervosa also was either not found or far less common (highest rate: 0.1 percent, Wittchen et al., 1998) than in girls. In the five studies that examined "lifetime" rates (ever having met criteria) of anorexia nervosa and bulimia nervosa, females' rates ranged from a low of 0 and 1 percent, respectively to a high of 3.9 percent (anorexia nervosa) and 3.2 percent (bulimia nervosa). Only three studies reported "lifetime" rates in males and of these one reported a rate of 0.1 percent (Wittchen et al., 1998) and two found no male cases of anorexia nervosa (Lewinsohn et al., 1993; Whitaker et al., 1990). Rates for bulimia nervosa were 0 (Wittchen et al., 1998), 0.14 percent (Lewinsohn et al., 1993) and 0.2 percent (Whitacker et al., 1990), in each case far lower than the rates reported for females in these same studies.

Third, a few studies reported "partial syndrome" (some but not all required symptoms are present), "subthreshold syndromes" (all symptoms are present but not at the required level of severity), or EDNOS, but the varying definitions and methods used to arrive at a count of such cases make an interpretation highly subjective. Not surprisingly, when these cases are added to the total count of "any eating disorder" the prevalence rates increase, but future studies are needed that use consistent criteria and assessment approaches to permit conclusions about the extent to which clinically significant eating syndromes are present in adolescent samples.

As a final observation, it is important to note that with the exception of the McKnight study which included girls from ethnic minority groups, the extant literature is based on samples representing Europeans or, if recruited outside of Europe, individuals of European ancestry. It is unknown, therefore, how many adolescents outside of Europe who represent different ethnic or national groups experience an eating disorder.

Natural course, outcome, and comorbidity

Although the mean age of onset for both anorexia nervosa and bulimia nervosa occurs during adolescence, few studies have documented the course, outcome, and comorbidity of these eating disorders using an adolescent sample. The few studies that have examined these issues will be summarized separately for anorexia nervosa and bulimia nervosa.

Course and outcome in adolescent anorexia nervosa

A review of the literature finds that approximately 50–70 percent of adolescents with anorexia nervosa recover, 20 percent are improved but continue to have residual symptoms, and 10–20 percent have chronic anorexia nervosa (Steinhausen, 2002). Across five European sites, Steinhausen and colleagues (2003) reported on 242 adolescent patients followed for 6.4 years into young adulthood; 70 percent recovered from the eating disorder. Herpertz-Dahlmann and colleagues (2001) followed 39 adolescent inpatients 3, 7, and 10 years after discharge and found that 69 percent met criteria for full recovery at the 10-year mark. Interestingly, long-term recovered patients did not differ from normal controls with regard to psychiatric morbidity or psychosocial functioning. Steinhausen et al. (2000) reported on a cohort of 60 adolescent eating disorder patients and found a trend of improvement as length of follow-up increased. Similarly, Strober et al. (1997) found that the calculated probability of reaching full recovery at 3 years was 1 percent versus 72 percent at 10 years in a follow-up of adolescent inpatients.

Although recovery rates appear optimistic, relapse rates are not insubstantial. In the Strober et al. (1997) study, for example, nearly one-third (30 percent) of those who had achieved weight recovery during hospitalization relapsed within the 10 to 15 years following discharge. Lower rates of relapse were found among adolescents considered partially recovered (10 percent) or fully recovered (0 percent) at discharge. In that same sample, course and outcome were compared between "typical" (restricting) and "atypical" cases of inpatient adolescent anorexia nervosa. Atypical anorexia nervosa was defined by "extreme weight loss without explanatory psychiatric (e.g., anorexia secondary to severe depression) or organic illness" in which weight phobia and body image disturbance were denied throughout treatment (Strober et al., 1997, p. 136). No significant difference in relapse rates or time to relapse between typical and atypical cases was found over the follow-up period (10 to 15 years).

Although anorexia nervosa has one of the highest mortality rates among psychiatric disorders (Sullivan, 1995), during adolescence, the mortality rate for anorexia nervosa is relatively low. Specifically, a mortality rate of 2 percent has been reported when anorexia nervosa begins during adolescence as compared to more than 5 percent for adolescent- and adult-onset combined (Steinhausen, 2002). Strober et al. (1997) found no deaths in their longitudinal study of anorexic inpatients followed 10–15 years post-discharge (ages 22–33 at follow-up). These data are consistent with the finding that adolescent onset appears to have a more positive course than adult onset cases (Fisher, 2003).

Patients with anorexia nervosa whose symptoms persist tend to manifest abnormalities with weight, eating behaviors, menstrual function, comorbid psychopathology, and difficulties with psychosocial functioning over time (Herpertz-Dahlmann et al., 2001; Steinhausen, 1997; Strober et al., 1997; Wentz et al., 2001). Few predictors of outcome have been found, but studies suggest that outcome is enhanced when duration of illness is short at time of presentation for treatment. Poor outcome is predicted by extremely low weight at presentation and vomiting. Data on predictors of mortality in AN have reported varied results. Some studies have found low weight at presentation, longer duration of illness, and severe alcohol use to be associated with higher risk of mortality (Keel et al., 2003; Patton, 1988), although these studies have been conducted only with adult samples that may (or may not) have had adolescent onset.

Comorbidity in anorexia nervosa

Few studies of comorbidity in eating disorders have utilized adolescent samples, with two exceptions. The first was a community-based epidemiological study reporting that more than 70 percent of adolescent full syndrome and partial syndrome eating disorder cases (both anorexia nervosa and bulimia nervosa) met criteria for an Axis I disorder in young adulthood (Lewinsohn et al., 2000). In addition, nearly 90 percent had concurrent comorbid disorders, with depression the most frequent psychiatric diagnosis. The second adolescent study followed over 2000 adolescents over 6 years and found that of the 8 percent who had a (partial or full syndrome) eating disorder over this time, nearly half had high levels of depression and anxiety. This was particularly so in those with partial syndrome bulimia nervosa in the teen years, and this same group also reported a high level of alcohol use at follow-up (Patton et al., 2003).

In adult samples, approximately 80 percent of anorexic patients have comorbid psychiatric disorders. The most common are affective disorders, anxiety disorders, substance use disorders, and personality disorders. Herpertz-Dahlmann et al. (2001) reported that 51 percent of anorexic subjects had an Axis I psychiatric disorder and nearly one-quarter (23 percent) met criteria for a personality disorder. In this small sample (N = 39), anxiety disorders, avoidant-dependent and obsessive-compulsive personality disorders were found most commonly. Herpertz-Dahlmann et al. (2001) also found that recovery from the eating disorder bodes well for recovery from other psychiatric disorders in adolescence, though the study is limited by the small sample size. A second study of adolescents meeting DSM-IV criteria for an eating disorder (63 restricting, 17 purging) found rates of substance use to be comparable between purgers and normal comparison subjects (Stock et al., 2002). However, adolescents with restricting eating disorders used substances to a lesser extent than purgers.

Course and outcome in bulimia nervosa

To our knowledge, there are no studies of course and outcome in an adolescent sample with bulimia nervosa. This may be due to the later age of onset of bulimia nervosa (APA, 1994) and the documented (Crow et al., 1999) delay in accessing treatment. However, the adult literature on course and outcome is extensive and provides some information that may be applicable to cases of adolescent bulimia nervosa.

In mixed studies that include both adolescent- and adult-onset bulimia nervosa, most are found to improve over time. Recovery rates are recorded to be from 35 percent to 75 percent at 5+ years of follow-up (Fairburn et al., 2000; Fichter and Quadflieg, 1997; Herzog et al., 1999). However, bulimia nervosa is known to be a chronic relapsing condition, with approximately one-third relapsing (Keel et al., 1999), often within one to two years of recovery (Herzog et al., 1996). In a study of 15–24 year olds, 50 percent recovered while the other half continued to be symptomatic, often with substantial impact on physical and psychosocial functioning (Herzog et al., 1999). In a longitudinal study of adolescents and adults (aged 16–35 years) followed prospectively over five years, only a minority continued to meet the DSM-IV criteria for BN, although a substantial number (one-half to two-thirds) had clinical significant eating disorder symptoms (Fairburn et al., 2000). Mortality is a rare outcome in BN, with mortality rates as low as 0.5 percent (Keel et al., 1999). Few prognostic factors in BN have been consistently reported across studies. Some of the factors that may be predictive of poor outcome include low self-esteem, longer duration of illness prior to presentation, higher frequency or severity of binge eating, substance abuse history, and a history of obesity (Bulik et al., 1998; Fairburn et al., 2003; Keel et al., 1999).

Comorbidity in bulimia nervosa

As noted earlier, few studies of bulimia have been undertaken with adolescent participants; thus we are left to note the comorbidity rates found in adult samples. It is possible that at least some comorbid disorders begin in adolescence, most notably depression; however, more research is needed to examine this speculation. One study (Le Grange and Lock, 2002) found that rates of comorbid depression were much higher in an adolescent sample (ages 13–19) than in a comparable sample of adults with bulimia nervosa, but the sample size was quite small ($N = 27$).

Nearly 83 percent of patients with bulimia nervosa have a lifetime history of a comorbid psychiatric disorder (Fichter and Quadflieg, 1997), most commonly affective disorders, anxiety disorders, substance use disorders (SUD), or personality disorders (Halmi et al., 2002; Herzog et al., 1992; Mitchell et al., 1991; Wonderlich and Mitchell, 1997). More than 50 percent of individuals with bulimia nervosa have a lifetime history of a mood disorder, with major depression occurring with the highest frequency. The lifetime prevalence of at least one anxiety disorder in clinical samples ranges from 13 percent to 65 percent (Herzog et al., 1992), with social phobia (17 percent) and obsessive-compulsive disorder (8–33 percent) most frequently diagnosed. Panic disorder is also commonly observed (Brewerton, 1995; von Ranson et al., 1999). Lifetime prevalence of substance use disorder is found in approximately 25 percent of patients with bulimia nervosa, with alcohol, cocaine, and marijuana the categories with highest use (Bulik et al., 1994). Multi-impulsivity, characterized by suicide attempts, self-injurious acts, and stealing, has been reported in patients with bulimia nervosa and the binge-purge form of anorexia nervosa who also have comorbid substance use disorders (Fichter et al., 1994; Nagata et al., 2000). Cluster B personality disorders (antisocial, borderline, histrionic, and narcissistic) are also prevalent in bulimia nervosa (Herzog et al., 1992).

Related issues

Three related issues have been studied recently in eating disorder samples. "Migration," the movement from one eating disorder subtype or eating disorder to another, has been studied; however, the available data include both adolescent and adult-onset cases. Although one study documented transitions from BN to AN (Kassett et al., 1988), the most common type of migration occurs in restricting anorexics (ANR) who develop bulimic symptomatology, shifting to the binge-purge subtype of anorexia nervosa, and in some cases, to bulimia nervosa. One prospective longitudinal study with frequent follow-up assessments found that more than 50 percent of ANRs developed bulimic symptomatology (Eddy et al., 2002), and only a small percent of the ANRs who continued to manifest symptoms of anorexia nervosa remained in the restricting subtype. In addition, nearly 20 percent of individuals with BN have a history of AN (Striegel-Moore et al., 2001).

Stability of eating disorders was examined with an epidemiological sample of nearly 800 children and their mothers (Kotler et al., 2001), in order to determine how stable eating disorder symptoms and diagnoses were over a 17-year period from childhood to adulthood. Stability was higher for bulimia nervosa than anorexia nervosa. Specifically, bulimia nervosa diagnosed in early adolescence was associated with a 9-fold increased risk for late adolescent bulimia nervosa and a 20-fold increase for adulthood. Late adolescent onset bulimia nervosa increased risk for adult bulimia nervosa by 35 times. For both eating disorders, eating symptoms (binge eating, dieting) in both early and late adolescence increased risk for young adult eating disorder symptoms. The authors concluded that eating problems in early childhood or an eating disorder during adolescence confers a strong risk for an eating disorder in young adulthood. Patton et al. (2003) followed 2032 adolescents over a period of 6 years, and reported that 11 percent of those with an eating disorder (partial or full syndrome) had a persisting disorder in young adulthood.

Finally, an interesting study found a number of differences between adolescents and young adults at presentation to an eating disorder clinic (Fisher et al., 2001). Of note, adolescents were more likely than adults to have a diagnosis of EDNOS and to have stronger denial of illness, greater weight loss and less wish for help. Young adults were more likely to have a history of binge eating, laxative, diuretic and ipecac use, a diagnosis of bulimia nervosa, and previous use of psychiatric medications. The authors suggested that such differences need to be considered when evaluating and treating patients with eating disorders. In a review of the literature, Fisher (2003) concluded that adolescents with eating disorders have a better prognosis than adult-onset eating disorders and that the difference increases with lengthier follow-up periods.

Risk factors

Research of the etiology of eating disorders is in the early stages. A comprehensive review by Jacobi et al. (2004) illustrates that most "risk factor" studies do not meet the fundamental methodological requirement of establishing temporal precedence of the hypothesized risk factor relative to the outcome of interest, onset of the eating disorder. Correlational studies serve only to generate hypotheses but cannot answer the question of "does exposure to X lead to Y?" As discussed in detail by Kraemer et al. (1997), to be considered a true risk factor (i.e., a variable that increases the probability of an adverse outcome), the variable should be measured prospectively and prior to onset of the outcome of interest, shown to precede the outcome of interest, and have some degree of specificity (i.e., does not merely increase risk for adverse outcomes in general). Finally, to establish causality, experimental evidence is required. Bulik (2003) has outlined two additional, related, methodological issues that often are not addressed adequately in risk factor research: timing of reporting and the nature of the outcome event. Specifically, information about risk factors (e.g., exposure to birth trauma) or outcomes (history of an adolescent eating disorder) has been measured retrospectively in some studies. Retrospective reporting of risk exposures or adverse outcomes likely is less accurate than reporting that occurs close in time to the actual events or experiences. The nature of the outcome refers to how the outcome is defined in risk research. Confronted with the challenge of finding only a handful (if any) of full syndrome cases even when following large samples over long time periods of time, some investigators have chosen to expand the adverse outcome category to include partial syndrome cases or focus on a specific symptom (e.g., weight concerns). There are at least two potential problems with this broad based approach to defining the adverse outcome. One, the outcome may be defined so broadly that the results of a significant factor no longer speak specifically to anorexia nervosa or bulimia nervosa. Two, a nonsignificant result may reflect, simply, that the outcome category was defined so broadly that the specific association between the particular variable of interest and the eating disorder was obscured by the "noise" created by defining the outcome too broadly. Clearly, the question of how to define the outcome category harkens back to the earlier discussion on how best to define the eating disorders.

In addition to methodological concerns, as pointed out by Pearson et al. (2002), a number of challenges limit the effort to identify risk factors for eating disorders. These include the absence of representative epidemiological data on full syndrome eating disorders, the infrequent occurrence of eating disorders in the population, and the multidimensional etiology of eating disorders. That being said, multiple studies have attempted to ascertain empirically based risk factors for eating disorders using a wide variety of methodologies, including cross-sectional, case control, and prospective designs (Franko and Orosan-Weine, 1998; Striegel-Moore and Cachelin, 2001; Steiner et al., 2003). In their comprehensive review, Striegel-Moore and Cachelin (2001) summarize what is currently known about risk factors into five categories: demographic, sociocultural, familial, constitutional, and personality variables. As can be seen in Table 7.1, relatively few risk variables have been found to predict full syndrome eating disorders. In a series of community-based case control studies, Fairburn and colleagues (1997, 1998, 2000) found that several risk factors differentiated those with anorexia nervosa or bulimia nervosa from comparison subjects. However, only two factors distinguished the AN cases from the psychiatric control cases: negative self-evaluation and perfectionism. Similarly, for the BN cases, only obesity risk and high parental expectations significantly differentiated eating disorder cases from the psychiatric control group.

As pointed out by Striegel-Moore and Cachelin (2001), because of the relatively low base rate of eating disorders, all of the published prospective studies of risk factors have used disordered eating or subthreshold eating disorders as the outcome variable. However, because the relationship between sub- and full-threshold eating disorders appears to be fairly strong (Crow et al., 2002), these prospective studies are useful for our emerging understanding of risk factors. Furthermore, such studies represent the most methodologically sound means by which to answer the question "does variable X lead to outcome Y?" Based on their review, Striegel-Moore and Cachelin (2001) concluded that "prospective studies have found support for the role of body image dissatisfaction and dieting in the development of disordered eating" (p. 655). Thus, we now summarize the studies that illustrate the risk conferred by these predictors.

169

Table 7.1 Risk factor variables (by domain) and corresponding study design(s)

Risk domain	Type of eating disorder	Type of study design
Demographic Characteristics		
Sex	AN, BN	Survey; family study; twin study
Age	AN, BN	Survey
Birth cohort	BN	Survey; prospective cohort
Parental socioeconomic status	AN, BN	Survey; twin study
Sociocultural context		
Acculturation	m.s.	Survey
Familial interpersonal and context		
Frequent house moves	n.s.	Case-control
Inadequate parenting	AN, BN, BED	Case-control
Parental psychopathology	BN	Family studies; case-control
Abuse (sexual, physical)	AN, BN, BED	Case-control; survey
Conflicted relationships with parents	DE	Prospective cohort
Parental high expectations	BN	Case-control
Parental concern with weight/eating	AN, BN, BED	Case-control
Familial eating disorders	AN, BN, BED	Family studies; twin studies; case-control
Parental obesity	BN	Case-control
No close friends	AN, BN	Case-control
Bullied by other children	BN, BED	Case-control
Constitutional vulnerability		
Premature birth	AN	Twin studies
Severe health problems	AN, BN	Case-control
Childhood obesity/body fat	AN, BN, BED	Case-control; prospective study
Early onset of menarche	BN, DE	Case-control; prospective study
Pregnancy (prior to onset)	BN, BED	Case-control
Perfectionism	AN, BN, BED	Case-control; prospective study
Personal vulnerability		
Psychopathology	AN, BN, BED	Case-control; prospective study
Negative affectivity	BN, BED	Case-control; prospective study
Social self-disturbance	BN	Case-control; prospective study
Low self-esteem	AN, BN, BED	Case-control; prospective study
Internalized thin ideal	DE	Prospective study
Body image concerns	DE	Case-control; prospective study
Dieting	DE	Prospective study

Source: Reprinted by permission of Sage Publications Inc., from Striegel-Moore and Cachelin (2001).
Note: AN = anorexia nervosa; BN = bulimia nervosa; BED = binge eating disorder;
DE = disordered eating; m.s. = mixed support; n.s. = not significant.

Body image is a multidimensional concept that includes how one thinks and feels about one's physical self (Cash and Deagle, 1997). Body dissatisfaction, an aspect of body image, refers to a perceived discomfort with one's body or appearance, or with a specific feature of the body, such as face, weight or shape. Body dissatisfaction is often not recognized as a serious risk factor but rather as a state of "normative discontent" that many people experience at some point in their lives (Rodin et al., 1984). Studies with adolescents conducted since the mid 1990s have consistently shown that up to 30 percent of boys and 60 percent of girls in the United States are dissatisfied with their bodies, for example, girls prefer to be thinner and boys prefer to be broader (Fisher et al., 1995; Schur et al., 2000). In a large epidemiological study, Field and her colleagues (1999a) found that 59 percent of fifth to twelfth grade girls reported body dissatisfaction.

Stice and Shaw (2002) reviewed the literature examining body dissatisfaction as a risk factor for eating pathology and found "mounting evidence" for this association. Highlighted are prospective studies in which body dissatisfaction was found to predict increases in eating disorder symptoms generally (Graber et al., 1994; Stice, 2001; Wertheim et al., 2001), as well as bulimic symptoms (e.g., vomiting and laxative abuse) (Field et al., 1999a; Stice and Agras, 1998; Stice et al., 2002) and full and partial diagnoses of bulimia nervosa (Killen et al., 1994, 1996). Stice and colleagues (Stice and Agras, 1998; Stice et al., 2001) also reported that body dissatisfaction predicted the onset of dieting in adolescent girls over and above the effects of other risk factors, including actual body mass, and concluded, "body dissatisfaction has emerged as one of the most robust risk factors for eating disturbances" (Stice, 2001, p. 55). Stice and Shaw (2002) further point out that dieting mediates the relationship between body dissatisfaction and eating pathology, as evidenced by studies finding that body dissatisfaction predicts dieting, and also that dieting has been shown to be associated prospectively with various forms of bulimic symptoms as well as the onset of eating disorders (Field et al., 1999b; Killen et al., 1994, 1996; Stice, 2001; Stice and Shaw, 2003).

Although it seems that both body dissatisfaction and dieting are important risk factors for eating disorders, risk factor research has been hampered by both methodological and conceptual difficulties. To advance the field, large-scale prospective studies are needed from childhood through young adulthood that assess full syndrome eating disorders. Moreover, research attempting to identify protective factors that contribute to risk resistance is lacking and would be welcomed, particularly with pre-adolescent samples.

Prevention

The prevention of eating disorders has been the focus of a growing literature (for excellent discussions of prevention in eating disorders, see Levine and Piran, 2001; Levine and Smolak, in press; Stice and Shaw, in press). The majority of published prevention programs are school-based universal approaches; however, the results of these studies have been to primarily affect knowledge, and to some extent attitudes (Levine and Piran, 2001). The limited findings from prevention interventions suggest that programs may need to be longer, more intensive, or include booster sessions. In addition, programs that target those at risk or those with early signs of eating disorders are needed; however, to our knowledge, none have yet been conducted with adolescents.

Several promising programs can be highlighted. A prevention-based curriculum geared toward both girls and boys that uses the basic principles of social cognitive theory is called "Everybody's Different" (O'Dea and Abraham, 2000). This program uses a self-esteem model to improve body image by enhancing student learning, behaviors, attitudes and skill development (O'Dea, 1995). Results indicated an improvement in body satisfaction and acceptance of normal weight increase in the intervention group, relative to control students, who exhibited significant weight decreases (O'Dea and Abraham, 2000). Additionally, this program also had a significant positive effect on students who were considered at risk for future eating disorders (i.e., high trait anxiety and low self-esteem), though it was designed as a universal, not a selected prevention program. A second program was integrated into a Girl Scouts group in an effort to prevent the development of disordered eating among preadolescent girls (Neumark-Sztainer et al., 2000). The program consisted of six 90-minute sessions that focused on both media literacy and advocacy skills. Although there were changes on media-related attitudes and behaviors, these were not maintained at three-month follow-up. Significant changes did not occur for dieting behaviors, but the data were in the predicted direction.

A "model" universal prevention program would include a number of components. First, in order to be a true preventive intervention, all participants would need to be screened for any eating disorder or disordered eating behaviors and excluded if such behaviors were found. The target of the preventive intervention should be clear. Although most studies purport to "prevent eating disorders," in fact most focus on the prevention of risk factors for the development of eating disorders. Stice and Shaw (2002) pointed out that successful prevention programs tend to be those that are focused on one risk factor, such as body dissatisfaction or media literacy, rather than an all-encompassing program.

It appears that information-giving classroom-style interventions have not, on the whole, been effective in changing behaviors. Future research should be directed toward developing and evaluating a wider array of preventive interventions. Specifically, researchers should develop innovative programs that are both creative and empirical, building on current research through revisions that address the weaknesses of published studies. Promising areas of research include the addition of multimedia technology (Winzelberg et al., 2000), the use of booster sessions (Varnado-Sullivan et al., 2001), and a focus on broad-based factors such as the development of self-esteem (O'Dea and Abraham, 2000). Learning from prevention interventions in other areas of adolescent health, such as tobacco and substance use, would be a positive innovation (Pearson et al., 2002). Thus, there is a pressing need for a time-effective delivery system of prevention that: (1) incorporates key features of empirically based risk factor research; (2) is developmentally appropriate;

(3) accounts for individual differences in risk; (4) tailors prevention information to students' characteristics; (5) is innovative so as to engage participants' attention, and (6) is cost effective and easy to administer in school and community settings.

Furthermore, finding the optimal match between level of risk and target for prevention is an important goal (Franko and Orosan-Weine, 1998). For example, early universal and selective prevention programs, aimed at increasing knowledge, are ideally targeted at younger individuals with nonsymptom risk factors (e.g., personality and psychological variables such as low self-esteem, perfectionism, and negative emotionality). Alternatively, indicated prevention programs aimed at normalizing eating, increasing coping skills, and changing subgroup norms are most suited for individuals with minimal, but detectable levels of symptoms (e.g., excessive dieting, internalization of the thin ideal). While it is difficult to develop and implement programs to prevent eating disorders when it is not yet clearly understood who is at risk or precisely how to intervene, the exchange of information between risk researchers and prevention researchers will, over time, illuminate the mechanisms by which preventive interventions can be most effectively developed.

Treatment

In its consensus statement, the Anorexia Nervosa Treatment Work Group (Agras et al., 2004) concluded that efficacy studies based on adolescent patients are almost non-existent in anorexia nervosa and bulimia nervosa. Consequently, current practice guidelines of organizations such as the American Psychiatric Association (2000), the Society for Adolescent Medicine (Golden et al., 2003), and the American Academy of Pediatrics (2003) are based on outcomes of randomized clinical trials with adults and the clinical experience of those working with adolescent patients. For example, a review of controlled treatment trials of individuals under 18 years of age found no studies on bulimia nervosa (Weisz and Hawley, 2002). Hence, clinical practice guidelines for adolescents rest on scant empirical evidence.

Experts further note that when treating adolescents, adaptations of treatments developed in adults need to be adjusted to accommodate several considerations. One, physical maturation is not yet complete in adolescent patients and variables such as immature neurotransmitter systems, rapid hepatic metabolism, and shifting hormone levels require specific data on the appropriate dosing in particular and overall safety of medications in adolescents. Two, although motivation to engage in treatment may be lacking among some adult patients as well, for adolescents issues of motivation to engage in treatment may be particularly challenging. Treasure et al. (1999) have described how to adapt Motivational Enhancement Therapy for the treatment of eating disorder patients. Vitousek et al. (1998) have discussed how CBT might be particularly well suited for the treatment of adolescents partly because this form of treatment makes no a priori assumption that the patient is committed to change and has specific strategies (e.g., decisional analysis; a collaborative therapeutic style) inherently conducive to enhancing motivation and overcoming resistance to change (see also Kazdin, 2003). Three, treatments for adolescents need to be tailored to their level of cognitive processing. Some have suggested that the more concrete thinking especially of young adolescents may make cognitive interventions less suitable for this age group than for adults (Weisz and Hawley, 2002). However, even among adults there is a range of responses to the cognitive techniques; CBT is to be implemented with some flexibility in any case and more behavioral procedures may be emphasized when cognitive techniques are thought to be less appropriate (Wilson et al., 1997). Recent iterations of CBT for eating disorders proscribe considerable flexibility in the implementation of CBT so that the particular strategies chosen for a given patient complement the person's cognitive capacity and behavioral skill level (Fairburn et al., 2003). Finally, the adolescent patient is dependent on her family (Kazdin, 2003) and more responsive to her immediate social context than is the case for adults and treatments need to consider this reality. For example, Weisz and Hawley (2002) have discussed in detail how "authoritative parenting" may enhance adolescent psychological adjustment. An adaptation of treatments that have proven effective in studies of adults thus may need to involve the adolescent's parent.

Expert consensus calls for a multidisciplinary, multimodal approach to the treatment of adolescent patients with an eating disorder, but it is unclear which disciplines need to be involved in the management of these disorders or how many components of a "multimodal" approach are essential.

Treatment of anorexia nervosa

Efficacy studies of anorexia nervosa are limited in several respects: only a handful of randomized clinical trials have been published to date, those studies have involved very small samples, assessment of outcome has relied upon unstandardized measures, the experimental treatment typically has been compared to treatments that lack credibility or are insufficiently different to permit clear conclusions about the efficacy of the treatment under study, and long-term outcome has not been determined. No study has included a delayed treatment condition, leaving unanswered the question of how much positive change might have occurred in the absence of any treatment.

What, then, are the modalities to be incorporated into the treatment of anorexia nervosa? Experts agree that refeeding is a key component to the treatment of anorexia nervosa. How this goal is best accomplished is less well agreed upon. Pike et al. (2003) found that nutritional therapy alone is not adequate in treating patients referred to a tertiary treatment center. In the absence of data concerning the efficacy of pharmacological treatments in adolescent patients, studies of adults need to be considered. To date, medication treatment has proven to produce disappointing results, despite the fact that a broad array of pharmacological approaches has been tried: antidepressants, mood stabilizers, anxiolytics, anticonvulsants, and antipsychotic drugs have been reported to be of little help in the effort to restore weight and improve dysfunctional body image in anorexia nervosa (Agras et al., 2004). There is some evidence that the malnourished state may interfere with the therapeutic action of Selective Serotonin Reuptake Inhibitors (SSRIs) (Attia et al., 1998) and that antidepressant medications such as SSRIs may be effective in reducing the risk of relapse when administered to weight restored patients (Kaye et al., 2001).

Despite the scant evidence, family therapy widely is considered the treatment of choice for adolescent anorexia nervosa (National Institute for Clinical Excellence, 2004). However, if experience based on clinical trials with adolescents suffering from other mental disorders (e.g., depressive or anxiety disorders) is any guide, other forms of treatment (e.g., cognitive behavior therapy) may prove efficacious in the treatment of anorexia nervosa.

Treatment of bulimia nervosa

As was true for studies of anorexia nervosa, few investigations of treatment for bulimia nervosa have utilized adolescent samples (Whittal et al., 1999). The main treatments that have been discussed, though primarily in theoretical terms, are cognitive behavior therapy, psychopharmacological interventions (particularly selective serotonin reuptake inhibitors), and most recently, family therapy (Phillips et al., 2003).

According to the guidelines set forth by the UK National Institute for Clinical Excellence (2004), older adolescents with bulimia nervosa can be treated using an adapted and developmentally appropriate version of cognitive behavior therapy. The authors suggest that the course of treatment should be 16–20 individual sessions over a period of 4 to 5 months. Furthermore, they find that the exception to this recommendation would be those bulimic patients with severe comorbidity or developmental problems "of a type that will interfere" with the benefits of CBT. Thus there is a need to design and test developmentally appropriate CBT protocols for adolescents with bulimia nervosa.

Psychopharmacologic treatments for bulimia nervosa have centered on the use of antidepressants (Zhu and Walsh, 2002). A review of the literature (Kotler and Walsh, 2000) concluded that evidence indicates that almost all classes of antidepressants are effective in the short-term treatment of bulimia nervosa in adolescents. However, it is noted that most studies have been conducted with adults, leaving open the question of whether results will generalize to adolescent samples. Kotler et al. (2003) conducted an open trial using fluoxetine with 10 adolescents (ages 12–18) diagnosed with bulimia nervosa. Each patient received 8 weeks of fluoxetine (60 mg/day) in conjunction with supportive psychotherapy. Results showed significant decreases in both weekly binge eating and purging behaviors and all subjects tolerated the dose and completed the trial. Overall, 20 percent were rated as much improved, 50 percent as improved, and 30 percent as slightly improved. Clearly additional double blind placebo controlled randomized trials are needed, with explicit attention to dosing, dropout rates, and side effects in adolescent samples.

Family therapy for bulimia nervosa has not yet been subjected to clinical trial (Le Grange et al., 2003); however, such studies are currently underway. Data from a small series of cases have demonstrated that family-based treatment may be of benefit to adolescents with bulimia nervosa (Le Grange et al., 2003). Lock (2002) describes a model for involving parents in CBT, suggesting that parents need to provide motivation, a supportive milieu that will encourage behavior change, and guidance and support to reduce the risk of relapse.

Conclusions

Several key issues have emerged based on this review:

- There is a lack of data on prevalence, treatment, and outcome with adolescent eating disorder samples.
- Studies that examine comorbidity with adolescent eating disorders would be of great clinical value.
- There may be key "curative factors" (e.g., increasing social support) that would be useful targets for both eating disorders and the disorders that are comorbid with them.
- Known risk factors, such as body dissatisfaction and dieting, should be the focus of future prevention trials. Outcomes may be improved by targeting broad-based psychological concerns, such as self-esteem, in prevention efforts.

References

Agras, W.S., Brandt, H.A., Bulik, C.M., Dolan-Sewell, R., Fairburn, C.G., Halmi, K.A., et al. (2004). Report of the National Institutes of Health workshop on overcoming barriers to treatment research in anorexia nervosa. *International Journal of Eating Disorders, 35*, 509–521.

American Academy of Pediatrics (AAP), Committee on Adolescence (2003). Identifying and treating eating disorders. *Pediatrics, 111*, 204–211.

American Psychiatric Association (1994). *Diagnostic and statistical manual of mental disorders*, 4th edn. Washington, DC: APA.

American Psychiatric Association (Work Group on Eating Disorders) (2000). Practice guideline for the treatment of patients with eating disorders (revision). *American Journal of Psychiatry, 157(1 Suppl)*, 1–39.

Attia, E., Haiman, C., Walsh, B.T., and Flater, S.R. (1998). Does fluoxetine augment the inpatient treatment of anorexia nervosa? *American Journal of Psychiatry, 155*, 548–551.

Attie, I. and Brooks-Gunn, J. (1992). Developmental issues in the study of eating problems and disorders. In J.H. Crowther and D.L. Tennenbaum (Eds.), *The etiology of bulimia nervosa: The individual and familial context*. London: Hemisphere.

Brewerton, T.D. (1995). Bulimia in children and adolescents. *Child and Adolescent Psychiatric Clinics of North America, 11*, 237–256.

Bulik, C.M. (2003). Eating disorders in adolescents and young adults. *Child and Adolescent Psychiatric Clinics of North America, 11*, 201–218.

Bulik, C.M., Sullivan, P.F., McKee, M., Weltzin, T.E., and Kaye, W.H. (1994). Characteristics of bulimic women with and without alcohol abuse. *American Journal of Drug and Alcohol Abuse, 20*, 273–283.

Bulik, C.M., Sullivan, P.F., Joyce, P.R., Carter, F.A., and McIntosh, V.V. (1998). Predictors of 1-year treatment outcome in bulimia nervosa. *Comprehensive Psychiatry*, *39*, 206–214.

Carlat, D.J., Camargo, C.A., and Herzog, D.B. (1997). Eating disorders in males: A report on 135 patients. *American Journal of Psychiatry*, *154*, 1127–1132.

Cash, T. and Deagle, E.A. (1997). The nature and extent of body-image disturbances in anorexia nervosa and bulimia nervosa: A meta-analysis. *International Journal of Eating Disorders*, *22*, 107–125.

Crow, S.J., Mussell, M.P., Peterson, C., Knopke, A., and Mitchell, J.E. (1999). Prior treatment received by patients with bulimia nervosa. *International Journal of Eating Disorders*, *25*, 39–44.

Crow, S.J., Agras, W.S., Halmi, K., Mitchell, J.E., and Kraemer, H.C. (2002). Full syndromal versus subthreshold anorexia nervosa, bulimia nervosa, and binge eating disorder: A multicenter study. *International Journal of Eating Disorders*, *32*, 309–318.

Eddy, K.T., Keel, P.K., Dorer, D.J., Delinsky, S.S., Franko, D.L., and Herzog, D.B. (2002). Longitudinal comparison of anorexia nervosa subtypes. *International Journal of Eating Disorders*, *31*, 191–201.

Emerson, E. (2003). Prevalence of psychiatric disorders in children and adolescents with and without intellectual disability. *Journal of Intellectual Disability Research*, *47*, 51–58.

Evans, D.L., Foa, E.B., Gur, G.R., Hendin, H., O'Brien, C.P., Seligman, M.E.P., et al. (Eds.) (2005). *Treating and preventing adolescent mental health disorders: What we know and what we don't know.* New York: Oxford University Press, Annenberg Foundation Trust at Sunnylands, and Annenberg Public Policy Centre, University of Pennsylvania, PA.

Fairburn, C.G., Welch, S.L., Doll, H.A., Davies, B.A., and O'Connor, M.E. (1997). Risk factors for bulimia nervosa: A community-based case-control study. *Archives of General Psychiatry*, *54*, 509–517.

Fairburn, C.G., Doll, H.A., Welch, S.L., Hay, P.J., Davies, B.A., and O'Connor, M.E. (1998). Risk factors for binge eating disorder: A community-based, case-control study. *Archives of General Psychiatry*, *55*, 425–432.

Fairburn, C.G., Cooper, Z., Doll, H.A., Norman, P., and O'Connor, M. (2000). The natural course of bulimia nervosa and binge eating disorder in young women. *Archives of General Psychiatry*, *57*, 659–665.

Fairburn, C.G., Cooper, Z., and Shafran, R. (2003). Cognitive behaviour therapy for eating disorders: A transdiagnostic theory and treatment. *Behaviour Research and Therapy*, *41*, 509–528.

Fichter, M. and Quadflieg, N. (1997). Six-year course of bulimia nervosa. *International Journal of Eating Disorders*, *22*, 361–384.

Fichter, M.M., Quadflieg, N., and Rief, W. (1994). Course of multi-impulsive bulimia. *Psychological Medicine*, *24*, 591–604.

Field, A.E., Camargo, C.A. Jr., Taylor, C.B., Berkey, C.S., Frazier, A.L., Gillman, M.W., et al. (1999a). Overweight, weight concerns, and bulimic behaviors among girls and boys. *Journal of the American Academy of Child and Adolescent Psychiatry*, *38*, 754–760.

Field, A.E., Camargo, C.A. Jr., Taylor, C.B., Berkey, C.S., and Colditz, G.A. (1999b). Relation of peer and media influences to the development of purging behaviors among preadolescent and adolescent girls. *Archives of Pediatric and Adolescent Medicine*, *153*, 1184–1189.

Fisher, M. (2003). The course and outcome of eating disorders in adults and in adolescents. *Adolescent Medicine, 14*, 149–158.

Fisher, M., Golden, N.H., Katzman, D.K., Kreipe, R.E., Rees, J., Schebendach, J., et al. (1995). Eating disorders in adolescents: A background paper. *Journal of Adolescent Health, 16*, 420–437.

Fisher, M., Schneider, M., Burns, J., Symons, H., and Mandel, F.S. (2001). Differences between adolescents and young adults at presentation to an eating disorders program. *Journal of Adolescent Health, 28*, 222–227.

Franko, D.L. and Orosan-Weine, P. (1998). Prevention of eating disorders: Empirical, methodological, and conceptual considerations. *Clinical Psychology: Science and Practice, 5*, 459–477.

Garfinkel, P.E., Kennedy, S.H., and Kaplan, A.S. (1995). Views on classification and diagnosis of eating disorders. *Canadian Journal of Psychiatry, 40*, 445–456.

Golden, N.H., Katzman, D.K., Kreipe, R.E., Stevens, S.L., Sawyer, S.M., Rees, J., et al. (2003). Eating disorders in adolescents: Position paper of the Society for Adolescent Medicine. *Journal of Adolescent Health, 33*, 496–503.

Graber, J.A., Brooks-Gunn, J., Paikoff, R.L., and Warren, M.P. (1994). Prediction of eating problems: An 8-year study of adolescent girls. *Developmental Psychology, 30*, 823–834.

Graber, J.A., Tyrka, A.R., and Brooks-Gunn, J. (2003). How similar are correlates of different subclinical eating problems and bulimia nervosa? *Journal of Child Psychology and Psychiatry, 44*, 262–273.

Halmi, K.A., Stewart, A., Mitchell, J., Wilson, T., Crow, S., Bryson, S.W., et al. (2002). Relapse predictors of patients with bulimia nervosa who achieved abstinence through cognitive behavioral therapy. *Archives of General Psychiatry, 59*, 1105–1109.

Herpertz-Dahlmann, B., Muller, B., Herpertz, S., Heussen, N., Hebebrand, J., and Remschmidt, H. (2001). Prospective 10-year follow-up in adolescent anorexia nervosa: Course, outcome, psychiatric comorbidity, and psychosocial adaptation. *Journal of Child Psychology and Psychiatry and Allied Disciplines, 42*, 603–662.

Herzog, D.B., Nussbaum, K.M., and Marmor, A.K. (1996). Comorbidity and outcome in eating disorders. *Psychiatric Clinics of North America, 19*, 843–859.

Herzog, D.B., Dorer, D.J., Keel, P.K., Selwyn, S.E., Ekeblad, E.R., and Flores, A.T. (1999). Recovery and relapse in anorexia and bulimia nervosa: A 7.5-year follow-up study. *Journal of the American Academy of Child and Adolescent Psychiatry, 38*, 829–837.

Herzog, D.B., Keller, M.B., Sacks, N.R., Yeh, C.J., and Lavori, P.W. (1992). Psychiatric comorbidity in treatment-seeking anorexics and bulimics. *Journal of American Academy of Child and Adolescent Psychiatry, 31*, 810–818.

Jacobi, C., Hayward, C., de Zwaan, M., Kraemer, H.C., and Agras, W.S. (2004). Coming to terms with risk factors for eating disorders: Application of risk terminology and suggestions for a general taxonomy. *Psychological Bulletin, 130*, 19–65.

Johnson, J.G., Cohen, P., Kasen, S., and Brook, J.S. (2002a). Eating disorders during adolescence and the risk for physical and mental disorders during early adulthood. *Archives of General Psychiatry, 59*, 545–552.

Johnson, J.G., Cohen, P., Kotler, L., Kasen, S., and Brook, J.S. (2002b). Psychiatric disorders associated with risk for the development of eating disorders during adolescence and early adulthood. *Journal of Consulting and Clinical Psychology, 70*, 1119–1128.

Kassett, J.A., Gwirtsman, H.E., Kaye, W.H., Brandt, H.A. and Jimerson, D.C. (1988). Pattern of onset of bulimic symptoms in anorexia nervosa. *American Journal of Psychiatry, 145*, 1287–1288.

Kaye, W.H., Nagata, T., Weltzin, T.E., Hsu, L.K.G., Sokol, M.S., McConaha, C., et al. (2001). Double-blind placebo-controlled administration of fluoxetine in restricting- and restricting-purging type anorexia nervosa. *Biological Psychiatry, 49*, 644–652.

Kazdin, A.E. (2003). Psychotherapy for children and adolescents. *Annual Review of Psychology, 54*, 253–276.

Keel, P.K., Mitchell, J.E., Miller, K.B., Davis, T.L., and Crow, S.J. (1999). Long-term outcome of bulimia nervosa. *Archives of General Psychiatry, 56*, 63–69.

Keel, P.K., Dorer, D.J., Eddy, K.T., Franko, D., Charatan, D.L., and Herzog, D.B. (2003). Predictors of mortality in eating disorders. *Archives of General Psychiatry, 60*, 179–183.

Kendler, K.S., MacLean, C., Neale, M., Kessler, R., Heath, A., and Eaves, L. (1991). The genetic epidemiology of bulimia nervosa. *American Journal of Psychiatry, 148*, 1627–1637.

Killen, J.D., Hayward, C., Wilson, D.M., Taylor, C.B., Hammer, L.D., Litt, I., et al. (1994). Factors associated with eating disorder symptoms in a community sample of 6th and 7th grade girls. *International Journal of Eating Disorders, 15*, 357–367.

Killen, J.D., Taylor, C.B., Hayward, C., Haydel, K.F., Wilson, D.M., Hammer, L., et al. (1996). Weight concerns influence the development of eating disorders: A 4-year prospective study. *Journal of Consulting and Clinical Psychology, 64*, 936–940.

Kotler, L.A. and Walsh, B.T. (2000). Eating disorders in children and adolescents: Pharmacological therapies. *European Child and Adolescent Psychiatry, 9 (Suppl. 5)*, I108–I116.

Kotler, L.A., Cohen, P., Davies, M., Pine, D.S., and Walsh, B.T. (2001). Longitudinal relationships between childhood, adolescent, and adult eating disorders. *Journal of the American Academy of Child and Adolescent Psychiatry, 40*, 1434–1440.

Kotler, L.A., Devlin, M.J., Davies, M., and Walsh, B.T. (2003). An open trial of fluoxetine for adolescents with bulimia nervosa. *Journal of Child and Adolescent Psychopharmacology, 13*, 329–335.

Kraemer, H.C., Kazdin, A.E., Offord, D.R., Kessler, R.C., Jensen, P.S., and Kupfer, D.J. (1997). Coming to terms with the terms of risk. *Archives of General Psychiatry, 54*, 337–343.

Le Grange, D. and Lock, J. (2002). Bulimia nervosa in adolescents: Treatment, eating pathology and comorbidity. *South African Psychiatry Review, 5*, 19–22, 24–25.

Le Grange, D., Lock, J., and Dymek, M. (2003). Family-based therapy for adolescents with bulimia nervosa. *American Journal of Psychotherapy, 57*, 237–251.

Levine, M.P. and Piran, N. (2001). The prevention of eating disorders: Towards a participatory ecology of knowledge, action, and advocacy. In R. Striegel-Moore and L. Smolak (Eds.), *Eating disorders: New directions for research and practice*. Washington, DC: American Psychological Association.

Levine, M.P. and Smolak, L. (in press). Primary prevention of body image disturbance and disordered eating in childhood and early adolescence. In J.K. Thompson and L. Smolak (Eds.), *Body image, eating disorders, and obesity in childhood and adolescence*. Washington, DC: American Psychological Association.

Lewinsohn, P.M., Hops, H., Roberts, R.E., Seeley, J.R., and Andrews, J.A. (1993). Adolescent psychopathology: I. Prevalence and incidence of depression and other

DSM-III-R disorders in high school students. *Journal of Abnormal Psychology, 102,* 133–144.

Lewinsohn, P.M., Striegel-Moore, R.H., and Seeley, J.R. (2000). Epidemiology and natural course of eating disorders in young women from adolescence to young adulthood. *Journal of the American Academy of Child and Adolescent Psychiatry, 39,* 1284–1292.

Lock, J. (2002). Treating adolescents with eating disroders in the family context: Empical and theoretical considerations. *Child and Adolescent Psychiatric Clinics of North America, 11,* 331–342.

McKnight Investigators (2003). Risk factors for the onset of eating disorders in adolescent girls: Results of the McKnight longitudinal risk factor study. *American Journal of Psychiatry, 160,* 248–254.

Mitchell, J.E., Specker, S.M., and de Zwaan, M. (1991). Comorbidity and medical complications of bulimia nervosa. *Journal of Clinical Psychiatry, 52,* 13–20.

Muise, A.M., Stein, D.G., and Arbess, G. (2003). Eating disorders in adolescent boys: a review of the adolescent and young adult literature. *Journal of Adolescent Health, 33,* 427–435.

Nagata, T., Kawarada, Y., Kiriike, N., and Iketani, T. (2000). Multi-impulsivity of Japanese patients with eating disorders: primary and secondary impulsivity. *Psychiatric Research, 94,* 239–250.

National Institute for Clinical Excellence (NICE) (2004). *Eating disorders: Core interventions in the treatment and management of eating disorders in primary and secondary care.* London: NICE.

Neumark-Sztainer, D., Sherwood, N.E., Coller, T., and Hannan, P.J. (2000). Primary prevention of disordered eating among preadolescent girls: Feasibility and short-term effect of a community-based intervention. *Journal of the American Dietetic Association, 100,* 1466–1473.

Newman, D.L., Moffitt, T.E., Caspi, A., Magdol, L., Silva, P.A., and Stanton, W.R. (1996). Psychiatric disorder in a birth cohort of young adults: Prevalence, comorbidity, clinical significance, and new case incidence from ages 11 to 21. *Journal of Consulting and Clinical Psychology, 64,* 552–562.

O'Dea, J.A. (1995). *Everybody's different: A self-esteem program for young adolescents.* Sydney: University of Sydney Press.

O'Dea, J.A. and Abraham, S. (2000). Improving the body image, eating attitudes and behaviors of young male and female adolescents: A new educational approach which focuses on self-esteem. *International Journal of Eating Disorders, 28,* 43–57.

Patton, G.C. (1988). Mortality in eating disorders. *Psychological Medicine, 18,* 947–951.

Patton, G.C., Selzer, R., Coffey, C., Carlin, J.B., and Wolfe, R. (1999). Onset of adolescent eating disorders: population based cohort study over 3 years. *British Medical Journal, 20,* 765–768.

Patton, G.C., Coffey, C., and Sawyer, S.M. (2003). The outcome of adolescent eating disorders: Findings from the Victorian adolescent health cohort study. *European Child and Adolescent Psychiatry, 12,* 25–29.

Pearson, J., Goldklang, D., and Striegel-Moore, R.H. (2002). Prevention of eating disorders: challenges and opportunities. *International Journal of Eating Disorders, 31,* 233–239.

Phillips, E.L., Greydanus, D.E., Pratt, H.D., and Patel, D.R. (2003). Treatment of bulimia nervosa: Psychological and psychopharmacologic considerations. *Journal of Adolescent Research, 18,* 261–279.

Pike, K.M., Walsh, B.T., Vitousek, K., Wilson, G.T., and Bauer, J. (2003). Cognitive behavior therapy in the posthospitalization treatment of anorexia nervosa. *American Journal of Psychiatry, 160,* 2046–2049.

Rathner, G. and Messner, K. (1993). Detection of eating disorders in a small rural town: An epidemiological study. *Psychological Medicine, 23,* 175–184.

Rodin, J., Silberstein, L., and Striegel-Moore, R.H. (1984). Women and weight: A normative discontent. *Nebraska Symposium on Motivation, 32,* 267–307.

Rome, E.S., Ammerman, S., Rosen, D.S., Keller, R.J., Lock, J., Mammel, K.A., et al. (2003). Children and adolescents with eating disorders: The state of the art. *Pediatrics, 111,* e98–e108.

Rosenvinge, J.H., Borgen, J.S., and Boerresen, R. (1999). The prevalence and psychological correlates of anorexia nervosa, bulimia nervosa and binge eating among 15-yr-old students: A controlled epidemiological study. *European Eating Disorders Review, 7,* 382–391.

Santonastaso, P., Zanetti, T., Sala, A., and Favaretto, G. (1996). Prevalence of eating disorders in Italy: A survey on a sample of 16-year-old female students. *Psychotherapy and Psychosomatics, 65,* 158–162.

Schur, E.A., Sanders, M., and Steiner, H. (2000). Body dissatisfaction and dieting in young children. *International Journal of Eating Disorders, 27,* 74–78.

Steiner, H., Kwan, W., Shaffer, T.G., Walker, S., Miller, S., Sagar, A., et al. (2003). Risk and protective factors for juvenile eating disorders. *European Child and Adolescent Psychiatry, 12* (Suppl), I38–I46.

Steinhausen, H.C. (1997). Outcome of anorexia nervosa in the younger patient. *Journal of Child Psychology and Psychiatry and Allied Disciplines, 38,* 271–276.

Steinhausen, H.C. (2002). The outcome in anorexia nervosa in the 20th century. *American Journal of Psychiatry, 159,* 1284–1293.

Steinhausen, H.C., Winkler, C., and Meier, M. (1997). Eating disorders in adolescence in a Swiss epidemiological study. *International Journal of Eating Disorders, 22,* 147–151.

Steinhausen, H.C., Seidel, R., and Winkler Metzke, C. (2000). Evaluation of treatment and intermediate and long-term outcome of adolescent eating disorders. *Psychological Medicine, 30,* 1089–1098.

Steinhausen, H.C., Boyadjieva, S., Griogoroiu-Serbanescu, M., and Neumarker, K.J. (2003). The outcome of adolescent eating disorders: Findings from an international collaborative study. *European Child and Adolescent Psychiatry, 12 (Suppl 1),* I91–I98.

Stice, E. (2001). Risk factors for eating pathology: Resent advances and future directions. In R.H. Striegel-Moore & L. Smolak (Eds.), *Eating Disorders: Innovative Directions for Research and Practice* (pp. 51–73). Washington, DC: American Psychological Association.

Stice, E. and Agras, W.S. (1998). Predicting onset and cessation of bulimic behaviors during adolescence: A longitudinal groups analysis. *Behavior Therapy, 29,* 257–276.

Stice, E. and Shaw, H. (2002). Role of body dissatisfaction in the onset and maintenance of eating pathology: A synthesis of research findings. *Journal of Psychosomatic Research, 53,* 985–993.

Stice, E. and Shaw, H. (2003). Prospective relations of body image, eating, and affective disturbances to smoking onset in adolescent girls: How Virginia slims. *Journal of Consulting and Clinical Psychology, 71,* 129–135.

Stice, E. and Shaw, H. (in press). Eating disorder prevention programs: A meta-analytic review. *Psychological Bulletin.*

Stice, E., Presnell, K., and Bearman, S.K. (2001). Relation of early menarche to depression, eating disorders, substance abuse, and comorbid psychopathology among adolescent girls. *Developmental Psychology*, *37*, 608–619.

Stice, E., Presnell, K., and Spangler, D. (2002). Risk factors for binge eating onset: A prospective investigation. *Health Psychology*, *21*, 131–138.

Stock, S.L., Goldberg, E., Corbett, S., and Katzman, D.K. (2002). Substance use in female adolescents with eating disorders. *Journal of Adolescent Health*, *31*, 176–182.

Striegel-Moore, R.H. and Cachelin, F.M. (2001). Etiology of eating disorders in women. *Counseling Psychologist*, *29*, 635–661.

Striegel-Moore, R.H. and Marcus, M. (1995). Eating disorders in women: Current issues and debate. In A. Stanton and S.J. Gallant (Eds.), *The psychology of women's health: Progress and challenges in research and application*. Washington, DC: American Psychological Association.

Striegel-Moore, R.H., Cachelin, F.M., Dohm, F.A., Pike, K.M., Wilfley, D.E., and Fairburn, C.G. (2001). Comparison of binge eating disorder and bulimia nervosa in a community sample. *International Journal of Eating Disorders*, *29*, 157–165.

Strober, M., Freeman, R., and Morrell, W. (1997). The long-term course of severe anorexia nervosa in adolescents: Survival analysis of recovery, relapse, and outcome predictors over 10–15 years in a prospective study. *International Journal of Eating Disorders*, *22*, 339–360.

Sullivan, P.F. (1995). Mortality in anorexia nervosa. *American Journal of Psychiatry*, *152*, 1073–1074.

Treasure, J.L., Katzman, M., Schmidt, U., Troop, N., Todd, G., and de Silva, P. (1999). Engagement and outcome in the treatment of bulimia nervosa: First phase of a sequential design comparing motivation enhancement therapy and cognitive behavioural therapy. *Behavior Research and Therapy*, *37*, 405–418.

Varnado-Sullivan, P.J., Zucker, N., Williamson, D.A., Reas, D., Thaw, J., and Netemeyer, S.B. (2001). Development and implementation of the Body Logic Program for adolescents: A two-stage prevention program for eating disorders. *Cognitive and Behavioral Practice*, *8*, 248–259.

Verhulst, F.C., van der Ende, J., Ferdinand, R.F., and Kasius, M.C. (1997). The prevalence of DSM-III-R diagnoses in a national sample of Dutch adolescents. *Archives of General Psychiatry*, *54*, 329–336.

Vitousek, K., Watson, S., and Wilson, G.T. (1998). Enhancing motivation for change in treatment-resistant eating disorders. *Clinical Psychology Review*, *18*, 391–420.

von Ranson, K.M., Kaye, W.H., Weltzin, T.E., Rao, R., and Matsunaga, H. (1999). Obsessive-compulsive disorder symptoms before and after recovery from bulimia nervosa. *American Journal of Psychiatry*, *156*, 1703–1708.

Walters, E.E. and Kendler, K.S. (1995). Anorexia nervosa and anorexic-like syndromes in a population-based female twin sample. *American Journal of Psychiatry*, *152*, 64–71.

Weisz, J.R. and Hawley, K.M. (2002). Developmental factors in the treatment of adolescents. *Journal of Consulting and Clinical Psychology*, *70*, 21–43.

Wentz, E., Gillberg, C., Gillberg, I.C., and Rastam, M. (2001). Ten-year follow-up of adolescent-onset anorexia nervosa: psychiatric disorders and overall functioning scales. *Journal of Child Psychology and Psychiatry and Allied Disciplines*, *42*, 613–622.

Wertheim, E.H., Koerner, J., and Paxton, S.J. (2001). Longitudinal predictors of restrictive eating and bulimic tendencies in three different age groups of adolescent girls. *Journal of Youth and Adolescence*, *30*, 69–81.

Whitaker, A., Johnson, J., Shaffer, D., Rapoport, J.L., Kalikow, K., Walsh, B.T., et al. (1990). Uncommon troubles in young people: Prevalence estimates of selected psychiatric disorders in a nonreferred adolescent population. *Archives of General Psychiatry*, *47*, 487–496.

Whittal, M.L., Agras, W.S., and Gould, R.A. (1999). Bulimia nervosa: A meta-analysis of psychosocial and pharmacological treatments. *Behavior Therapy*, *30*, 117–135.

Wilson, G.T., Fairburn, C.G., and Agras, W.S. (1997). Cognitive-behavioral therapy for bulimia nervosa. In D.M. Garner (Ed). *Handbook of treatment for eating disorders*, 2nd edn (pp. 67–93). New York: Guilford.

Winzelberg, A.J., Eppstein, D., Eldredge, K.L., Wilfley, D., Dasmahapatra, R., Dev, P., et al. (2000). Effectiveness of an Internet-based program for reducing risk factors for eating disorders. *Journal of Consulting and Clinical Psychology*, *68*, 650–657.

Wittchen, H.-U., Nelson, C.B., and Lanchner, G. (1998). Prevalence of mental disorders and psychosocial impairments in adolescents and young adults. *Psychological Medicine*, *28*, 109–126.

Wlodarczyk-Bisaga, K. and Dolan, B. (1996). A two-stage epidemiological study of abnormal eating attitudes and their prospective risk factors in Polish schoolgirls. *Psychological Medicine*, *26*, 1021–1032.

Wolraich, M.L., Felice, M.E., and Drotar, D. (eds) (1996). *The classification of child and adolescent mental diagnosis in primary care: Diagnosis and statistical manual for primary care (DSM-PC) child and adolescent version*. Elk Grove Village, IL: American Academy of Pediatrics.

Wonderlich, S.A. and Mitchell, J.E. (1997). Eating disorders and comorbidity: Empirical, conceptual, and clinical implications. *Eating Disorders Research*, *33*, 381–388.

Zhu, A.J. and Walsh, B.T. (2002). Pharmacologic treatment of eating disorders. *Canadian Journal of Psychiatry*, *47*, 227–234.

183

8

SUBSTANCE USE DISORDERS

Paul Rohde and Judy A. Andrews

The purpose of this chapter is to describe the epidemiology, comorbidity, course and consequences of adolescent substance use and substance use disorders (SUDs). Substance use and abuse in adolescents encompasses using tobacco (primarily cigarettes), drinking alcohol, smoking marijuana, and using other illicit drugs. Although there is a high degree of co-occurrence among the use of substances, with some similarity in causes and consequences, each substance is unique, with a unique developmental trajectory. Wherever possible, our review will look at tobacco, alcohol, cannabis, and hard drug use disorders separately.

Substance use and abuse appear to develop in relatively consistent stages (e.g., Chassin et al., 1985; Flay, 1993) that include initiation (first use), experimentation, progression to regular use, and finally to problematic use, including a diagnosis of psychoactive substance abuse or dependence, followed by maintenance, recovery, or relapse. Our review will focus predominantly on substance use at the diagnostic levels of abuse and dependence, a topic that has received surprisingly little attention.

A major source of data for this review will be the Oregon Adolescent Depression Project (OADP; Lewinsohn et al., 1993), which initially consisted of a cohort of 1709 community adolescents from schools in western Oregon (ages 14–18) who were first assessed (T1) in the mid 1980s on a host of psychosocial and diagnostic measures. Approximately one year later (T2), 1507 participants (88 percent) returned for a re-administration of the interview and questionnaire (mean T1–T2 interval = 13.8 months, *SD* = 2.3). Between 1993 and 1999, all individuals with a history of psychopathology (N = 644) and a randomly selected set of participants with no history of mental disorder (N = 457) were invited to a T3 interview when they turned 24 years of age. T3 data were obtained from 941 individuals (85 percent participation of selected T2 sample). A total of 57 percent of the T3 participants were female, 89 percent were Caucasian, 54 percent had lived with both biological parents at T1, and 45 percent had one or more parents with a college education.

Given that very few community-based studies have examined the use of substances by children younger than 12, we will also report data from the Oregon Youth Substance Use Project (OYSUP; Andrews et al., 2003). This study used a cohort-sequential design wherein 1075 first through fifth grade students from one school district in Western Oregon were assessed at annual intervals over a four year period. An average of 215 students per grade (first through fifth) participated in the study at T1, with an even distribution by gender (50 percent female). The sample was primarily Caucasian (86 percent) and 40 percent of the sample was eligible for free or reduced lunch for low-income families. At T4, the sample size was 1031 (5 percent attrition). T4 participants were comparable to non-participants on all demographic variables and attitudes regarding substance use, intention to use substances, and use of substances.

Adolescent substance use

Substance use in adolescence has been assessed by two extensive national epidemiologic studies of drug use: the *Monitoring the Future* study (MTF; Johnston et al., 2003) and the *National Survey on Drug Use and Health* (NSDUH; Substance Abuse and Mental Health Services Administration, 2003), which was previously called the National Household Survey on Drug Abuse. For the MTF study, more than 43,000 US students in grades 8, 10, and 12 were surveyed in 2002. By twelfth grade, approximately 78 percent of the adolescents had used alcohol, 57 percent had tried smoking cigarettes, and 53 percent had used an illicit drug, most often marijuana (48 percent). Other drugs that were frequently used included inhalants and hallucinogens (12 percent each), tranquilizers (11 percent), and MDMA (10 percent).

For the NSDUH study, 68,126 interviews were completed with residents aged 12 and older of households across the 50 states. The prevalence of current alcohol use increased with age, from 2 percent among 13 year olds to 50 percent at age 21. Current cigarette use also increased from 2 percent at age 12 to 46 percent at age 21. After age 21, rates for both alcohol and cigarette use generally declined. Among youth aged 12 or 13, 4 percent reported current illicit drug use, with illicit use peaking at age 18 to 20 (22 percent) and declining with age. Marijuana was the most prevalent illicit drug.

Definition of substance use disorders

According to DSM-IV criteria (APA, 1994), substance dependence or abuse is a maladaptive pattern of use leading to significant impairment or distress. To meet the criteria for dependence, three or more of the following symptoms must be present: tolerance, withdrawal, more use of the drug than intended, a persistent desire or unsuccessful effort to control use, spending a great deal of time in activities necessary to obtain the substance, and continued use despite recurrent problems associated with use. A diagnosis of substance abuse requires one of the following four symptoms: recurrent use interfering with role obligations at school or home, recurrent use in physically hazardous situations, recurrent substance-related legal problems, and continued use despite recurrent social or interpersonal problems. A diagnosis of abuse is pre-empted by dependence if the individual has ever met the diagnostic criteria for dependence.

Although the specific DSM criteria for dependence and abuse were developed for adults, these criteria are used for both adolescents and adults. However, symptoms may vary depending on whether the user is a child, adolescent or an adult (Newcomb and Bentler, 1989). Compared to adults, adolescents typically use substances in a social context, use more episodically, use greater quantities, and more frequently binge (e.g., Bailey et al., 2000). SUD symptoms may also vary by gender (Haver, 1986; Wagner et al., 2002).

Substance use disorders in adolescence and young adulthood

While large long-term studies have tracked the rates of substance use among adolescents, surprisingly little is known regarding the natural course of SUDs in the general population. Knowledge of the longitudinal course of SUDs is essential to determine the prognosis of these disorders and to understand the continuities and discontinuities between adolescent and adult psychopathology. Although the majority of adolescents who use drugs do not progress to abuse or dependence (Newcomb, 1995), rates of SUDs in adolescents appear to be high. Key findings from the largest and most representative studies of SUD among non-patient samples of adolescents are shown in Table 8.1.

To briefly summarize the pattern of findings from these various projects, adolescence is the primary period of onset for most SUDs. Substance use prior to age 15 very seldom meets diagnostic criteria for abuse or dependence, but rates increase very quickly during the high school and college years, with many of these patterns of problematic use continuing into young adulthood. Daily smoking and nicotine dependence are among the first disorders to develop, emerging around age 16 (in approximately 15 percent of youth). By young adulthood, one-quarter of the population will have developed nicotine dependence. Alcohol use disorders appear in less than 5 percent of the population by age 16, but increase to 10 percent or more by the end of high school and may reach 15–30 percent by young adulthood. Marijuana use disorders also tend to develop after age 15, although rates by the end of high school appear to be between 3 and 14 percent. Unlike alcoholism, rates of marijuana abuse/dependence do not continue to escalate and appear to be about 5 percent among young adults. Hard drug use disorders are rare in adolescents, occurring in 1–4 percent of youth, although they may eventually affect one in ten adults. Contrary to common perceptions, SUDs are not exclusively a problem for men. Young men may have somewhat higher rates of alcohol and cannabis use disorders, but rates of nicotine dependence and most hard drug use disorders are more fairly similar across genders.

Substance use and SUDs in the Oregon samples

Using data from the OADP and OYSUP samples, we next examine the developmental progression of SUDs from adolescence to young adulthood. Issues of initiation, progression, and continuity are examined separately for tobacco, alcohol,

Table 8.1 Major recent epidemiological studies on substance use disorders

Study	Study design	Major findings
National Household Studies (Kandel, 2000)	Used data from 1991–1993 surveys to estimate substance dependence, according to DSM-IV criteria among adolescents.	• 8 percent had alcohol dependence, 20 percent tobacco dependence, 14 percent marijuana dependence, 11 percent cocaine dependence. • Gender differences nonsignificant, except higher cocaine dependence among female, compared to male, users (17.5 percent versus 4.7 percent).
National Comorbidity Survey (Kessler et al., 1994; Anthony et al., 1994; Nelson et al., 1998; Breslau et al., 2001)	Nationally representative sample of US adolescents. Estimated lifetime prevalence of DSM-III-R disorders in over 8000 respondents 15–54 years of age. Youngest cohort was 15–24 years of age.	• 24 percent of entire sample developed nicotine dependence, 14 percent alcohol dependence, 7.5 percent hard drug dependence (most often, cannabis dependence 4.2 percent). • Youngest cohort (15–24 years) had highest 12-month SUD prevalence rate. • Alcohol abuse symptoms emerged around age 16, escalated rapidly to approximately 20 percent of sample by their mid-twenties. • Half had month or more of daily smoking. Daily smoking almost always began prior to age 25. 24 percent became nicotine dependent.
National Survey of Adolescents (Kilpatrick et al., 2000)	First project assessing DSM-IV SUDs in national representative sample of adolescents. Over 4000 adolescents (ages 12–17) assessed for alcohol, marijuana, and hard drug abuse/ dependence in past year.	• 8 percent had alcohol use disorders by age 16, 11 percent by age 17. • Marijuana use disorders emerged around age 15 (6 percent; increased to 7 percent at ages 16 and 17). • 2 percent had hard drug use disorders by ages 16 and 17. • Controlling for demographics, familial SUD, and victimization, SUD rates were 3–9 times higher in Caucasians compared to African Americans (differences compared to Hispanics and Native Americans nonsignificant).

Table 8.1 (continued)

Study	Study design	Major findings
Boston College Students Study (Deykin et al., 1987)	One of earliest studies of SUD and comorbid psychopathology. SUD assessed in 424 college students aged 16–19.	• 8 percent lifetime prevalence of alcohol use disorders; 9 percent lifetime prevalence of other drug use disorders. • Both alcohol and other drug use disorders associated with depression (ORs ~ 3.0).
Christchurch Health and Development Study (Fergusson et al., 1993, 2003)	Began with a cohort of 1265 children born in Christchurch, New Zealand in 1977. Latent class analysis method combined self and maternal report to estimate SUD rates; 930 of participants followed to age 26.	• At 15, 3 percent had nicotine dependence, 4 percent alcohol abuse, 1.7 percent other substance abuse (primarily marijuana) by self-report. Maternal report rates lower. • Estimated SUD prevalence higher for females than males (7 percent versus 4 percent). • By 26, two-thirds had tried cannabis, with 5 percent reporting heavy lifetime use by age 21. • Among those who used cannabis before 16, 22 percent met DSM-IV cannabis dependence by age 21.
Dunedin Multi-disciplinary Health and Development Study (Newman et al., 1996)	Began with over 1000 New Zealand children born during 1972–1973. Mental health data obtained at ages 11, 13, 15, 18, and 21.	• By age 21, one-year prevalence rates for alcohol and cannabis dependence were 10 percent. • Rates of both disorders higher for males than females (14 percent versus 6 percent and 14 percent versus 5 percent). • Majority with SUD had comorbid disorder(s). • Of participants with SUD at age 21, 78 percent had been diagnosed with SUD at age 18.
Children in the Community Study (Cohen et al., 1993a, 1993b; D.W. Brook et al., 2002)	Began with children from 776 families from upstate New York. Examined prevalence rates of alcohol, marijuana, and hard drug abuse in three groups: 10–13, 14–16, and 17–20 years of age. Sample followed to 27 years of age.	• Alcohol abuse nonexistent in 10–13 year-olds, 4 percent in 14–16 year-olds, and 15 percent in 17–20 year-olds (9 percent females; 20 percent males). • Marijuana abuse disorders increased from 0.2 percent at ages 10–13 to 1.4 percent at ages 14–16 to 3 percent at ages 17–20.

188

		• Hard drug abuse rates in three age groups were 0.2 percent, 0.7 percent, and 1.1 percent, respectively. • 48 percent of alcohol abuse disorders persisted over 2.5 year period. • Use of all substances in early twenties predicted alcohol dependence and other SUD by age 27.
Boston Longitudinal Study (Reinherz et al., 1993; Giaconia et al., 1994, 2001)	Began when participants were 5 years of age. Additional assessments occurred at ages 6, 9, 15, 18, and 21, for a final sample of 375 (28 percent attrition in the targeted sample over 17 years).	• At age 18, alcohol abuse/dependence had lifetime prevalence rate at 32 percent. Lifetime drug abuse/dependence rate was 10 percent. • Male gender associated with alcohol use disorders (38 percent males versus 27 percent females) but not drug use disorders (11 percent versus 9 percent). • Hazard rates for alcohol and drug use disorders peaked at ages 14–17 and dropped sharply by age 18. • Earlier onset of alcohol use disorder associated with greater disorder severity. • Significant continuity of SUDs from 18 to 21.
Great Smokey Mountain Study (Costello et al., 1999, 2003)	Longitudinal community study assessing prevalence and development of psychiatric disorders from age 9 to 16. Sample began with 1420 participants ages 9–13 from North Carolina, who were assessed annually until 16 years of age.	• Boys more likely than girls to use chewing tobacco, cannabis, snuff, and crack cocaine. • SUDs basically nonexistent from 9–13 (0.3 percent at age 13), increasing to 3-month prevalence rates of 1.4 percent, 5 percent, and 8 percent at ages 14, 15, and 16, respectively. Gender differences nonsignificant. • By age 16, estimated cumulative SUD prevalence was 12 percent (10 percent girls; 14 percent boys). • Past SUDs strongly associated with increased odds of future SUDs (OR = 26).
Minnesota Student Survey (Harrison et al., 1998)	Assessed by survey over 74,000 students in ninth and twelfth grades in Minnesota.	• Half of ninth grade students and 70 percent of twelfth grade students reported substance use in prior 12 months.

189

Table 8.1 (*continued*)

Study	Study design	Major findings
		• Among students who reported recent substance use, 14 percent of ninth graders and 23 percent of twelfth graders met criteria for substance abuse (8 percent and 10 percent for dependence, respectively).
Center for Antisocial Drug Dependence Study (Young et al., 2002)	Examined the rates of SUD among 3072 adolescents ages 12–18 selected from three communities in Colorado.	• Tobacco dependence uncommon to age 16 (≤4 percent), although nicotine dependence rates were 15 percent and 17 percent in 17 and 18 year olds. Among daily smokers, half had nicotine dependence. • Rates of alcohol abuse low to age 16. By ages 17–18, one in six had alcohol abuse, and 6 percent had alcohol dependence. • Rates of marijuana abuse and dependence in older participants were 11 percent and 8 percent, respectively. • Dependence on illicit drugs other than marijuana was low, reaching maximum of 3 percent. • Across all substances, one in four 18 year olds met criteria for abuse and one in five met criteria for dependence. • Rates fairly similar for males and females.
Early Developmental Stages of Psychopathology Study (von Sydow et al., 2001)	Reported on the rates of cannabis use disorders among 2446 German adolescents ages 14–24, who were followed for an average of 42 months.	• At first assessment, 2 percent had cannabis abuse and 1.4 percent dependence. Disorders usually developed after age 15. • Symptoms of cannabis use disorder emerged, on average, 2–3 years after first use. • Rates of abuse/dependence lower for women than men. • Half with cannabis abuse improved during 12 month follow-up interval. Remaining adolescents remained abusers (41 percent) or developed dependence (2 percent).

- 19 percent with cannabis dependence remained dependent 12 months later, 21 percent moved to the abuse category, 16 percent stopped using cannabis completely.
- Participants who stopped using cannabis did not shift to using other licit or illicit substances at greater rate.

marijuana, and hard drugs. We present data from the OYSUP study describing the use of individual substances and use without parent's knowledge among children in the first through the eighth grade. Since intention to use substances is theoretically predictive of subsequent onset of substance use (Ajzen, 1988, 1991) and suggested as the first step in the substance use initiation process (Pierce et al., 1996), we also present data on intentions from this study.

Cigarette use

Initiation

Data from the Oregon Youth Substance Use Project (Andrews et al., 2003) show that 18 percent of first graders report intention to smoke when older; 16 percent of fourth graders report intention to smoke and report a lifetime use of cigarettes (2 percent without parent's knowledge); and by eighth grade, 29 percent report lifetime use of cigarettes. A significantly greater proportion of eighth grade girls than boys (29 percent versus 16 percent) reported smoking without parents' knowledge.

Rates of smoking initiation in the OADP were higher for males at all three assessments. Approximately half of the sample had tried smoking by the first assessment (51 percent of males; 46 percent of females). The rate increased to 63 percent by age 24. The mean age of first smoking was 13.8 years ($SD = 3.5$).

Progression to daily smoking

Rates of lifetime daily smoking for the OADP were 8 percent at T1, 11 percent at T2, and 20 percent by T3. Females had a higher rate of daily smoking at T1 (10 percent versus 7 percent), although males had a higher lifetime rate by the third assessment (25 percent versus 17 percent). One-fifth of the sample had smoked daily for at least a month by age 24. Among those who had tried smoking, however, more than half (53 percent) reported daily tobacco use by age 24. The mean onset age of daily smoking was 17.3 years ($SD = 3.1$). Among OADP participants who had begun smoking daily in adolescence, 64 percent met full criteria for lifetime nicotine dependence and 38 percent reported having had nicotine withdrawal (Rohde et al., 2004). Progression from smoking initiation to daily smoking was associated with lower parental education, MDD, alcohol and drug use disorders, ADHD/disruptive behavior disorders, antisocial personality disorder symptoms, regular smoking by father (but not mother or sibling), and the presence of externalizing disorders in family members.

Smoking cessation

Most individuals smoke for 15 to 20 years before they quit smoking and the median age of smoking cessation for individuals who began smoking as adolescents is 33 years of age for men and 37 years of age for women (Pierce and Gilpin, 1996). Thus, information on tobacco cessation in young people is limited. However, we showed that among those OADP participants who had begun daily smoking prior to turning age 24, 22 percent reported that they had not smoked at all during the 12 previous months (Rohde et al., 2004). The median length of longest quit attempt was 365 days, with 39 percent of daily smokers reporting that they had made at least one quit attempt. The median length of time from beginning daily smoking to making a quit attempt (of at least 24 hours) was 27 months.

Two of the eight lifetime psychiatric categories were associated significantly with reduced odds of quitting by age 25: MDD and elevated antisocial personality disorder scores. The odds of successful cessation were 2.5 times greater if the daily smoker did not have a history of MDD compared to daily smokers who had a history of MDD. Similarly, the odds of cessation were 3.3 times higher if the daily smoker did not have an elevated antisocial personality disorder score.

Tobacco cessation may be particularly difficult for adult women. Women make successful quit attempts less frequently than men and relapse more frequently than men (Blake et al., 1989; Swan et al., 1993; Ward et al., 1997). This gender difference could be due to at least two factors. First, a review of the psychobiology of smoking suggests that nicotine has antidepressant properties. Thus, abrupt cessation may cause a rebound effect, increasing depression and anxiety immediately following cessation. Women may relapse to cope with this negative affect (Carmody, 1989). Second, some women tend to gain weight following tobacco cessation (Jeffery et al., 2000).

Alcohol use

Experimentation

In the OYSUP sample (Andrews et al., 2003), 33 percent of first grade boys and 22 percent of girls reported that they intended to drink when older. This proportion increases to 38 percent of both genders, by fourth grade; 20 percent of first grade boys and 4 percent of girls had used alcohol in their lifetime. By fourth grade, approximately 20 percent of both genders reported lifetime use and by eighth grade, approximately 65 percent reported lifetime use, with 21 percent of boys and 32 percent of girls using without parents' knowledge.

In the OADP, three-quarters of the sample had tried alcohol during adolescence. Almost the entire sample (94 percent) had tried alcohol by young adulthood. Adolescent alcohol use was not a frequent occurrence, but when they drank, adolescents often consumed large quantities of alcohol (e.g., 9 percent of females and 23 percent of males consumed five or more drinks per drinking occasion) (Lewinsohn et al., 1996).

Progression to alcohol use disorders

Problematic alcohol consumption tends to begin early in life. Among adults in the Epidemiologic Catchment Area study with a lifetime diagnosis of alcohol use disorder, over 80 percent developed their first symptoms of the disorder before age 30, and over 35 percent had developed at least one symptom of alcohol use disorder between the ages of 15 and 19 (Helzer and Burnam, 1991). In the OADP study (Lewinsohn et al., 1996), 7 percent met criteria for a lifetime diagnosis of alcohol use disorder by T2 (i.e., ages 15 to 19), with an additional 17 percent having problematic alcohol use, as indicated by the occurrence of behaviors meeting criteria for one or two DSM-IV symptoms of alcohol dependence but not diagnosis. Gender differences in the OADP sample at T1 and T2 were nonsignificant. By T3, rates of alcohol use disorder had increased substantially (30 percent). Almost one-fourth of young women (23 percent) and 37 percent of young men met criteria for an alcohol use disorder by age 24.

In Rohde et al. (2001), we examined the degree that alcohol use disorders in adolescence (defined at T2) predicted course of alcoholism to age 24. Three groups of adolescents who had tried alcohol were compared: (1) 75 percent who had non-problematic alcohol use, (2) 16 percent who had one or two symptoms of alcohol dependence but no diagnosis, and (3) 9 percent who met lifetime criteria for a DSM-IV diagnosis of alcohol use disorder. Overall, rates of alcohol use disorder between T2 and T3 in the sample of adolescent alcohol users were high (55 percent in those with adolescent alcohol use disorder, 37 percent in those with one or two symptoms, and 23 percent in those who drank in adolescence but had no diagnostic symptoms by T2). Given that the average time interval between T2 and T3 was 6.8 years, the rates of alcohol use disorder translate into an annual recurrence rate of approximately 8 percent for the adolescent alcohol disorder group, and annual first incidence rates of 5 percent in the adolescent problematic use and 3 percent in the non-problematic use groups.

193

Marijuana use

Initiation

Marijuana use was negligible in the early grade in the OYSUP sample. By fourth grade, 5 percent intended to use marijuana when older with 1 percent of both genders reporting lifetime use. By eighth grade, 18 percent reported lifetime use of marijuana, all without parent's knowledge. There were no gender differences in marijuana use.

In the OADP, approximately 40 percent of the sample had tried marijuana in adolescence (38 percent at T1, 39 percent by T2), with rates approaching 60 percent by age 24. Gender differences were nonsignificant.

Progression to marijuana use disorders

In the OADP data (Lewinsohn et al., 1993), the lifetime prevalence of marijuana abuse/dependence was 5 percent at T1; rates were significantly higher for males compared to females (7 percent versus 4 percent). The point prevalence of marijuana abuse/dependence was 1.7 percent at T1 and 1.3 percent approximately one year later (T2). The one-year first incidence rate of marijuana abuse/dependence from T1 to T2 was 1.3 percent. For those adolescents who already experienced an episode of marijuana abuse/dependence at T1, the relapse rate between T1 and T2 was 4 percent. Differences in rates for boys and girls tended to be small and none were statistically significant. By T3, 22 percent of the men and 14 percent of the women met criteria for either marijuana abuse or dependence.

Course of marijuana use disorders from T2 to T3

We examined whether the presence of marijuana abuse/dependence in adolescence would predict substance use disorders by age 24. Almost two-thirds of the adolescents with marijuana use disorder by T2 (62 percent) continued to have an SUD by age 24 (compared to 29 percent among the remaining participants; OR = 4.1; CI = 2.5–6.7).

Use of other illicit substances

Initiation

The use of illicit substances other than marijuana at the first and second assessments were relatively infrequent. The most frequently used substances were hallucinogens (16 percent by T2) and amphetamines (12 percent by T2). Gender differences in use during adolescence were nonsignificant. By age 24, experimentation had increased with young men reporting significantly higher rates of hallucinogen (34 percent), cocaine (22 percent), and opioid use (10 percent; comparable rates for young women were 27 percent, 17 percent, and 5 percent, respectively). These were among the most frequently used substances, in addition to inhalants.

Progression to hard drug use disorders

Problematic use of substances other than cigarettes, alcohol, and marijuana are infrequent in adolescence (3 percent at T1, 4 percent at T2), although one in ten young adults uses hard drugs in a problematic manner by age 24. The most commonly diagnosed hard drug use disorders at T3 were amphetamine (5 percent), hallucinogen (6 percent), and cocaine (2 percent) abuse/dependence. Unlike smoking, alcohol, and marijuana, the rates of hard drug use disorders in young men and women did not differ, with the one exception of hallucinogen disorders, which were more common among men (6 percent versus 2 percent).

Course of hard drug use disorders from T2 to T3

The presence of a hard drug use disorder by T2 significantly increased the probability of both alcohol use disorders (42 percent versus 26 percent; OR = 2.1; CI = 1.2–3.7) and SUDs (56 percent versus 30 percent; OR = 2.9, CI = 1.6–5.2) by T3. However, adjusting for demographic factors and a history of either alcohol or drug use disorders in adolescence eliminated the ability of hard drug use disorders to predict onset of new SUDs in young adulthood.

The issue of comorbidity

Comorbidity within SUDs

There is substantial comorbidity within the various types of SUD. For example, in previous research, primarily with adult samples, heavy alcohol consumption and alcohol use disorder have been found to be comorbid with other SUDs, including nicotine dependence (e.g., Costello et al., 1999; Kandel et al., 1997; Kessler et al., 1997b; Merikangas et al., 1998). In Kilpatrick et al. (2000), 7 percent of the more than 4000 adolescents met criteria for an SUD: 58 percent met criteria for only one SUD (41 percent for alcohol, 3 percent for marijuana, 14 percent for hard drug); the remaining 42 percent met criteria for two or three SUD categories.

Using the OADP sample, we found that level of problematic alcohol use was associated with both daily smoking and drug use disorders during adolescence (Rohde et al., 1996). For example, the rates of daily tobacco use were 3 percent in the alcohol abstainers, 10 percent in experimenters, 22 percent in social drinkers, 39 percent in problem drinkers, and 59 percent in adolescents with a diagnosis of alcohol use disorder. Rates of drug use disorder were 42 percent among those with alcohol use disorder at T2 versus 12 percent among those who had tried alcohol but had no symptoms of abuse or dependence. Alcohol and drug use disorders in adolescence were predictive of nicotine dependence by age 24 (Rohde et al., 2004).

Lewinsohn et al. (1999) examined the relation between adolescent cigarette use (measured at T1 and T2) and the occurrence of SUDs during young adulthood. Daily smoking in adolescence was associated with increased risk of future cannabis, hard drug, and multiple drug use disorders. For instance, 27 percent of the adolescent daily smokers developed cannabis use disorders compared to 8 percent of those who had never smoked by adolescence; comparable rates of hard drug use disorders were 18 percent versus 4 percent. Quitting smoking did not reduce the risk of future SUD, although having maintained smoking cessation for more than 12 months was associated with significantly lower rates of future alcohol use disorder. These previously published findings highlight the strong degree of comorbidity across various categories of substance abuse and dependence.

Unpublished results from the OADP also illustrate the magnitude of comorbidity between adolescent SUDs through an examination of the occurrence of various SUDs by T2 given the presence of another SUD by T2. Among those who were daily smokers, 22 percent had alcohol use disorders, 28 percent had marijuana use disorders, and 19 percent had hard drug use disorders (comparable rates for the non-smokers were 5 percent, 4 percent, and 2 percent). Among those who had alcohol use disorders by T2, 50 percent also had marijuana use disorders and 34 percent had hard drug use disorders (versus 4 percent and 2 percent among participants who did not have an alcohol use disorder). Lastly, among those who had marijuana use disorders, 37 percent had another hard drug use disorder (compared to only 1.7 percent of those who did not have a marijuana use disorder). All of these associations were highly significant ($p < 0.0001$). Clearly, adolescents and young adults who abuse one substance are extremely likely to abuse other substances either concurrently or in the future.

Comorbidity of SUDs with other disorders

The comorbidity of SUDs and other psychiatric disorders represents an important public health challenge. Comorbid psychiatric conditions typically are more chronic and severe, associated with greater functional impairment, and derive less benefit from available treatments (Hirschfeld et al., 1990; Kessler, 1995; Lewinsohn et al., 1995).

Conduct disorder (CD) has been found in previous research to increase the risk of drug use in adolescence (e.g., Slutske et al., 1998). Disruptive behavior problems often predict an early onset and faster progression of problematic levels of alcohol use (e.g., Costello et al., 1999; Windle and Davies, 1999). With the OADP sample, we found that the presence of CD or oppositional defiant disorder doubled the probability of future alcohol use disorder (Rohde et al., 2001). *ADHD* appears to be associated with SUDs (Biederman et al., 1995; Loney, 1988), although the association may be moderated by CD (Disney et al., 1999; Pihl and Peterson, 1991).

Depression, both at the level of diagnosis and at the level of symptoms (subsyndromal depression), appears to have one of the strongest and most consistent associations with SUD (e.g., Brook et al., 1996; Helzer and Pryzbeck, 1988; Hesselbrock et al., 1985). The occurrence of early-onset *bipolar disorder* is much less frequent but may also be at risk for SUD (Wilens et al., 1999). The presence of depression greatly reduces the ability of smokers to quit (e.g., Breslau and Klein, 1999; Glassman et al., 1990), and several models have been proposed to account for the association between negative affect and smoking (Kassel et al., 2003). The model that appears to most directly account for the role of depression is the nicotine withdrawal escape model (e.g., Parrott, 1999), in which smokers achieve a reduction in negative affect through relief of nicotine withdrawal symptoms.

Although not universally found (e.g., Schuckit and Hesselbrock, 1994), a significant association between alcoholism and *anxiety disorders* has been reported in several studies (e.g., Helzer and Pryzbeck, 1988; Kessler et al., 1996; Kushner et al., 1999; Regier et al., 1990; Merikangas et al., 1998). Of the various anxiety disorders, *post-traumatic stress disorder* (PTSD) has been found to have the strongest association with substance abuse (e.g., Chilcoat and Breslau, 1998; Giaconia et al., 2000).

Although the prevalence of *schizophrenia* is low, drug use and SUDs may precipitate the development of psychosis in vulnerable individuals (Buckley, 1998; Strakowski et al., 1993). In addition, the vast majority of individuals with schizophrenia abuse psychoactive substances and 50 percent or more have a comorbid SUD (Buckley, 1998; Fowler et al., 1998).

The association between *eating disorders* and SUD is inconsistent. Holderness et al. (1994) found a significant association between SUD and eating disorders, especially bulimia, whereas Zaider et al. (2000) found no significant comorbidity between adolescent eating disorders with either alcohol or hard drug dependence.

Lastly, the rates of *personality disorders* are significantly elevated among adults who seek drug and alcohol treatment, with rates generally between 50 and 80 percent (e.g., Van Horn and Frank, 1998; Weiss et al., 1993). Rates of personality disorders are especially elevated among adult patients with multiple SUDs (O'Boyle, 1993). Numerous classification systems for alcoholism distinguish groups on the basis of antisocial personality disorder features (e.g., Babor et al., 1992; Cloninger, 1987; Hesselbrock et al., 1985; Zucker, 1987). Almost all of these typologies suggest that adult alcoholics with comorbid antisocial personality disorder have a more pernicious outcome.

Gender appears to moderate the pattern of many comorbid associations (Kandel et al., 1997; Robins, 1989). Several studies have found that SUDs are significantly associated with lifetime CD in men (e.g., Kessler et al., 1994, 1997b); and with affective and anxiety disorders in women (Kessler et al., 1994, 1997b; Turnbull and Gomberg, 1988).

Temporal order of comorbid SUD and psychopathology

The majority of adult patients with comorbid SUD/psychiatric disorder experienced the psychiatric disorder prior to abuse of substances (e.g., Kessler et al., 1996; Ross et al., 1988). This is not surprising, given that many psychiatric disorders emerge in childhood or early adolescence, prior to the period of highest risk for SUD. For example, in the Dunedin Study, several psychiatric disorders at age 18 preceded occurrence of SUD at age 21 included history of conduct disorder (present in 43 percent of SUD cases), depressive disorder (38 percent), anxiety disorder (29 percent), and ADHD (11 percent). However, the patterns are far from clear-cut. In the Epidemiological Catchment Area (ECA) study, MDD preceded alcoholism in 36 percent of adults, began concomitantly in 19 percent of adults, and followed the alcoholism in the remaining 45 percent of adults (Merikangas et al., 1996). Temporal relations probably vary as a function of the nature of the psychiatric diagnosis (Merikangas and Gelernter, 1990) and gender (Hesselbrock et al., 1985).

Brook et al. (1998) reported that, after controlling for other psychiatric disorders, drug *use* in adolescence was predictive of depressive, anxiety, and antisocial personality disorders in young adulthood. Conversely, psychiatric disorders did not predict escalation in drug use in young adulthood. The authors suggest that once an adolescent is using drugs, prior psychopathology is not significantly related to escalation of substance use. Other studies have suggested that adolescent substance use precedes onset of the psychiatric disorder (Johnson and Kaplan, 1990; Kandel et al., 1986).

Risk factors associated with substance use and abuse

Early use of substances is one of the primary predictors of substance abuse in adolescence and young adulthood (Hawkins et al., 1992; Hesselbrock et al., 1985). Thus, risk factors of substance abuse throughout adolescence and early adulthood may be derived from the adolescence substance use literature. Risk factors of substance use and abuse are comprised of variables from multiple domains, which, as suggested by Rutter (1982), are complex, multiple and interacting. Domains include genetic factors, biological factors, individual factors, and cognitive factors. Additionally, within an ecological approach (Bronfenbrenner, 1988) several domains encompass the context in which the adolescent or young adult develops, including peer factors, family factors, and neighborhood or community factors. In Table 8.2, we have listed empirically supported examples from the literature of risk factors within each of these domains.

The consequences of adolescent SUDs

The transition from adolescence to young adulthood is a critical period when the young person is expected to assume a number of adult responsibilities, including

Table 8.2 Examples of risk factors associated with substance use and abuse

Domains	Examples of risk factors
Genetic factors	• Through reward-deficiency pathways of addiction (Koob and LeMoal, 2001; Robinson and Berridge, 2001)
Biological factors	• Early biological maturation, particularly for girls (Graber et al., 1997; Stice et al., 2001) • Direct and indirect influences of hormonal levels including testosterone (Booth et al., 1999; Martin et al., 2001), estradiol (Inoff-Germain et al., 1988), and cortisol (Susman and Pajer, 2004)
Individual factors	• Poor social skills (Dishion, 1990) • Poor self-esteem (Connor, 1994; Kaplan et al., 1982) • Stressful life events (Wills et al., 2002) • Sensation seeking (Simon et al., 1995; Wills et al., 2002) • Antisocial behaviour (Jessor, 1987; Severson et al., 2003) • Academic underachievement (Kandel and Davies, 1992) • Child temperament (Caspi et al., 1997)
Cognitive factors	• Social images of substance users (Gibbons and Gerrard, 1997) • Subjective norms regarding use (Ajzen and Fishbein, 1980) • Attitude toward use (Ajzen and Fishbein, 1980)
Peer factors	• Association with substance-using peers (Andrews et al., 2002; Patterson et al., 2000) • Peer rejection (Dishion et al., 1994) • Peer encouragement (Duncan et al., 1994)
Family factors	• Parental substance use and abuse (Andrews et al., 1997; Chassin et al., 1991; Merikangas et al., 1998) • Poor parenting skills (Dishion et al., 1988) • Low level of monitoring (Dishion and Loeber, 1985) • Poor family relationships (Brook et al., 1988; Duncan et al., 1994) • Parental psychopathology (Brook et al., 1983; Schwartz et al., 1990)
Neighbourhood/ community factors	• Neighbourhood disadvantage (Crum et al., 1996) • Low socioeconomic status (Smart et al., 1994) • High neighbourhood density (Ennett et al., 1997) • Low neighbourhood social cohesion (Duncan et al., 2002)

completion of education, obtaining a job, developing a relationship and becoming married, and (often) becoming a parent. The extent to which SUDs impairs this transition can have important long-term implications for the individual. This association would also have implications for treatment and prevention of psycho-social impairments.

While the consequences of drug experimentation or low level use may be relatively harmless (e.g., Shedler and Block, 1990), the consequences of substance abuse or dependence are deleterious and costly. SUD appears to have a negative effect on physical and psychological development and family relationships, and has been associated with conflicts with authority figures, school failure, criminal behavior, unwanted pregnancy, accidents and injuries, homicides, and suicides (e.g., Centers for Disease Control and Prevention, 1997; Kokotailo et al., 1995; McKeown et al., 1997; O'Hara et al., 1998). The economic costs of drug abuse to society amount to nearly half a trillion dollars each year (Harwood, 2001). The negative consequences of substance abuse increase given earlier onset (e.g., Fergusson, and Horwood, 2001; Windle, 1994) and chronicity of disorder (Fergusson et al., 2002; MacKenzie and Kipke, 1992).

Impact on academic/occupational functioning

Research has shown that substance use is associated with dropping out of school (Newcomb and Bentler, 1988), delayed entry into the labor force (Kandel et al., 1987) and job instability (Kandel et al., 1986). Giaconia et al. (2001) found that problems in the academic and occupational functioning were uniquely associated with SUDs (as opposed to also being a negative consequence of depression).

Marijuana use among heavy users may also result in an "amotivational syndrome," which is characterized by an inability to sustain goal-directed activity leading to marked deterioration in academic, vocational, and social spheres (J.S. Brook et al., 2002a; Schonberg, 1992). However, these consequences could be explained by other variables. For example, Andrews and Duncan (1997) showed that the significant relation between substance use, including cigarette, alcohol and marijuana use, and subsequent academic motivation in adolescence could be explained by the general deviance of the adolescent.

For this chapter, we conducted preliminary analyses in the OADP sample examining the degree that SUD by age 19 was associated with negative functioning by age 24. Those with adolescent SUD had completed fewer years of education (13.5 versus 14.3 years) and had a lower annual household income ($24,000 versus $29,000). These differences remained significant after adjusting for demographic differences.

Impact on marriage and parenting

Several studies have documented the pernicious impact of substance use during adolescence on the psychosocial functioning of individuals as they become young adults (e.g., Bachman et al., 1997; Chassin et al., 1996; Kandel et al., 1986; Newcomb and Bentler, 1987). Two processes have been proposed to explain the relation. First, the concept of "pseudo-maturity" proposed by Newcomb and Bentler (1988) predicts a positive relation between substance use and early entry into adult roles. This is supported by data that show that substance use and SUDs are associated with early onset of sexual activity, teenage parenthood, and early marriage (e.g., Kessler et al., 1997a; Krohn et al., 1997). In contrast, Yamaguchi and Kandel (1984a, 1984b) emphasize the concept of "role incompatibility" in which (a) drug use disrupts the normative transitions to adult roles, and (b) the adoption of adult roles discourages the initiation or continuation of drug use. This hypothesis has been supported by studies which show that adolescent drug use disrupts or delays age-appropriate transitions to parenthood and marriage (e.g., Kandel and Yamaguchi, 1985; Kandel et al., 1986). Brook et al. (1999) examined the consequences of marijuana use and the assumption of adult roles from childhood to the late twenties. Past marijuana use was predictive of adopting a more unconventional adult role, which the authors defined as delay of marriage, having children out of wedlock, and unemployment.

Compared to OADP participants who did not experience an SUD by age 19, those who did were less likely to be married by age 24 (28 percent versus 35 percent), although, if married, they were more likely to have been divorced (8 percent versus 2 percent). The presence of adolescent SUD was not significantly associated with early parenting (25 percent among those with SUD versus 22 percent among those without adolescent SUD).

Impact on health-risk behaviors

Substance abuse is one of the most significant factors in the spread of HIV infection, serving as both a direct (i.e., through injection drug use) and indirect risk factor (i.e., through impaired judgment, disinhibition) (National Institute on Drug Abuse (NIDA), 2003). Adolescent substance abuse treatment, therefore, presents a prime opportunity for intervention on HIV/AIDS risk behaviors within this population (Rounds-Bryant and Staab, 2002). Various findings suggest that significant reductions in HIV/AIDS risk behavior can be achieved among adolescents in treatment for SUD (e.g., Jainchill, 1999; Joshi et al., 2002).

The health consequences of SUDs

The majority of health consequences associated with substance use develop following long-term use but effects have been noted even after five years of use (Aarons et al., 1999). Both tobacco and cannabis smoking have detectable effects on decreased lung capacity by the mid-twenties (Taylor et al., 2002). Alcohol and drug use is associated with future respiratory disease and impaired neuropsychological functioning, including headaches, dizziness, and vision problems (J.S. Brook et al., 2002b). Adverse physical effects from marijuana smoking include bronchitis and other respiratory disease, increased blood pressure, endocrine changes, and decreases in male fertility (MacKenzie and Kipke, 1992). J.S. Brook et al. (2002b) noted that SUDs may be linked with subsequent health problems because of specific toxic effects of substance use or because of associations with either risk-taking behaviors in general or psychopathology specifically, which in turn leads to negative health behaviors and physical problems.

Gender differences have been noted in these health effects, with findings suggesting that women may experience a broader range of smoking-related diseases (US Department of Health and Human Services (USDHHS), 1989) and may develop physical illnesses as a result of alcohol consumption more rapidly than men (Blume, 1992).

Clinical implications for assessment

Four general recommendations can be made regarding the assessment of SUDs in adolescents and young adults. Given the frequency and negative consequences of SUDs, our first recommendation is that adolescents be routinely screened for substance use and problematic use at the levels of abuse and dependence. This recommendation includes the need for systematic screening of subthreshold tobacco, alcohol, and drug use problems. The fact that even the presence of a single symptom of alcoholism in adolescence increases the likelihood of alcohol abuse/dependence by young adulthood (Rohde et al., 2001) emphasizes the important public health implications of assessment.

Second, given the high probability that young people with SUD will also have comorbid psychiatric disorders, clinicians are advised to thoroughly probe for the presence of psychiatric disorders in any adolescent seeking treatment for SUD and to probe for SUD among those seek treating for other psychiatric disorders.

Third, we suggest that assessment procedures employed in research trials be used in clinical practice. This includes the use of various self-report questionnaires and structured or semi-structured diagnostic interviews. Weinberg et al. (1998) reviewed various methods for assessing substance use and SUDs in young people. She noted that although many self-report questionnaires and diagnostic interviews were initially developed and normed on adult samples, several psychometrically sound self-report screening instruments have been created to assess adolescent SUD, including the Problem Oriented Screening Instrument for Teenagers (POSIT; Rahdert, 1991), Personal Experience Screening Questionnaire (PESQ; Winters, 1991), and Substance Abuse Subtle Screening Inventory (SASSI; Miller, 1990). Diagnostic instruments for adolescents include the Adolescent Diagnostic Interview Schedule (Winters and Henly, 1993), and the Teen Addiction Severity Index (TASI, Kaminer et al., 1991). In addition, various lab measures are available to assess substance use. Urinalysis is the most widely used biological measure because of its accuracy when reliable samples are collected (Cone, 1997). Urinalysis is limited, however, by relatively short detection periods: between one and three days for heroin, amphetamine, and cocaine, and up to thirty days after chronic use of marijuana. Hair, saliva, and sweat analyses represent promising alternatives.

Finally, we recommend changes in the diagnostic system that may make it more developmentally appropriate for adolescents and even young adults and more consistent across genders. Our own research, and the work of others (e.g., Pollock and Martin, 1999), suggests that the distinction between substance abuse versus dependence may be more problematic with adolescents than with adults. Several investigators have questioned the validity of some DSM criteria for the diagnosis of abuse in girls and women (Haver, 1986). For example, adolescent girls tend to have a lower occurrence of recurrent use associated with legal problems and in hazardous situations than boys (Wagner et al., 2002). Gender differences in symptom prevalence could affect the relative prevalence of a diagnosis of abuse and dependence. However, the notion of gender-specific criteria for abuse and dependence has yet to be explored.

Clinical implications for prevention

Four broad recommendations in the area of prevention are offered. First, prevention must occur prior to the development of an SUD. It is clear that SUD is the final stage of the progression of behaviors starting with substance intentions, followed by initiation, sporadic experimentation, regular use, and finally substance abuse or dependence. Age of initiation is a significant risk factor for regular substance use and subsequent problem use (Breslau and Peterson, 1996; Yamaguchi and Kandel, 1984a, 1984b). Thus delaying initiation is a reasonable prevention goal. Furthermore, problematic adolescent substance use at subthreshold levels should not be ignored, and reducing adolescent use will prevent the development of an SUD. We strongly support the conclusion of Sobell and Sobell (1993) that individuals experiencing subdiagnostic levels of problematic alcohol use often require treatment to prevent the development of an SUD.

Second, substance use in prevention must focus on the adolescent and their interaction with their peer group, the family and the community. Most of the currently available prevention programs aimed at delaying onset or decreasing adolescent substance use are school-based. School-based programs that are interactive as opposed to didactic (Tobler and Stratton, 1997) and that target normative (e.g., peer resistance) and informational social influences (e.g., changing evaluation of and attitudes toward substance use) have been shown to be effective (Flay, 1986; Tobler 1986). Furthermore, program components based on the physical consequences of problem substance use delivered in an interactive format have been shown to be effective (Hirschman and Leventhal, 1989; Sussman et al., 1995). School-based interventions, however, only have the potential of impacting adolescents who are attending school. In addition, fidelity of implementation in schools is problematic. For example, an evaluation of the effective Life Skills Training Program showed that 60 percent of the students did not receive the program (Botvin et al., 1995). Dishion and Andrews (1995) argue effectively for a prevention program which incorporates the family and demonstrate the efficacy of a family-based prevention program. Biglan (1995) has demonstrated the importance of the community and changing community norms in youth substance use prevention.

Third, the preventionist must keep in mind the comorbidity between substances and between SUD and other psychiatric disorders. For example, since substance use progresses from smoking to the use of other substances, prevention of smoking has the potential of preventing other SUDS as well. As another example, treating child disorders, such as externalizing behaviors, may prevent the onset of alcohol use disorders in young adulthood (Rohde et al., 2001). Conversely, the treatment of adolescent SUDs may prevent onset or escalation of comorbid psychiatric disorders. Consistent with this recommendation, Kessler and Price (1993) have called for interventions in which the treatment of one disorder is conceptualized as a prevention intervention for a secondary, comorbid condition.

Fourth, we recommend the development and evaluation of gender-specific prevention programs. Whereas a broad program aimed at changing antisocial behavior in general may be an appropriate substance use prevention program for boys, programs targeting girls may often need to be more focused. For example, programs specifically for early maturing girls are needed. One approach to prevention of substance use in girls is to improve their emotional well-being and to teach them effective coping skills for the new situations they encounter as they transition to adolescence. These skills could potentially prevent the use of substances as a form of self-medication in response to the stress associated with adolescence.

Clinical implications for treatment

The majority of adolescents with SUDs do not receive treatment. Given what is known regarding the continuity of SUDs, for many adolescents, SUD and problematic substance use are not benign conditions that self-resolve. Instead they are often indicators of persistent and recurrent psychopathology, resulting in significant and potentially long-term dysfunction. Therefore, strong consideration should be given to the appropriate referral and treatment of these problems in order to prevent or at least reduce the severity of subsequent pathology.

Family-based therapies appear to be the most efficacious treatments for adolescent SUD (Deas and Thomas, 2001; Muck et al., 2001; Williams et al., 2000). Family approaches view substance abuse as a problem that develops and is maintained in the context of maladaptive family relationships (Ozechowski and Liddle, 2000). The approach proposes that correcting faulty family interaction patterns (e.g., improving communication, parental supervision) will, in turn, reduce adolescents' involvement with illicit drugs. Several theory-based models of family therapy have been shown to be efficacious in reducing adolescent drug use, including structural-strategic family therapy (SSFT; Joanning et al., 1992; Lewis et al., 1990; Szapocznik et al., 1988), multidimensional family therapy (MDFT; Liddle and Diamond, 1991), multisystemic family therapy (MSFT; Pickrel and Henggeler, 1996), and Functional Family Therapy (FFT; Alexander and Barton, 1981; Alexander and Parsons, 1982, 1998; Waldron and Slesnick, 1996). Reviews of formal clinical trials of family therapy have consistently found that more drug-abusing adolescents enter, engage in, remain in, and respond to family therapy compared to nonfamily-based treatments (Liddle and Dakof, 1995; Stanton and Shadish, 1997; Waldron, 1997).

Adolescent-focused approaches have received less research attention although a few approaches appear promising, including adolescent peer group therapy (Fisher and Bentley, 1996), cognitive-behavioral treatments (Azrin et al., 1994), problem-solving and coping skills training (Hawkins et al., 1991), and relapse-prevention techniques (Catalano et al., 1990; Myers and Brown, 1993). Pharmacotherapy interventions also exist for certain SUDs (e.g., methadone for heroin addiction; naltrexone for alcohol addition) but almost all research of these approaches has been conducted with adult patients. Lastly, it should be noted that little research has evaluated the efficacy of 12-step programs (i.e., Alcoholics Anonymous, Narcotics Anonymous) with either adolescent or adult addicts, although they are a very common (and inexpensive) treatment approach.

Impact of comorbidity

Comorbidity complicates the selection and sequencing of treatment. Which disorder should be treated first? Should disorders be treated separately, or can a single treatment be directed at both? Answers to basic clinical questions such as these are currently unknown. Given the high degree of comorbidity and risk for future other psychopathology, greater efforts are needed to develop empirically supported treatments for the dual diagnosis patient. The presence of comorbid psychiatric disorders with alcohol use disorder has been shown to be associated with poorer treatment outcome, greater suicidality, disability, and functional impairment (e.g., Regier et al., 1990).

Regarding the impact of MDD/SUD comorbidity on treatment, the vast majority of studies have examined the role of depression among adults treated for alcohol/drug addictions; almost nothing is known regarding the impact of depression on treatment of the addicted adolescent. Some studies find that depression in adult patients with SUD is associated with lower substance recovery rates (Mueller et al., 1994; Ritsher et al., 2002), higher relapse rates (Greenfield et al., 1998; McKay et al., 2002), and significantly higher SUD treatment costs (Westermeyer et al., 1998). Others, however, report that depression in addicts is either unrelated to treatment response (Araujo et al., 1996; Charney et al., 2001) or associated with better outcomes (Charney et al., 1998; Hasin et al., 1996), perhaps due to higher treatment attendance or the fact that depression indicates a less severe form of SUD. Explanations for these contradictory findings are unknown, although the impact of comorbid depression on SUD may vary as a function of gender (Westermeyer et al., 1997). Among adolescents, Kaminer and others have shown that conduct-disordered, substance-abusing youth are at increased risk of not completing treatment (Kaminer et al., 1994; Myers et al., 1998). This is true in particular with those who do not also have comorbid diagnoses of depression or anxiety disorders (Kaminer et al., 1994).

Four basic models could account for the associations between depression and SUDs. First, many clinicians and patients have adopted the *self-medication model*, which proposes that drug abuse is a maladaptive coping mechanism used to mitigate the symptoms of depression (e.g., Khantzian, 1985). Second, the *affective consequences model*, proposes that drug abuse creates or exacerbates psychopathology, including depression, either due to the biological effects of the substance or to increases in life stress and functional difficulties. Several studies report that depression often remits in adult addicts after alcohol detoxification or abstinence (e.g., Brown and Schuckit, 1988; Brown et al., 1995), although this effect appears to be less pronounced with substance-dependence adolescents compared to adults (Riggs et al., 1995). A third model, *reciprocal relations*, suggests that each disorder contributes to the maintenance of the other disorder. Lastly, the *independent factors model* posits that independent factors promote and maintain SUD and depression.

Conclusions and future directions

This review has documented the frequency and significance of SUDs in adolescence and young adulthood. From our review, several directions for future research and clinical work appear particularly compelling.

First, there is a need for larger, more representatives studies of the natural history, incidence, prevalence, and comorbidity patterns of adolescent substance abuse and dependence. A good deal of information has been collected and continues to be obtained regarding the initiation and frequency of substance use in the general population. More research needs to focus on substance use at the level of abuse and dependence. In an effort to add to this gap in the literature, Peter Lewinsohn and his colleagues are currently in the process of completing analyses on a fourth panel of assessments (T4) with the OADP participants after they become 30 years of age.

Second, although the diagnostic criteria contained in the DSM have greatly facilitated the comparison of findings across research projects, concerns regarding the optimal method of defining and categorizing adolescent SUDs remain, including the value of distinguishing between substance abuse and dependence (Harrison et al., 1998).

Third, several empirically based treatment approaches exist and several prevention interventions appear promising. Research needs to move to the next stage, in which empirically supported treatments are disseminated and implemented in real-world treatment settings, including schools, community clinics, and juvenile correction facilities. In addition, given the high degree of continuity of alcohol problems from adolescence to young adulthood, treatment recommendations should include the development of booster or maintenance treatments.

Fourth, research on the treatment of the dual diagnosis adolescent is a major area in need of attention.

Fifth, we know that adolescents with SUD shown numerous negative consequences in young adulthood. Further research must focus on the processes or mediational mechanisms which explain the occurrence of these consequences and the protective processes that prevent these consequences from necessarily occurring.

Sixth, research findings need to be translated into theory building and intervention development. Although this chapter has focused primarily on the epidemiology, rather than etiology, of substance use and abuse, numerous studies have investigated the factors that explain the development and maintenance of SUDs. For example, several theories address the familial transmission of SUDs. While it is well-established that SUDs aggregate in families (e.g., Hesselbrock, 1995; Kendler et al., 1997), the factors accounting for this intergenerational transmission of substance abuse may include genetic components, modeling of parental behavior, or impairments in parenting as a result of substance abuse. One of the most influential theories addressing the etiology of SUDs is Problem Behavior Theory (e.g., Jessor, 1987), in which substance use is a part of an underlying "problem behavior syndrome" along with antisocial behavior and conduct disorders. Two additional theoretical frameworks – the Theory of Reasoned Action (Ajzen and Fishbein, 1980) and the Theory of Planned Behavior (Ajzen, 1988) – have related cognitions to subsequent health behavior, including substance use. Lastly, Wills (1987, 1990; Wills et al., 2002) has written on the impact of perceived stress in relation to subsequent substance use, positing that individuals with ineffective coping skills use substances as a form of self-medication in reaction to stress. Prevention interventions need to address processes that lead to the initiation of substance use or SUD whereas treatment interventions need to address factors that maintain SUDs and prevent relapse. These two sets of processes are not necessarily the same.

Acknowledgments

This work was partially supported by National Institute of Mental Health Grant MH 56238 (PI: P. Rohde) and National Institute on Drug Abuse Grants DA10767 (PI: J. Andrews) and DA12951 (PI: P.M. Lewinsohn).

References

Aarons, G.A., Brown, S.A., Coe, M.T., Myers, M.G., Garland, A.F., Ezzet-Lofstram, R., et al. (1999). Adolescent alcohol and drug abuse and health. *Journal of Adolescent Health*, *24*, 412–421.

Ajzen, I. (1988). *Attitudes, personality and behavior*. New York: Open University Press.

Ajzen, I. (1991). The theory of planned behavior. *Organizational Behavior and Human Decision Processes*, *50*, 179–211.

Ajzen, I. and Fishbein, M. (1980). *Understanding attitudes and predicting social behavior*. Englewood Cliffs, NJ: Prentice-Hall.

Alexander, J.F. and Barton, C. (1981). Methodological issues in systems-behavioral family intervention. In J.L. Vincent (Ed.), *Family assessment and research: Volume I*. New York: JAI Press.

Alexander, J.F. and Parsons, B.V. (1982). *Functional family therapy*. Monterey, CA: Brooks/Cole.

Alexander, J.F. and Parsons, B.V. (1998). Functional family therapy: Implementation in Washington. Presentation at the Violence Prevention Communication Plan for Preventing Youth Violence: The Best Practices Project meeting, Washington, DC, July.

American Psychiatric Association (1987). *Diagnostic and statistical manual of mental disorders*, 3rd edn revised (DSM-III-R). Washington, DC: APA.

American Psychiatric Association (1994). *Diagnostic and statistical manual of mental disorders*, 4th edn (DSM-IV). Washington, DC: APA.

Andrews, J.A. and Duncan, S.C. (1997). Examining the reciprocal relation between academic motivation and substance use: Effects of family relationships, self-esteem and general deviance. *Journal of Behavioral Medicine, 20*, 523–549.

Andrews, J.A., Hops, H., and Duncan, S.C. (1997). Adolescent modeling of parent substance use: The moderating effect of the relationship with the parent. *Journal of Family Psychology, 11*, 259–270.

Andrews, J.A., Tildesley, E., Hops, H., Duncan, S., and Severson, H.H. (2003). Elementary school age children's future intentions and use of substances. *Journal of Clinical Child and Adolescent Psychology, 32(4)*, 556–567.

Anthony, J.C., Warner, L.A., and Kessler, R.C. (1994). Comparative epidemiology of dependence on tobacco, alcohol, controlled substances and inhalants: Basic findings from the National Comorbidity Survey. *Clinical and Experimental Psychopharmacology, 2*, 244–268.

Araujo, L., Goldberg, P., Eyma, J., Madhusoodanan, S., Buff, D.D., Shamim, K., et al. (1996). The effect of anxiety and depression on completion/withdrawal status in patients admitted to substance abuse detoxification program. *Journal of Substance Abuse Treatment, 13*, 61–6.

Azrin, N.H., McMahon, P.T., Donohue, V.A., Besalel, V., Lapinski, K.J., Kogan, E., et al. (1994). Behavior therapy for drug abuse: A controlled treatment outcome study. *Behavior Research and Therapy, 32*, 857–866.

Babor, T.F., Hofmann, M., DelBoca, F.K., Hesselbrock, V., Meyer, R., Dolinsky, Z.S., et al. (1992). Types of alcoholics, I: Evidence for an empirically derived typology based on indicators of vulnerability and severity. *Archives of General Psychiatry, 49*, 599–608.

Bachman, J.G., Wadsworth, K.N., O'Malley, P.M., Johnston, L.D., and Schulenberg, J.E. (1997). *Smoking, drinking, and drug use in young adulthood: The impacts of new freedoms and new responsibilities*. Mahwah, NJ: Erlbaum.

Bailey, S.L., Martin, C.S., Lynch, K.G. and Pollock, N.K. (2000). Reliability and concurrent validity of DSM-IV subclinical symptom ratings for alcohol use disorders among adolescents. *Alcoholism, Clinical and Experimental Research, 24*, 1795–1802.

Biederman, J., Wilens, T., Mick, E., and Milberger, S. (1995). Psychoactive substance use disorders in adults with attention deficit hyperactivity disorder (ADHD): Effects of ADHD and psychiatric comorbidity. *American Journal of Psychiatry, 152*, 1652–1658.

Biglan, A. (1995). *Changing cultural practices: A contextualist framework for intervention research*. Reno, NV: Context Press.

Blake, S.M., Klepp, K.-I., Pechacek, T.F., Folsom, A.R., Luepker, R.V., Jacobs, D.R., et al. (1989). Differences in smoking cessation strategies between men and women. *Addictive Behaviors, 14*, 409–418.

Blume, S.B. (1992). Alcohol and other drug problems in women. In J.H. Lowinson, P. Ruiz, R.B. Millman, and J.G. Langrod (Eds.), *Substance abuse: A comprehensive textbook*, 2nd edn (pp. 794–807). Baltimore, MD: Williams and Wilkins.

Booth, A., Johnson, D., and Granger, D.A. (1999). Testosterone and men's depression: The role of social factors. *Journal of Health and Social Behavior, 40*, 130–140.

Botvin, G. J., Baker, E., Dusenbury, L., Botvin, E.M., and Diaz, T. (1995). Long-term follow-up results of a randomized drug abuse prevention trial in a white middle-class population. *Journal of the American Medical Association, 273*, 1106–1112.

Breslau, N. and Klein, D.F. (1999). Smoking and panic attacks: An epidemiologic investigation. *Archives of General Psychiatry, 56,* 1141–1147.

Breslau, N. and Peterson, E.L. (1996). Smoking cessation in young adults: Age at initiation of cigarette smoking and other suspected influences. *American Journal of Public Health, 86,* 214–220.

Breslau, N., Johnson, E.O., Hiripi, E., and Kessler, R. (2001). Nicotine dependence in the United States. *Archives of General Psychiatry, 58,* 810–816.

Bronfenbrenner, U. (1988). Interacting systems in human development. Research paradigms: Present and future. In N. Bolger, A. Caspi, G. Downey, and M. Moorehouse (Eds.), *Persons in context: Developmental processes* (pp. 25–49). Cambridge: Cambridge University Press.

Brook, D.W., Brook, J.S., Zhang, C., Cohen, P., and Whiteman, M. (2002). Drug use and the risk of major depressive disorder, alcohol dependence, and substance use disorders. *Archives of General Psychiatry, 59,* 1039–1044.

Brook, J.S., Whiteman, M., and Gordon, A.S. (1983). Stages of drug use in adolescence: Personality, peer, and family correlates. *Developmental Psychology, 19,* 269–277.

Brook, J.S., Whiteman, M., Nomura, C., Gordon, A.S., and Cohen, P. (1988). Personality, family, and ecological influences on adolescent drug use: A developmental analysis. *Journal of Chemical Dependency Treatment, 1(2), 123–161.*

Brook, J.S., Whiteman, M., Finch, S.J., and Cohen, P. (1996). Young adult drug use and delinquency: Childhood antecedents and adolescent mediators. *Journal of the American Academy of Child and Adolescent Psychiatry, 35,* 1584–1592.

Brook, J.S., Cohen, P., and Brook, D.W. (1998). Longitudinal study of co-occurring psychiatric disorders and substance use. *Journal of the American Academy of Child and Adolescent Psychiatry, 37,* 322–330.

Brook, J.S., Richter, L., Whiteman, M., and Cohen, P. (1999). Consequences of adolescent marijuana use: Incompatibility with the assumption of adult roles. *Genetic, Social, and General Psychology Monographs, 125,* 193–207.

Brook, J.S., Adams, R.E., Balka, E.B., and Johnson, E. (2002a). Early adolescent marijuana use: Risks for the transition to young adulthood. *Psychological Medicine, 32,* 79–91.

Brook, J.S., Finch, S.J., Whiteman, M., and Brook, D.W. (2002b). Drug use and neuro-behavioral, respiratory, and cognitive problems: Precursors and mediators. *Journal of Adolescent Health, 30,* 433–441.

Brown, S.A. and Schuckit, M.A. (1988). Changes in depression among abstinent alcoholics. *Journal of Studies on Alcohol, 49,* 412–417.

Brown, S.A., Inaba, R.K., Gillin, J.C., Schuckit, M.A., Stewart, M.A., and Irwin, M.R. (1995). Alcoholism and affective disorder: Clinical course of depressive symptoms. *American Journal of Psychiatry, 152,* 45–52.

Buckley, P.E. (1998). Substance abuse in schizophrenia: A review. *Journal of Clinical Psychiatry, 59,* 26–30.

Carmody, T.P. (1989). Affect regulation, nicotine addiction, and smoking cessation. *Journal of Psychoactive Drugs, 21,* 331–342.

Caspi, A., Begg, D., Dickson, N., Harrington, H., Langley, J., Moffitt, T.E., et al. (1997). Personality differences predict health-risk behaviors in young adulthood: Evidence from a longitudinal study. *Journal of Personality and Social Psychology, 73,* 1052–1063.

Catalano, R.F., Hawkins, J.D., Wells, E.A., Miller, J.L., and Brewer, D.D. (1990). Evaluation of the effectiveness of adolescent drug abuse treatment, assessment of risks for relapse, and promising approaches for relapse prevention. *International Journal of Addiction*, *25*, 1085–1140.

Centers for Disease Control and Prevention (1997). *Youth Risk Behavior Survey, 1997*. Washington, DC: US Department of Health and Human Services.

Charney, D.A., Paraherakis, A.M., Negrete, J.C., and Gill, K.J. (1998). The impact of depression on the outcome of addictions treatment. *Journal of Substance Abuse Treatment*, *15*, 123–130.

Charney, D.A., Paraherakis, A.M., and Gill, K.J. (2001). Integrated treatment of comorbid depression and substance use disorders. *Journal of Clinical Psychiatry*, *62*, 672–677.

Chassin, L.A., Presson, C.C., and Sherman, S.J. (1985). Stepping backward in order to step forward: An acquisition-oriented approach to primary prevention. *Journal of Consulting and Clinical Psychology*, *53*, 612–622.

Chassin, L., Rogosch, F., and Barrera, M. (1991). Substance use and symptomatology among adolescent children of alcoholics. *Journal of Abnormal Psychology*, *100*, 449–463.

Chassin, L., Presson, C.C., Rose, J.S., and Sherman, S.J. (1996). The natural history of cigarette smoking from adolescence to adulthood: Demographic predictors of continuity and change. *Health Psychology*, *15*, 478–484.

Chilcoat, H.D. and Breslau, N. (1998). Posttraumatic stress disorder and drug disorders. *Archives of General Psychiatry*, *55*, 913–917.

Cloninger, C.R. (1987). Neurogenetic adaptive mechanisms in alcoholism. *Science*, *236*, 410–416.

Cohen, P., Cohen, J., and Brook, J. (1993a). An epidemiological study of disorders in late childhood and adolescence: II. Persistence of disorders. *Journal of Child Psychology and Psychiatry*, *34*, 869–877.

Cohen, P., Cohen, J., Kasen, S., Velez, C. N., Hartmark, C., Johnson, J., et al. (1993b). An epidemiological study of disorders in late childhood and adolescence: I. Age- and gender-specific prevalence. *Journal of Child Psychology and Psychiatry*, *34*, 851–867.

Cone, E. J. (1997). New developments in biological measures of drug prevalence. In L. Harrison and A. Hughes (Eds.), *The validity of self-reported drug use: Improving the accuracy of survey estimates* (NIDA Research Monograph 167, pp. 108–129). Rockville, MD: US Department of Health and Human Services.

Connor, M.J. (1994). Peer relations and peer pressure. *Educational Psychology in Practice*, *9(4)*, 207–215.

Costello, E.J., Erkanli, A., Federman, E., and Angold, A. (1999). Development of psychiatric comorbidity with substance abuse in adolescents: Effects of timing and sex. *Journal of Clinical Child Psychology*, *28*, 298–311.

Costello, E.J., Mustillo, S., Erkanli, A., Keeler, G., and Angold, A. (2003). Prevalence and development of psychiatric disorders in childhood and adolescence. *Archives of General Psychiatry*, *60*, 837–844.

Crum, R.M., Lillie-Blanton, M., and Anthony, J.C. (1996). Neighborhood environment and opportunity to use cocaine and other drugs in late childhood and early adolescence. *Drug and Alcohol Dependence*, *43*, 155–161.

Deas, D. and Thomas, S.E. (2001). An overview of controlled studies of adolescent substance abuse treatment. *American Journal on Addictions*, *10*, 178–189.

210

Deykin, E.Y., Levy, J.C., and Wells, V. (1987). Adolescent depression, alcohol and drug abuse. *American Journal of Public Health, 77*, 178–182.

Dishion, T.J. (1990). The peer context of troublesome child and adolescent behavior. In P.E. Leone (Ed.), *Understanding troubled and troubling youth* (pp. 128–153). Beverly Hills, CA: Sage.

Dishion, T.J. and Andrews, D.W. (1995). Preventing escalation in problem behaviors with high-risk young adolescents: Immediate and 1-year outcomes. *Journal of Consulting and Clinical Psychology, 63*, 538–548.

Dishion, T.J. and Loeber, R. (1985). Adolescent marijuana and alcohol use: The role of parents and peers revisited. *American Journal of Drug and Alcohol Abuse, 11*, 11–25.

Dishion, T.J., Patterson, G.R., and Reid, J.B. (1988). Parent and peer factors associated with early adolescent drug use: Implications for treatment. In E. Rahdert and J. Grabowski (Eds.), *Adolescent drug abuse: Analyses of treatment research* (NIDA Research Monograph 77, pp. 69–93). Washington, DC: US Government Printing Office.

Dishion, T.J., Patterson, G.R., and Griesler, P.C. (1994). Peer adaptations in the development of antisocial behavior: A confluence model. In L.R. Huesmann (Ed.), *Current perspectives on aggressive behavior*. New York: Plenum.

Disney, E.R., Elkins, I.J., McCue, M., and Iacono, W.G. (1999). Effects of ADHD, conduct disorder, and gender on substance use and abuse in adolescence. *American Journal of Psychiatry, 156*, 1515–1521.

Duncan, S.C., Duncan, T.E., and Strycker, L.A. (2002). A multilevel analysis of neighborhood context and youth alcohol and drug problems. *Prevention Science, 3*, 125–134.

Duncan, T.E., Duncan, S.C., and Hops, H. (1994). The effect of family cohesiveness and peer encouragement on the development of adolescent alcohol use: A cohort-sequential approach to the analysis of longitudinal data. *Journal of Studies on Alcohol, 55*, 588–599.

Ennett, S.T., Flewelling, R.L., Lindrooth, R.C., and Norton, E.C. (1997). School and neighborhood characteristics associated with school rates of alcohol, cigarette, and marijuana use. *Journal of Health and Social Behavior, 38*, 55–71.

Fergusson, D.M. and Horwood, L.J. (2001). Cannabis use and traffic accidents in a birth cohort of young adults. *Accident Analysis and Prevention, 33*, 703–711.

Fergusson, D.M., Horwood, L.J., and Lynskey, M.T. (1993). Prevalence and comorbidity of DSM-III-R diagnoses in a birth cohort of 15 year olds. *Journal of the American Academy of Child and Adolescent Psychiatry, 32*, 1127–1134.

Fergusson, D.M., Horwood, L.J., and Swain-Campbell, N.R. (2002). Cannabis use and psychosocial adjustment in adolescence and young adulthood. *Addiction, 97*, 1123–1135.

Fergusson, D.M., Swain-Campbell, N.R., and Horwood, L.J. (2003). Arrests and convictions for cannabis related offences in a New Zealand birth cohort. *Drug and Alcohol Dependence, 70*, 53–63.

Fisher, M.S. and Bentley K.J. (1996). Two group therapy models for clients with a dual diagnosis of substance abuse and personality disorder. *Psychiatric Services, 47*, 1244–1250.

Flay, B.R. (1986). Efficacy and effectiveness trials (and other phases of research) in the development of health promotion programs. *Preventive Medicine, 15*, 451–474.

Flay, B.R. (1993). Youth tobacco use: Risks, patterns, and control. In C.T. Orleans and J. Slade (Eds.), *Nicotine addiction: Principles and management* (pp. 365–384). New York: Oxford University Press.

Fowler, I.L., Carr, V.J., Carter, N.T., and Lewin, T.J. (1998). Patterns of current and lifetime substance use in schizophrenia. *Schizophrenia Bulletin, 24*, 443–455.

Giaconia, R.M., Reinherz, H.Z., Silverman, A.B., Pakiz, B., Frost, A.K., and Cohen, E. (1994). Ages of onset of psychiatric disorders in a community population of older adolescents. *Journal of the American Academy of Child and Adolescent Psychiatry, 33*, 706–717.

Giaconia, R.M., Reinherz, H.Z., Hauf, A.C., Paradis, A.D., Wasserman, M.S., and Langhamer, D.M. (2000). Comorbidity of substance use and post-traumatic stress disorders in a community sample of adolescents. *American Journal of Orthopsychiatry, 70*, 253–262.

Giaconia, R.M., Reinherz, H.Z., Paradis, A.D., Hauf, A.M.C., and Stashwick, C.K. (2001). Major depression and drug disorders in adolescence: General and specific impairments in early adulthood. *Journal of the American Academy of Child and Adolescent Psychiatry, 40*, 1426–1433.

Gibbons, F.X. and Gerrard, M. (1997). Health images and their effects on health behavior. In B.P. Buunk and F.X. Gibbons (Eds.), *Health, coping, and well-being: Perspectives from social comparison theory* (pp. 63–94). Mahwah, NJ: Erlbaum

Glassman, A.H., Helzer, J.E., Covey, L.S., Cottler, L.B., Stetner, F., Tipp, J.E., et al. (1990). Smoking, smoking cessation, and major depression. *Journal of the American Medical Association, 264*, 1546–1549.

Graber, J.A., Lewinsohn, P.M., Seeley, J.R., and Brooks-Gunn, J. (1997). Is psychopathology associated with the timing of pubertal development? *Journal of the American Academy of Child and Adolescent Psychiatry, 36*, 1768–1776.

Greenfield, S.F., Weiss, R.D., Muenz, L.R., Vagge, L.M., Kelly, J.F., Bello, L.R., et al. (1998). The effect of depression on return to drinking: A prospective study. *Archives of General Psychiatry, 55*, 259–265.

Harrison, P.A., Fulkerson, J.A., and Beebe, T.J. (1998). DSM-IV substance use disorder criteria for adolescents: A critical examination based on a statewide school survey. *American Journal of Psychiatry, 155*, 486–492.

Harwood, H.J. (2001). Overview of the economic costs of alcohol, tobacco, and other drug abuse, updated to 2001. Unpublished manuscript.

Hasin, D.S., Tsai, W.Y., Endicott, J., Mueller, T.I., Coryell, W., and Keller, M. (1996). Five-year course of major depression: Effects of comorbid alcoholism. *Journal of Affective Disorders, 41*, 63–70.

Haver, B. (1986). The DSM-III diagnosis of alcohol use disorders in women: Findings from a follow-up study of 44 female alcoholics. *Acta Psychiatrica Scandinavica, 73*, 22–30.

Hawkins, J.D., Jensen, J.M., Catalano, R.F., and Wells, E.A. (1991). Effects of a skills training intervention with juvenile delinquents. *Research on Social Work Practices, 1*, 107–121.

Hawkins, J.D., Catalano, R.F., and Miller, J. (1992). Risk and protective factors for alcohol and other drug problems in adolescence and early adulthood: Implications for substance abuse prevention. *Psychological Bulletin, 112*, 64–105.

Helzer, J.E. and Burnam, A. (1991). Epidemiology of alcohol addiction: United States. In N.S. Miller (Ed.), *Comprehensive handbook of drug and alcohol addiction* (pp. 9–38). New York: Marcel Dekker.

Helzer, J.E. and Pryzbeck, T.R. (1988). The co-occurrence of alcoholism with other psychiatric disorders in the general population and its impact on treatment. *Journal of Studies on Alcohol, 49*, 219–224.

Hesselbrock, M.N. (1995). Genetic determinants of alcoholic subtypes. In H. Begleiter and B. Kissin (Eds.), *The genetics of alcoholism* (pp. 40–69). New York: Oxford University Press.

Hesselbrock, V., Hesselbrock, M., and Stabenau, J. (1985). Alcoholism in men patients subtyped by family history and antisocial personality. *Journal of Studies on Alcohol, 46*, 59–64.

Hirschfeld, R.M.A., Hasin, D., Keller, M.B., Endicott, J., and Wunder, J. (1990). Depression and alcoholism: Comorbidity in a longitudinal study. In J.D. Maser and C.R. Cloninger (Eds.), *Comorbidity of mood and anxiety disorders* (pp. 293–304). Washington, DC: American Psychiatric Press.

Hirschman, R.S. and Leventhal, H. (1989). Preventing smoking behavior in school children: An initial test of a cognitive-development program. *Journal of Applied Social Psychology, 19*, 559–583.

Holderness, C., Brooks-Gunn, J., and Warren, M. (1994). Comorbidity of eating disorders and substance abuse: Review of the literature. *International Journal of Eating Disorders, 16*, 1–34.

Inoff-Germain, G., Arnold, G.S., Nottelmann, E.D., Susman, E.J., Cutler, G.B., and Chrousos, G.P. (1988). Relations between hormone levels and observational measures of aggressive behavior of young adolescents in family interactions. *Developmental Psychology, 24*, 129–139.

Jainchill, N. (1999). Adolescent admission to residential drug treatment: HIV risk behaviors pre- and post-treatment. *Psychology of Addictive Behaviors, 13*, 163–173.

Jeffrey, R.W., Hennrikus, D.J., Lando, H.A., Murray, D.M., and Liu, J.W. (2000). Reconciling conflicting findings regarding postcessation weight concerns and success in smoking cessation. *Health Psychology, 19*, 242–246.

Jessor, R. (1987). Problem behavior theory, psychosocial development, and adolescent problem drinking. *British Journal of Addiction, 82*, 331–342.

Joanning, H., Quinn, T.F., and Mullen, R. (1992). Treating adolescent drug abuse: A comparison of family systems therapy, group therapy, and family drug education. *Journal of Marital Family Therapy, 18*, 345–356.

Johnson, R.J. and Kaplan, H.B. (1990). Stability of psychological symptoms: Drug use consequences and intervening processes. *Journal of Health and Social Behavior, 31*, 277–291.

Johnston, L.D., O'Malley, P.M., and Bachman, J.G. (2003). *Monitoring the future national results on adolescent drug use: Overview of key findings 2002*. Rockville, MD: US Department of Health and Human Services.

Joshi, V., Hser, Y-I., Grella, C.E., and Houlton, R. (2002). Sex-related HIV risk reduction behavior among adolescents in DATOS-A. *Journal of Adolescent Research, 16*, 642–660.

Kaminer, Y., Bukstein, O., and Tarter, R.E. (1991). The Teen-Addiction Severity Index: Rationale and reliability. *International Journal of Addiction, 26*, 219–226.

Kaminer, Y., Tarter, R.E., Bukstein, O.G., and Kabene, M. (1994). Adolescent substance abuse treatment: Staff, treatment completers', and noncompleters' perceptions of the value of treatment variables. *American Journal on Addictions, 1*, 115–120.

Kandel, D.B. (2000). Gender differences in the epidemiology of substance dependence in the United States. In E. Frank (Ed.), *Gender and its effects on psychopathology* (pp. 231–252). Washington, DC: American Psychiatric Press.

Kandel, D.B. and Davies, M. (1992). Progression to regular marijuana involvement: Phenomenology and risk factors for near-daily use. In M. Glantz and R. Pickens (Eds.), *Vulnerability to drug abuse* (1) (pp. 211–253). Washington, DC: American Psychological Association.

Kandel, D. and Yamaguchi, K. (1985). Developmental patterns of the use of legal, illegal, and medically prescribed psychotropic drugs from adolescence to young adulthood. In C.L. Jones and R. Battjes (Eds.), *Etiology of drug abuse: Implications for prevention* (pp. 193–235). Rockville, MD: National Institute on Drug Abuse.

Kandel, D.B., Davies, M., Karus, D., and Yamaguchi, K. (1986). The consequences in young adulthood of adolescent drug involvement. *Archives of General Psychiatry, 43*, 746–754.

Kandel, D.B., Mossel, P., and Kaestner, R. (1987). Drug use, the transition from school to work and occupational achievement in the United States. *European Journal of Psychology of Education, 2*, 337–363.

Kandel, D.B., Johnson, J.G., Bird, H.R., Canino, G., Goodman, S.H., Lahey, B.B., et al. (1997). Psychiatric disorders associated with substance use among children and adolescents: Findings from the Methods for the Epidemiology of Child and Adolescent Mental Disorders (MECA) Study. *Journal of Abnormal Child Psychology, 25*, 121–132.

Kaplan, H.B., Martin, S.S., and Robbins, C. (1982). Application of a general theory of deviant behavior. *Journal of Health and Social Behavior, 23*, 274–294.

Kassel, J.D., Stroud, L.R., and Paronis, C.A. (2003). Smoking, stress, and negative affect: Correlation, causation, and context across stages of smoking. *Psychological Bulletin, 129*, 270–304.

Kendler, K.S., Davis, C.G., and Kessler, R.C. (1997). The familial aggregation of common psychiatric and substance use disorders in the National Comorbidity Survey: A family history survey. *British Journal of Psychiatry, 170*, 541–548.

Kessler, R.C. (1995). Epidemiology of psychiatric comorbidity. In M.T. Tsuang, M. Tohen, and G.E.P. Zahner (Eds.), *Textbook in psychiatric epidemiology* (pp. 179–209). New York: Wiley-Liss.

Kessler, R.C. and Price, R.H. (1993). Primary prevention of secondary disorders: A proposal and agenda. *American Journal of Community Psychology, 21*, 607–633.

Kessler, R.C., McGonagle, K.A., Zhao, S., Nelson, C.B., Hughes, M., Eshleman, S., et al. (1994). Lifetime and 12-month prevalence of DSM-III-R psychiatric disorders in the United States: Results from the National Comorbidity Survey. *Archives of General Psychiatry, 51*, 8–19.

Kessler, R.C., Nelson, C.B., McGonagle, K.A., Edlund, M.J., Frank, R.G., and Leaf, P.J. (1996). The epidemiology of co-occurring addictive and mental disorders in the National Comorbidity Survey: Implications for prevention and service utilization. *American Journal of Orthopsychiatry, 66*, 17–31.

Kessler, R.C., Berglund, P.A., Foster, C.L., Saunders, W.B., Stang, P.E., and Walters, E.E. (1997a). Social consequences of psychiatric disorders: II. Teenage parenthood. *American Journal of Psychiatry, 154*, 1405–1411.

Kessler, R.C., Crum, R.M., Warner, L.A., Nelson, C.B., Schulenberg, J., and Anthony, J.C. (1997b). Lifetime co-occurrence of DSM-III-R alcohol abuse and dependence with other psychiatric disorders in the National Comorbidity Survey. *Archives of General Psychiatry, 54*, 313–321.

Khantzian, E.J. (1985). The self-medication hypothesis of addictive disorders: Focus on heroin and cocaine dependence. *American Journal of Psychiatry, 142*, 1259–1264.

Kilpatrick, D.G., Acierno, R., Saunders, B., Resnick, H.S., Best, C.L., and Schnurr, P.P. (2000). Risk factors for adolescent substance abuse and dependence: Data from a national sample. *Journal of Consulting and Clinical Psychology, 68*, 18–30.

Kokotailo, P.K., Fleming, M.F., and Koscik, R.L. (1995). A model alcohol and other drug use curriculum for pediatric residents. *Academic Medicine, 70*, 495–498.

Koob, G.F. and LeMoal, M. (2001). Drug addiction, dysregulation of reward and allostatis. *Neuropsychopharmacology, 24*, 97–129.

Krohn, M.D., Lizotte, A., and Perez, C. (1997). The interrelationship between substance use and precocious transitions to adult statuses. *Journal of Health and Social Behavior, 38*, 87–103.

Kushner, M.G., Sher, K.J., and Erickson, D.J. (1999). A prospective analysis of the relation between DSM-III anxiety disorders and alcohol use disorders. *American Journal of Psychiatry, 156*, 723–732.

Lewinsohn, P.M., Hops, H., Roberts, R.E., Seeley, J.R., and Andrews, J.A. (1993). Adolescent psychopathology: I. Prevalence and incidence of depression and other DSM-III-R disorders in high school students. *Journal of Abnormal Psychology, 102*, 133–144.

Lewinsohn, P.M., Rohde, P., and Seeley, J.R. (1995). Adolescent psychopathology: III. The clinical consequences of comorbidity. *Journal of the American Academy of Child and Adolescent Psychiatry, 34*, 510–519.

Lewinsohn, P.M., Rohde, P., and Seeley, J.R. (1996). Alcohol consumption in high school adolescents: Frequency of use and dimensional structure of associated problems. *Addiction, 91*, 375–390.

Lewinsohn, P.M., Rohde, P., and Brown, R.A. (1999). Level of current and past adolescent cigarette smoking as predictors of future substance use disorders in young adulthood. *Addiction, 94*, 913–921.

Lewis, R.A., Peircy, F., Sprenkle, D., and Trepper, T. (1990). Family-based interventions and community networking for helping drug abusing adolescents: The impact of near and far environments. *Journal of Adolescent Research, 5*, 82–95.

Liddle, H.A. and Dakof, G.A. (1995). Family-based intervention for adolescent drug abuse: State of the science. In E. Rahdert and D. Czechowicz (Eds.), *Adolescent drug abuse: Clinical assessment and therapeutic interventions* (NIDA Research Monograph 156, DHHS Publication 95–3908). Rockville, MD: National Institutes of Health.

Liddle, H.A. and Diamond, G. (1991). Adolescent substance abusers in family therapy: The critical initial phase of treatment. *Family Dynamics and Addiction, 1*, 55–68.

Loney, J. (1988). *Substance abuse in adolescents: Diagnostic issues derived from studies of attention deficit disorder with hyperactivity.* Washington, DC: US Government Printing Office.

McKay, J.R., Pettinati, H.M., Morrison, R., Feeley, M., Mulvaney, F.D., and Gallop, R. (2002). Relation of depression diagnoses to 2-year outcomes in cocaine-dependent patients in a randomized continuing care study. *Psychology of Addictive Behaviors, 16*, 225–235.

MacKenzie, R.G. and Kipke, M.D. (1992). Substance use and abuse. In S.B. Friedman, M. Fisher, and S.K. Schonberg (Eds.), *Comprehensive adolescent health care* (pp. 765–786). St Louis, MO: Quality Medical.

McKeown, R.E., Jackson, K.L., and Valois, R.F. (1997). The frequency and correlates of violent behaviors in a statewide sample of high school students. *Family and Community Health, 20*, 38–53.

Martin, C.A., Logan, T.K., Portis, C., Leukefled, C.G., Lynam, D., Staton, M., et al. (2001). The association of testosterone with nicotine use in young adult females. *Addictive Behaviors*, *26*, 279–283.

Merikangas, K.R., and Gelernter, C.S. (1990). Comorbidity for alcoholism and depression. *Psychiatric Clinics of North America*, *13*, 613–632.

Merikangas, K.R., Angst, J., Eaton, W., Canino, G., Rubio-Stipec, M., Wacker, H., et al. (1996). Comorbidity and boundaries of affective disorders with anxiety disorders and substance misuse: Results of an international task force. *British Journal of Psychiatry*, *168*, 58–67.

Merikangas, K.R., Stevens, D.E., Fenton, B., Stolar, M., O'Malley, S., Woods, S.W., et al. (1998). Comorbidity and familial aggregation of alcoholism and anxiety disorders. *Psychological Medicine*, *28*, 773–788.

Miller, G. (1990). *The Substance Abuse Subtle Screening Inventory-Adolescent Version*. Bloomington, IN: SASSI Institute.

Muck, R., Zempolich, K.A., Titus, J.C., Fishman, M., Godley, M.D., and Schwebel, R. (2001). An overview of the effectiveness of adolescent substance abuse treatment models. *Youth and Society*, *33*, 143–168.

Mueller, T.I., Lavori, P.W., Keller, M.B., Swartz, A., Warshaw, M., Hasin, D., et al. (1994). Prognostic effect of the variable course of alcoholism on the 10-year course of depression. *American Journal of Psychiatry*, *151*, 701–706.

Myers, M.G. and Brown, S.A. (1993). Coping as a predictor of adolescent substance abuse treatment outcome. *Journal of Substance Abuse*, *5*, 15–29.

Myers, M.G., Stewart, D.G., and Brown, S.A. (1998). Progression from conduct disorder to antisocial personality disorder following treatment for adolescent substance abuse. *American Journal of Psychiatry*, *155*, 479–485.

National Institute on Drug Abuse (NIDA) (2003). *Director's Report to the National Advisory Council on Drug Abuse* – February, 2003. Washington, DC: US Department of Health and Human Services.

Nelson, C.B., Heath, A.C., and Kessler, R.C. (1998). Temporal progression of alcohol dependence symptoms in the US household population: Results from the National Comorbidity Study. *Journal of Consulting and Clinical Psychology*, *66*, 474–483.

Newcomb, M.D. (1995). Identifying high-risk youth: prevalence and patterns of adolescent drug abuse. In E. Rahdert and D. Czechowicz (Eds.), *Adolescent drug abuse: Clinical assessment and therapeutic interventions* (NIDA Research Monograph 156, pp. 7–38). Rockville, MD: US Department of Health and Human Services.

Newcomb, M.D. and Bentler, P.M. (1987). The impact of late adolescent substance use on young adult health status and utilization of health services: A structural-equation model over four years. *Social Science and Medicine*, *24*, 71–82.

Newcomb, M.D. and Bentler, P.M. (1988). *Consequences of adolescent drug use: Impact on the lives of young adults*. Beverly Hills, CA: Sage.

Newcomb, M.D. and Bentler, P.M. (1989). Substance use and abuse among children and teenagers. *American Psychologist*, *44*, 242–248.

Newman, D. L., Moffitt, T. E., Caspi, A., Magdol, L., and Silva, P.A. (1996). Psychiatric disorder in a birth cohort of young adults: Prevalence, comorbidity, clinical significance, and new case incidence from age 11 to 21. *Journal of Consulting and Clinical Psychology*, *64*, 552–562.

O'Boyle, M. (1993). Personality disorder and multiple substance dependence. *Journal of Personality Disorders*, *7*, 342–347.

O'Hara, P., Parris, D., Fichtner, R.R., and Oster, R. (1998). Influence of alcohol and drug use on AIDS risk behavior among youth in dropout prevention. *Journal of Drug Education, 28,* 159–168.

Ozechowski, T.J. and Liddle, H.A. (2000). Family-based therapy for adolescent drug abuse: Knowns and unknowns. *Clinical Child and Family Psychology Review, 3(4),* 269–298.

Parrott, A. C. (1999). Does cigarette smoking cause stress? *American Psychologist, 54,* 817–820.

Patterson, G.R., Dishion, T.J., and Yoerger, K. (2000). Adolescent growth in new forms of problem behavior: Macro- and micro-peer dynamics. *Prevention Science, 1,* 3–13.

Pickrel, S.G. and Henggeler, S.W. (1996). Multisystemic therapy for adolescent substance abuse and dependence. *Child and Adolescent Psychiatric Clinic of North America, 5,* 201–211.

Pierce, J.P. and Gilpin, E.A. (1996). How long will today's new adolescent smoker be addicted to cigarettes? *American Journal of Public Health, 86,* 253–256.

Pierce, J.P., Choi, W.S., Gilpin, E.A., Farkas, A.J., and Merritt, R.K. (1996). Validation of susceptibility as a predictor of which adolescents take up smoking in the United States. *Health Psychology, 15,* 355–361.

Pihl, R. and Peterson, J. (1991). Attention deficit hyperactivity disorder, childhood conduct disorder, and alcoholism. *Alcohol Health and Research World, 15,* 25–31.

Pollock, N.K. and Martin, C.S. (1999). Diagnostic orphans: Adolescents with alcohol symptomatology who do not qualify for DSM-IV abuse or dependence diagnoses. *American Journal of Psychiatry, 156,* 897–901.

Rahdert, E. (1991). *The adolescent assessment and referral manual* (DHHS Publication ADM-91-1735). Rockville, MD: National Institute on Drug Abuse.

Regier, D.A., Farmer, M.E., Rae, D.S., Locke, B.Z., Keith, S.J., Judd, L.L., et al. (1990). Comorbidity of mental disorders with alcohol and other drug abuse: Results from the Epidemiologic Catchment Area (ECA) study. *Journal of the American Medical Association, 264,* 2511–2518.

Reinherz, H.Z., Giaconia, R.M., Lefkowitz, E.S., Pakiz, B., and Frost, A.K. (1993). Prevalence of psychiatric disorders in a community population of older adolescents. *Journal of the American Academy of Child and Adolescent Psychiatry, 32,* 369–377.

Riggs, P.D., Baker, S., Mikulich, S.K., Young, S.E., and Crowley, T.J. (1995). Depression in substance-dependent delinquents. *Journal of the American Academy of Child and Adolescent Psychiatry, 34,* 764–771.

Ritsher, J.B., McKellar, J.D., Finney, J.W., Otilingam, P.G., and Moos, R.H. (2002). Psychiatric comorbidity, continuing care and mutual help as predictors of five-year remission from substance use disorders. *Journal of Studies on Alcohol, 63,* 709–715.

Robins, L.N. (1989). Diagnostic grammar and assessment: Translating criteria into questions. *Psychological Medicine, 19,* 57–68.

Robinson, T.E. and Berridge, K.C. (2000). The psychology and neurobiology of addiction: An incentive-sensitization view. *Addiction, 95*(Suppl. 2), S91–S117.

Rohde, P., Lewinsohn, P.M., and Seeley, J.R. (1996). Psychiatric comorbidity with problematic alcohol use in high school adolescents. *Journal of the American Academy of Child and Adolescent Psychiatry, 35,* 101–109.

Rohde, P., Lewinsohn, P.M., Kahler, C.W., Seeley, J.R., and Brown, R.A. (2001). Natural course of alcohol use disorders from adolescence to young adulthood. *Journal of the American Academy of Child and Adolescent Psychiatry, 40,* 83–90.

Rohde, P., Kahler, C.W., Lewinsohn, P.M., and Brown, R.A. (2004). Psychiatric disorders, familial factors, and cigarette smoking: II. Associations with progression to daily smoking. *Nicotine and Tobacco Research, 6,* 119–132.

Ross, H.E., Glaser, F.B., and Germanson, T. (1988). The prevalence of psychiatric disorders in patients with alcohol and other drug problems. *Archives of General Psychiatry, 45,* 1023–1031.

Rounds-Bryant, J.L. and Staab, J. (2002). Patient characteristics and treatment outcomes for African American, Hispanic, and White adolescents in DATOS-A. *Journal of Adolescent Research, 16,* 624–641.

Rutter, M. (1982). Prevention of children's psychosocial disorders: Myth and substance. *Pediatrics, 70,* 883–894.

Schonberg, S.K. (1992). Substance use and abuse. In E.R. McAnarney, R.E. Kreipe, D.P. Orr, and G.D. Comerci (Eds.), *Textbook of adolescent medicine* (pp. 1063–1077). Philadelphia, PA: W.B. Saunders

Schuckit, M.A. and Hesselbrock, V. (1994). Alcohol dependence and anxiety disorders: What is the relationship? *American Journal of Psychiatry, 12,* 1723–1734.

Schwartz, C.E., Dorer, D.J., Beardslee, W.R., and Lavori, P.W. (1990). Maternal expressed emotion and parental affective disorder: Risk for childhood depressive disorder, substance abuse, or conduct disorder. *Journal of Psychiatric Research, 24,* 231–250.

Severson, H.H., Andrews, J.A., and Walker, H.M. (2003). Screening and early intervention for antisocial youth within school settings as a strategy for reducing substance use. In D. Romer (Ed.), *Reducing adolescent risk: Toward an integrated approach.* Thousand Oaks, CA: Sage.

Shedler, J. and Block, J. (1990). Adolescent drug use and psychological health: A longitudinal perspective. *American Psychologist, 45,* 612–629.

Simon, T.R., Sussman, S., Dent, C.W., Burton, D. and Flay, B. (1995). Prospective correlates of exclusive or combined adolescent use of cigarettes and smokeless tobacco: A replication-extension. *Addictive Behaviors, 20(4),* 517–524.

Slutske, W.S., Heath, A.C., Dinwiddie, S.H., Madden, P.A.F., Bucholz, K.K., Dunne, M.P., et al. (1998). Common genetic risk factors for conduct disorder and alcohol dependence. *Journal of Abnormal Psychology, 107,* 363–374.

Smart, R.G., Adlaf, E.M., and Walsh, G.W. (1994). The relationships between declines in drinking and alcohol problems among Ontario students: 1979–1991. *Journal of Studies on Alcohol, 55, 3,* 338–341.

Sobell, M.B. and Sobell, L.C. (1993). Treatment for problem drinkers: A public health priority. In J.S. Baer, G.A. Marlatt, and R.J. McMahon (Eds.), *Addictive behaviors across the life span* (pp. 138–157). Newbury Park, CA: Sage.

Stanton, M.D. and Shadish, W.R. (1997). Outcome, attrition, and family-couples treatment for drug abuse: A meta-analysis and review of the controlled, comparative studies. *Psychological Bulletin, 122,* 170–191.

Stice, E., Presnell, K., and Bearman, S. K. (2001). Relation of early menarche to depression, eating disorders, substance abuse, and comorbid psychopathology in adolescent girls. *Developmental Psychology, 37,* 608–619.

Strakowski, S.M., Tohen, M., Stoll, A.L., Faedda, G.L., Mayer, P.V., Kolbrener, M.L., et al. (1993). Comorbidity in psychosis at first hospitalization. *American Journal of Psychiatry, 150,* 752–757.

Substance Abuse and Mental Health Services Administration (2003). *Results from the 2002 National Survey on Drug Use and Health*. Office of Applied Studies, NHSDA Series. Rockville, MD: US Department of Health and Human Services.

Susman, E.J. and Pajer, K. (2004) Biology-behavior integration and antisocial behavior in girls. In K. Bierman and M. Putallaz (Eds.), *Aggression, antisocial behavior and violence among girls: A developmental perspective*. New York: Guilford.

Sussman, S., Dent, C.W., Burton, D., Stacy, A.W., and Flay, B.R. (1995). *Developing school-based tobacco use prevention and cessation programs*. Thousand Oaks, CA: Sage.

Swan, G.E., Ward, M.M., Carmelli, D., and Jack, L.M. (1993). Differential rates of relapse in subgroups of male and female smokers. *Journal of Clinical Epidemiology, 46*, 1041–1053.

Szapocznik, J., Perez-Vidal, A., Brickman, A.L., Foote, F.H., Santisteban, D., Hervis, O., et al. (1988). Engaging adolescent drug abusers and their families in treatment: A strategic structural systems approach. *Journal of Consulting and Clinical Psychology, 56*, 552–557.

Taylor, D.R., Fergusson, D.M., Milne, B.J., Horwood, L.J., Moffitt, T.E., Sears, M.R., et al. (2002). A longitudinal study of the effects of tobacco and cannabis exposure on lung function in young adults. *Addiction, 97*, 1055–1061.

Tobler, N.S. (1986). Meta-analysis of 143 adolescent drug prevention programs: Quantitative outcomes results of program participants compared to a control or comparison group. *Journal of Drug Issues, 16*, 535–567.

Tobler, N.S. and Stratton, H.S. (1997). Effectiveness of school-based drug prevention programs: A meta-analysis of the research. *Journal of Primary Prevention, 18*, 71–128.

Turnbull, J. and Gomberg, E. (1988). Impact of depressive symptomatology and alcohol problems in women. *Alcoholism: Clinical and Experimental Research, 12*, 374–381.

US Department of Health and Human Services (USDHHS) (1989). *The health consequences of smoking: Nicotine addiction. A report of the Surgeon General, 1988*. Atlanta, GA: USDHHS.

Van Horn, D.H.A. and Frank, A.E. (1998). Substance-use situations and abstinence predictions in substance abusers with and without personality disorders. *American Journal of Drug and Alcohol Abuse, 24*, 395–404.

von Sydow, K., Lieb, R., Pfister, H., Hofler, M., Sonntag, H., and Wittchen, H. (2001). The natural course of cannabis use, abuse and dependence over four years: A longitudinal community study of adolescents and young adults. *Drug and Alcohol Dependence, 64*, 347–361.

Wagner, E.F., Lloyd, D.A., and Gil, A.G. (2002). Racial/ethnic and gender differences in the incidence and onset age of DSM-IV alcohol use disorder symptoms among adolescents. *Journal of Studies on Alcohol, 63*, 609–619.

Waldron, H.B. (1997). Adolescent substance abuse and family therapy outcome: A review of randomized trials. In T.H. Ollendick and R.J. Prinz (Eds.), *Advances in clinical child psychology* (Vol. 19). New York: Plenum.

Waldron, H.B. and Slesnick, N. (1996). Treating the family. In W.R. Miller and N. Heather (Eds.), *Treating addictive behaviors*, 2nd edn. New York: Plenum.

Ward, K.D., Klesges, R.C., Zbikowski, S.M., Bliss, R.E., and Garvey, A.J. (1997). Gender differences in the outcome of an unaided smoking cessation attempt. *Addictive Behaviors, 22*, 521–533.

Weinberg, N.Z., Rahdert, E., and Glantz, M.D. (1998). Adolescent substance abuse: A review of the past 10 years. *Journal of the American Academy of Child and Adolescent Psychiatry, 37,* 252–260.

Weiss, R.D., Mirin, S.M., Griffin, M.L., Gunderson, J G., and Hufford, C. (1993). Personality disorders in cocaine dependence. *Comprehensive Psychiatry, 34,* 145–149.

Westermeyer, J., Kopka, S., and Nugent, S. (1997). Course and severity of substance abuse among patients with comorbid major depression. *American Journal on Addictions, 6(4),* 284–292.

Westermeyer, J., Eames, S., and Nugent, S. (1998). Comorbid dysthymia and substance disorder: Treatment history and cost. *American Journal of Psychiatry, 155,* 1556–1560.

Wilens, T.E., Biederman, J., Millstein, R.B., Wozniak, J., Hahesy, A.L., and Spencer, T.J. (1999). Risk for substance use disorders in youths with child- and adolescent-onset bipolar disorder. *Journal of the American Academy of Child and Adolescent Psychiatry, 38,* 680–685.

Williams, R.J., Chang, S.Y., and Group, A.C.A.R. (2000). A comprehensive and comparative review of adolescent substance abuse treatment outcome. *Clinical Psychology: Science and Practice, 7,* 138–166.

Wills, T.A. (1987). Downward comparison as a coping mechanism. In C.R. Snyder and C. Ford (Eds.), *Coping with Negative Life Events: Clinical and Social Psychological Perspectives.* New York: Plenum.

Wills, T.A. (1990). Stress and coping factors in the epidemiology of substance use. In L.T. Kozlowski, H.M. Annis, H.D. Cappell, F.B. Glaser, M.S. Goodstadt, Y. Israel, et al. (Eds.), *Research advances in alcohol and drug problems,* Vol. 10 (pp. 215–250). New York: Plenum.

Wills, T.A., Sandy, J.M., and Yaeger, A. (2002). Stress and smoking in adolescence: A test of directional hypotheses. *Health Psychology, 21,* 122–130.

Windle, M. (1994). Substance use, risky behaviors, and victimization among a US national adolescent sample. *Addiction, 89,* 175–182.

Windle, M. and Davies, P.T. (1999). Depression and heavy alcohol use among adolescents: Concurrent and prospective relations. *Development and Psychopathology, 11,* 823–844.

Winters, K.C. (1991). *The Personal Experience Screening Questionnaire and Manual.* Los Angeles, CA: Western Psychological Services.

Winters, K.C. and Henly G.A. (1993). *The Adolescent Diagnostic Interview Schedule and User's Manual.* Los Angeles, CA: Western Psychological Services.

Yamaguchi, K. and Kandel, D.B. (1984a). Patterns of drug use from adolescence to young adulthood: II. Sequences of progression. *American Journal of Public Health, 74,* 668–672.

Yamaguchi, K. and Kandel, D.B. (1984b). Patterns of drug use from adolescence to young adulthood: III. Predictors of progression. *American Journal of Public Health, 74,* 673–681.

Young, S.E., Corley, R.P., Stallings, M.C., Rhee, S.H., Crowley, T.J., and Hewit, J.K. (2002). Substance use, abuse and dependence in adolescence: Prevalence, symptom profiles and correlates. *Drug and Alcohol Dependence, 68,* 309–322.

Zaider, T.I., Johnson, J.G., and Cockell, S.J. (2000). Psychiatric comorbidity associated with eating disorder symptomatology among adolescents in the community. *International Journal of Eating Disorders, 28,* 58–67.

Zucker, R.A. (1987). The four alcoholisms: A developmental account of the etiologic process. In P.C. Rivers (Ed.), *Nebraska Symposium on Motivation, 1986: Alcohol and addictive behavior* (pp. 27–83). Lincoln, NE: University of Nebraska Press.

9

SOMATOFORM DISORDERS

Cecilia A. Essau

Children and adolescents often express physical complaints and worries about their health (Taylor et al., 1996). Up to 50 percent of children and adolescents reported having had at least one physical symptoms without any physical basis (Garber et al., 1991). These symptoms tend to follow a developmental sequence. Recurrent abdominal pain and headaches are the most common physical complaints among school-age children, whereas complaints related to limb pain, aching muscles, fatigue, and neurological symptoms generally increase in frequency with age (Walker and Greene, 1991). In some children and adolescents, these physical complaints may spontaneously disappear, or are "cured" with medical treatment. In some children, however, these symptoms tend to persist and cause a significant impairment. These persistent and pervasive physical complaints are categorized as somatoform disorders.

The central feature of somatoform disorders is the presence of physical symptoms which are not fully explained by a known medical condition. The symptoms must cause significant distress or impairment, and may not be primarily due to substance use or another psychiatric disorder (American Psychiatric Association (APA), 1994). Somatoform disorders first appeared as a class of psychiatric disorders in DSM-III (APA, 1980) in order to facilitate the differential diagnosis of disorders which have been characterized by physical symptoms suggestive of physical disorder for which no organic findings or known physiological mechanism can be found. Furthermore, there is a positive evidence, or a strong assumption that the symptoms are associated to psychological factors or conflicts (APA, 1980). Except for some minor modifications, this category reminds the same in DSM-III-R and DSM-IV. In DSM-IV (APA, 1994), the somatoform disorders include pain disorder, conversion disorder, somatization disorder, dysmorphic disorder, undifferentiated somatoform disorders, hypochondriasis, and somatoform disorder not otherwise specified. These disorders are assumed to share clinical utility, which consists of an overriding diagnostic concern, namely, the exclusion of occult physical or organic pathology underlying the symptoms (Martin and Yutzy, 1994).

The grouping of the specific disorders in the somatoform category has been regarded as heterogenous in terms of its focus and overall presentation (Martin and Yutzy, 1994). The major focus in somatization, undifferentiated somatoform, conversion, and pain disorders, is on the symptoms themselves. In hypochodriasis, the preoccupation is with the interpretation and implications of bodily symptoms, and in body dysmorphic disorder, the preoccupation is related to an imagined or exaggerated defect in appearance. Thus, hypochondriasis and body dysmorphic disorder seem to closely resemble the characteristics of obsessive-compulsive disorder than the characteristics of somatoform disorder.

In the International Classification of Diseases (ICD), a somatoform grouping was not incorporated into the international system until its tenth version (ICD-10: WHO, 1992). ICD-10 includes a medical utilization specification which requires a "repeated presentation" of symptoms, persistent requests for medical investigation, and resistance to consideration of "psychological causation" despite repeated negative findings and reassurances by doctors that the "symptoms have no physical basis" (WHO, 1992, p. 161). In ICD-10 somatoform disorders include somatization disorder, undifferentiated somatoform disorder, hypochondriacal disorder, somatoform autonomic dysfunction, persistent somatoform pain disorder, other somatoform disorder, and somatoform disorder, unspecified. Conversion disorder is subsumed under dissociative (conversion) disorder, and not under somatoform disorders as is the case in DSM-IV. ICD-10 also includes neurasthenia with chronic fatigue as the defining symptom. This is now more commonly referred to as chronic fatigue syndrome (CFS).

In this chapter, a brief description of each type of somatoform disorder will be presented. Since most studies of somatoform disorders in children and adolescents generally used DSM-IV criteria, we will focus our description on the main characteristics of the somatoform disorders according to DSM-IV. It should be noted that the same diagnostic criteria are required for a diagnosis of somatoform disorders in adults, adolescents, and children (APA, 1994). The use of the same diagnostic criteria was the result of a lack of a child-specific research base and a developmentally appropriate alternative system.

After a short description of the main features of somatoform disorders, recent child and adolescent literature on somatoform disorders (somatization disorder, conversion disorder, pain disorder, hypochondriasis, and body dysmorphic disorder) will be reviewed. The literature on somatoform disorders in children and adolescents is rare, therefore, adult studies will be cited when relevant. Treatment approaches are reviewed collectively for the various specific disorders.

Features of somatoform disorders

Somatization disorder

The main feature of somatization disorder (historically known as hysteria or Briquet's syndrome) is recurrent multiple physical complaints that are not fully explained by physical factors and result in medical attention or significant impairment. It is a polysymptomatic disorder which affects multiple body system. In DSM-IV (APA, 1994), a diagnosis of somatization disorder requires at least

- pain symptoms on at least four different sites or functions such as head, abdomen, back, joints, chest, during sexual intercourse, during menstruation, or during urination
- two gastrointestinal symptoms other than pain (e.g., nausea, bloating, diarrhea, intolerance of several different foods, vomiting other than during pregnancy)
- one sexual symptom other than pain such as sexual indifference, erectile or ejaculatory dysfunction, irregular menses, and excessive menstrual bleeding
- one pseudoneurological symptom that suggests a neurological disorder not limited to pain (e.g., dissociative symptom such as amnesia, impaired coordination or balance, paralysis or localized weakness, double vision, blindness, seizures).

These medically unexplained complaints of multiple physical symptoms begin before age 30 years and occur over a period of several years. None of these symptoms can be fully explained by a known general medical condition, or the direct effects of a substance.

The symptoms of somatization disorder are often nonspecific and may overlap with various medical disorders. Somatization disorder can be discriminated from physical illness by considering the following factors: involvement of multiple organ system; early onset and chronic course; absence of characteristic laboratory abnormalities of the suggested physical disorder (Cloninger, 1986). In addition, three psychiatric disorders need to be considered in the differential diagnosis of somatization disorders: anxiety and mood disorders, and schizophrenia.

Conversion disorder

The main feature of conversion disorder is the presence of "one or more symptoms or deficits which effect voluntary motor or sensory function that suggest a neurological or other general medical condition" (APA, 1994, p. 457). Specific symptoms include

- motor symptoms such as impaired coordination balance, difficulty swallowing or lump in throat
- sensory symptoms including blindness and deafness
- seizures or convulsions with voluntary motor or sensory components
- symptoms with mixed presentation.

Additionally, psychological stressors must precede the development or exacerbation of the conversion symptoms. In order to meet the diagnostic criteria, the symptom is not fully explained as a culturally sanctioned behavior or experience, such as behaviour related with certain religious ceremonies (e.g., "seizure-like episodes"). The symptoms cannot be fully explained by a general medical condition, or by the direct effects of a substance. In addition, the symptoms must cause significant distress or impairment in several important areas of functioning.

Hypochondriasis

The essential feature of hypochondriasis is not preoccupation with symptoms themselves, but rather with the fear or ideas of having a serious disease. This fear is based on misinterpretation of one or multiple physical symptoms (e.g., headache is believed to be associated with brain tumor) and it persists despite evidence to the contrary and reassurance from physicians that there is no underlying disease which justifies the intense distress. The preoccupation must be present for at least six months, and causes significant distress or impairment. In order to meet the diagnostic criteria, the symptoms are not accounted for by generalized anxiety disorder, obsessive-compulsive disorder, panic disorder, major depressive episode, separation anxiety disorder, or another somatoform disorder. Hypochondriasis is often associated with dissatisfaction regarding medical care, doctor shopping, and the risk of iatrogenic complication as a result of excessive or repeated diagnostic procedures.

There has been much debate in the adult literature about the status of hypo-chondriasis and obsessive-compulsive disorder (Fritz et al., 1997). Both disorders involve intense fears of illness or contamination, and they tend to co-occur highly (Barsky et al., 1992).

Body dysmorphic disorder

The diagnostic criteria for body dysmorphic disorder (BDD) was not introduced until the introduction of DSM-III, although the concept of BDD had been identified by an Italian psychiatrist Enriquo Morseli as early as 1891 (cited in Phillips, 1991). At that time, the term "dysmorphophobia" was used to describe a subjective feeling of ugliness despite a normal outward appearance (Phillips, 1991). Dysmorpho-phobia was briefly noted in DSM-III and in DSM-III-R, the term was changed to BDD because the term dysmorphobia was thought to overemphasize phobic avoidance (Carroll et al., 2002). The popularity of BDD has been attributed to the publication of Katharine Phillips' book *The broken mirror: Understanding and treating body dysmorphic disorder* in 1996.

BDD is defined in DSM-IV as the preoccupation with imagined defects in appearance, or a markedly excessive concern with a minor physical anomaly. Such preoccupation persists even after medical reassurances. In order to fulfil the diagnostic criteria, the preoccupation must also cause clinically significant distress or impairment in social, occupational or other important areas of functioning. The preoccupation must not be better accounted for by another mental disorder such as the dissatisfaction which occurs in anorexia nervosa.

Children and adolescents with BDD have excessive concern about various parts of the body, but overwhelmingly involved the skin, weight, teeth, legs, and nose (Albertini and Phillips, 1999). Studies conducted among adults showed significant gender differences in their areas of concern: females compared to males were more concerned with their weight and hips; generally, they believe that they were too large or fat. Males were more preoccupied with body build, and they generally think of their body as too small, skinny, or not muscular.

Children with BDD spend an average of three hours or more per day thinking about their perceived defects (Albertini and Phillips, 1999). This preoccupation often leads to obsessional thinking and compulsive behaviours (e.g., mirror-checking, camouflaging, and avoidance of daily activities) which may cause impairment in social relations, academic performance, and role functions (Phillips, 1991). The distress experienced may be so intense and may result in unnecessary medical procedures, suicidal ideations, suicide attempts, hospitalization, and acts of self-mutilation (Phillips, 1991). Self-mutilation in BDD can take various forms. Because of intensive hate of their appearance they purposely mutilate the body part such as slashing their face with a razor blade or compulsively picking their skin to remove minor imperfections (Phillips, 1996; Phillips and Diaz, 1997). In an attempt to remove a perceived deformity, some patients even do self-surgery such as cutting off their nipples or attempting a facelift with a staple gun (Phillips, 1996; Veale, 2000).

There is a considerable debate and research on the comorbidity between BDD, social phobia, and OCD. That is, although BDD has been categorized under somatoform disorders, it shows several features of social phobia and obsessive-compulsive disorder (Carroll et al., 2002). Similar to patients with social phobia, BDD patients tend to fear and avoid situations which may expose them to scrutiny and negative evaluation. As reported by some authors (e.g., Horowitz et al., 2002), some BDD patients hid under the bed or in the closet for fear that others were looking at their face and body. At school they sometimes hide in the bathroom or walk the hallway pressed up against the walls. BDD is also similar to obsessive-compulsive disorder in that it is characterized by recurrent, intrusive thoughts about one's ugliness which are difficult to resist and which prompt checking (e.g., looking in mirrors) and excessive grooming.

Pain disorder

Pain disorder is characterized by complaints of pain in one or more anatomical sites in the absence of a somatic explanation for the pain or for its intensity (APA, 1994). Like other somatoform disorders, pain causes significant distress and impairment in the person's important areas of functioning. Children with pain disorder often miss school and other activities, and many of them go from doctor to doctor in an attempt to find the cause of the disorder (Campo and Fritsch, 1994). Pain may interfere with the child's concentration and cause irritability, which may contribute to social isolation and low self-esteem in some children (Campo and Fritsch, 1994). Furthermore, psychological factors are judged to have an important role in the onset, severity, exacerbation, or maintenance of the pain. The pain is neither feigned nor part of a mood, anxiety, or psychotic disorder. If pain disorder co-occurs with actual physical problems, the following diagnosis will be given: "pain associated with both psychological factors and a general medical condition". Pain disorder which does not co-occur with actual physical problems will be given a diagnosis of "pain disorder associated with psychological factors".

Undifferentiated somatoform disorder

The essential aspect of undifferentiated somatoform disorder is the presence of one or more physical complaints such as fatigue, loss of appetite, and gastrointestinal complaints (APA, 1994). The symptoms must have lasted for at least six months, and are not better accounted for by another mental disorder such as mood or anxiety disorders or another somatoform disorder. This category serves to capture syndromes which resemble somatization disorder but do not meet the full criteria. As with the other somatoform disorders, the symptoms cause significant distress or impairment in social, occupational, or other important areas of functioning. The final diagnostic criteria states that the symptom is not produced on purpose, or feigned.

Somatoform disorder not otherwise specified (NOS)

Somatoform disorder NOS is a residual category for the somatoform disorder. This disorder is characterized by the presence of somatic symptoms which do not meet diagnostic criteria for any of the specified somatoform disorders (APA, 1994). An example of a symptom which has been listed under this somatoform disorder is pseudocyesis, defined as a false belief of being pregnant together with the presence of objective signs of pregnancy. The symptoms last for less than six months and are not caused by another mental disorder. Another criterion involves the presence of non-psychotic hypochondrical symptoms.

Physical symptoms

Some evidence suggests that physical symptoms are quite common in children and adolescents. An early study by Offord et al. (1987) has shown recurrent distressing symptoms to be present in 11 percent of girls and 4 percent of boys aged 12 to 16 years. A study by Perquin et al. (2000) indicated that 53.7 percent of the children and adolescents reported having experienced a pain in the previous three months. Among these children, 25 percent reported chronic pain (i.e., pain existing recurrently or continuously for more than three months) and 24.2 percent reported non-chronic pain (i.e., pain lasting less than three months). About 49 percent of the chronic pain sufferers reported the occurrence of pain at least once a week, in 21 percent less than once a month, and in 30 percent somewhere in between. Children who had chronic pains also reported chronic disability and emotional distress as a result of the recurrent or persistent pain (Bursch et al., 1998).

Recurrent abnormal pain (RAP) is defined as pain without any known organic cause which occurs at least three times over a period longer than three months, and which is severe enough to interfere with the child's activities (Aro et al., 1987). RAP is among one of the most common pain symptoms in children and adolescents.

Between 10 and 30 percent of children and adolescents have been reported to suffer from RAP. In Perquin et al.'s (2000) study, 22 percent of the children and adolescents had chronic abdominal pain, with significantly more girls than boys affected. This pain was also the most common among children aged up to 8 years. Children with RAP were three times more likely to have similar complaints when being re-interviewed six years later (Borge et al., 1994), and they had higher use of health care services than controls (Walker et al., 1995).

Limb pain is also known as growing pain because it usually occurs in the limbs during a period of skeletal growth in the absence of organic disease or physical injury (Goodman and McGrath, 1991). However, no empirical evidence is available on the association between growth and limb pain. According to some early studies, between 5 and 20 percent of youth reported having frequent or at least weekly limb pains (Garber et al., 1991; Larsson, 1991). In a study by Perquin et al. (2000), 22 percent of the children and adolescents reported having had limb pain. Significantly more boys than girls reported chronic limb pain; this study also indicated limb pain to be more common among those older than 8 years old. Headaches are also common physical complaints in children and adolescents, the two most common being that of migraine and tension headaches. Tension headaches have been described as non-paroxysmal, frequent, and bilateral, and are associated with dizziness, whereas migraine tends to be periodic, severe, and unilateral (Garralda, 1999). Migraine is often associated with visual aura, nausea, and vomiting. The presence of migraine headache has been reported in 2.5 percent to 22 percent of children and adolescents in community and school settings (see review by Goodman and McGrath, 1991). Unlike migraine headache, little is known about tension headache. The prevalence of unspecified headaches which occur at least once a week has been reported in 7 percent to 29 percent of school children (see review by P.J. McGrath and Larsson, 1997).

Studies have also examined the prevalence of pseudoseizures, in which cultural differences could be found. Pehlivantürk and Unal (2002) reported higher rates of pseudoseizures in children and adolescents in Turkey than in Western countries (Goodyer, 1981; Turgay, 1990). It was argued that the high rate of pseudoseizures in Turkey may be due to cultural influence (Pehlivantürk and Unal, 2002). Because of the association with death, fainting and seizures may be perceived as life threatening symptoms by the environment. It can also be speculated that pseudo-seizures, because of their secondary gain potential and episodic nature, may be unconsciously preferred as a symptom. These factors may contribute to the high rate of this symptom, in addition to the possible referral bias.

Chronic fatigue syndrome (CFS) is characterized by debilitating fatigue, which is unexplained by medical or psychiatric disorders (Garralda and Rangel, 2002). Fatigue tends to get worse following minor exertion. In addition to fatigue, children and adolescents with this syndrome experience numerous symptoms such as headache, sore throat, muscle pain, sleep disturbance, and cognitive dysfunction. About 2 percent of the children and adolescents have been reported to have CFS-like illness (Bell et al., 1991; Jordan et al., 2000). Higher rates have been reported among females than males, and among those of Latino origins compared to those from other ethnic groups (Jordan et al., 2000). Physical illness (e.g., flu-type illness, glandular fever) has been found to be a common precipitant of CFS (Bell et al., 2001). A study by Garralda and Rangel (2004) compared impairment, illness attitudes and coping mechanisms in childhood CFS and in other pediatric disorders. Children with CFS reported significantly more illness impairment, especially in school attendance, than those with other pediatric disorders (idiopathic arthritis and emotional disorders). They had more worries about illness, and had an illness coping pattern which involved reduced active strategies. During its worst episode (Rangel et al., 2000), most children with CFS had stopped socializing with their friends and family members. Half had been bedridden for prolonged periods and some were even in wheelchairs, two-thirds were unable to attend school with a mean time out of school of one year. CFS seems to have a favorable outcome. In most studies, about half to three-quarters of the cases have full recovery or showed significant reduction in CFS symptoms (Carter et al., 1996; Feder et al., 1994; Krilov et al., 1998; Rangel et al., 2000). In a study by Garralda and Rangel (2001), two-thirds of the cases had recovered and resumed normal activities at an average of 45 months after illness onset. Factors related to negative outcome of CFS included low socio-economic status, chronic maternal health problems, and the lack of acute physical triggers (Rangel et al., 2000).

Epidemiology of somatoform disorders

Studies examining the prevalence of somatoform disorders in children and adolescents are rare, and the few existing studies are difficult to compare because of methodological differences and/or limitations. In fact, somatoform disorders have been regarded as one of the least explored areas in child and adolescent psychopathology (Fritz et al., 1997). The lack of attention may be due to the ill-defined nature of the disorders – at least before the introduction of the DSM-III. That is, the problem with studying somatoform disorders has been due to the unresolved problems at the borderland between psychiatry and medicine (Lipowski, 1987).

The Bremen Adolescent Study (Essau et al., 1999) is among one of the few large-scale studies in which the prevalence and comorbidity of somatoform disorders have been explored in detail. In this study, 13.1 percent of the adolescents, aged 12 to 17 years, met the DSM-IV criteria for somatoform disorders. When considering the subtypes of somatoform disorders, undifferentiated somatoform disorder was the most frequent with 11 percent of all the adolescents reporting having had this disorder sometimes in their lives. The next most frequent was that of pain disorder (1.7 percent), followed by conversion disorder (1.4 percent). None of the subjects had somatization disorder or hypochondriasis. In the Early Developmental Stages of Psychopathology project, 12 percent of the 14 to 24 year olds met the diagnosis of at least one somatoform disorders (Lieb et al., 2000). The 12-month incidence was 7.2 percent. The most common somatoform disorder was pain (lifetime = 1.7 percent, 12-month = 0.9 percent), and conversion disorder (0.4 percent, 12-month

0.2 percent). None of these young adults met the criteria for a somatization disorder, and only one fulfilled the criteria for hypochondriasis. Undifferentiated somatoform disorder, which is a residual form of a disorder, occurred rather frequently, with a lifetime prevalence of 9.1 percent.

Somatization disorder among children and adolescents is rare. The low prevalence of somatization disorder in these studies (Essau et al., 1999; Lieb et al., 2000) could be directly attributable to the diagnostic criteria requiring 13 physical symptoms from a list of 35, of which 8 are appropriate only for postpubertal and/or sexually active individuals. Furthermore, the pattern and number of symptoms experienced, the language used to describe symptoms and the associated functional impairment may differ across the lifespan. All these could be a reflection that the somatization criteria may not be developmentally appropriate for use in children and adolescents. In this respect, the criteria may need to be revised in children (Fritz et al., 1997).

Somatoform disorders such as undifferentiated somatoform disorder, pain disorder, and conversion disorder were significantly more common in females than in males (Essau et al., 1999; Lieb et al., 2000). The frequency of any somatoform disorders increased with age: 8.9 percent of the 12 to 13 year olds met the diagnosis of somatoform disorder, compared to 13.7 percent in the 14 to 15 year olds, and 17.7 percent of the 16 to 17 year olds (Essau et al., 1999). The subtypes of somatoform disorders with the greatest increase with age were of undifferentiated somatoform disorder and pain disorder, whereas the frequency of conversion disorder is equally distributed across age. Somatoform disorders, with the exception of pain disorder, were generally found among those in the low socio-economic status. Pain disorder was mostly associated with higher education (Lieb et al., 2000).

The prevalence of the specific types of somatoform disorders have been reported in some small-scale studies. The prevalence of BDD among adolescents was 2.3 percent in a community sample (Mayville et al., 1999), and among young adults in university settings, the lifetime rates have been reported to range from 5.3 percent to 13 percent (Biby, 1998; Bohne et al., 2002). The high prevalence of BDD has been reported in specialized medical settings. In studies that involved adult females seeking cosmetic surgery (e.g., Sarwer et al., 1998a, 1998b), between 7 percent and 16 percent of them met criteria for BDD. With regards to conversion disorder, 4.7 percent of the adolescents who attended a child psychiatric outpatient clinic met the diagnosis of this disorder (Murase et al., 2000). More than half of these patients were classified as polysymptomatic (57 percent) and 43 percent were monosymptomatic. Among adolescents who are in treatment for conversion disorder, the most common symptoms were that of pseudoseizures (82.5 percent) (Pehlivantürk and Unal, 2002). The average age of onset for the conversion symptoms was 12 years. Fifteen (37.5 percent) of these patients were referred to child psychiatry within one month from onset (Pehlivantürk and Unal, 2002).

Comorbidity

Pure somatoform disorders were rare. In a study by Essau and colleagues (1999), only one-third of the adolescents with these disorders did not meet the diagnoses of other disorders. About 46.3 percent had one additional disorder, 22 percent had two, and 3.7 percent had three additional disorders. As a whole, the most frequent comorbidity pattern was that of somatoform and anxiety disorders (Table 9.1). Within the somatoform disorders, half of the adolescents with pain and conversion disorders also met the diagnosis of depressive disorders (Essau et al., 1999). Pain disorder also co-occurred frequently with anxiety and substance use disorders, with one-third of those with pain disorder meeting the criteria for the latter disorders. Undifferentiated somatoform disorder co-occurred most frequently with anxiety, followed by depressive disorders. However, the patterns of comorbidity seemed to differ with age and gender. Among females, somatoform disorder highly co-occurred with anxiety and depressive disorders. Among males, especially the 16 to 17 year olds, a high comorbidity rate was found for somatoform disorders and

Table 9.1 Comorbidity patterns in somatoform disorders

	Undifferentiated somatoform disorder (N = 114) N (%)	Conversion disorder (N = 14) N (%)	Pain disorder (N = 18) N (%)
Depressive disorders	41 (35.9)	9 (50.0)	8 (57.1)
• Major depression	32 (28.1)	8 (44.4)	7 (50.0)
• Dysthymic disorder	14 (12.3)	3 (16.7)	3 (21.4)
Anxiety disorders	42 (36.8)	6 (33.3)	4 (28.6)
• Panic disorder	1 (0.9)	1 (5.6)	0 (0)
• Agoraphobia	7 (6.1)	2 (11.1)	1 (7.1)
• Social phobia	5 (4.4)	1 (5.6)	1 (7.1)
• Specific phobia	10 (8.8)	0 (0)	2 (14.3)
• Obsessive-compulsive disorder	1 (0.9)	0 (0)	2 (14.3)
• Generalized anxiety disorder	1 (0.9)	0 (0)	0 (0)
• Post-traumatic stress disorder	5 (4.4)	0 (0)	1 (7.1)
• Anxiety not otherwise specified	21 (18.4)	3 (16.7)	2 (14.3)
Substance use disorders	27 (23.7)	6 (33.3)	3 (21.4)
• Alcohol abuse/dependence	20 (17.5)	2 (11.1)	2 (14.3)
• Cannabis abuse/dependence	16 (14.0)	4 (22.2)	1 (7.1)
• Opiate abuse/dependence	3 (2.6)	0 (0)	0 (0)
• Amphetamine abuse/dependence	3 (2.6)	0 (0)	0 (0)
• Hallucinogen abuse/dependence	1 (0.9)	0 (0)	0 (0)
• Other substance abuse/dependence	0 (0)	0 (0)	0 (0)

Source: Essau et al. (1999). http://www.tandf.co.uk

substance use disorders. Pure somatoform disorders most commonly occurred in the younger than older age groups.

In Lieb et al.'s (2000) study, the most common comorbid pattern was between conversion/dissociative disorder NOS and eating disorders, as well as between pain and major depression, panic disorder and posttraumatic stress disorder. Among those with comorbid disorder, pain disorder and abridged somatization disorder (SS14.6) begin before symptoms of other psychiatric disorders, whereas, conversion disorder generally begin after the occurrence of other disorders. Within the somatoform disorders, BDD co-occurred highly with major depression, followed by obsessive compulsive disorder and social phobia (Albertini and Phillips, 1999). In clinical settings, 45 percent of the children with conversion disorder had a comorbid diagnosis of major depression and/or anxiety disorders, and 35 percent had premorbid conduct problems (Pehlivantürk and Unal, 2002).

Benjamin and Eminson (1992) found positive associations between somatic symptoms and affective disorders. It was suggested that depression and anxiety could possibly lower the threshold at which minor symptoms are perceived, which may enhance perceptions of an increase in bodily complaints. It could also be that chronic physical symptoms may initiate depression and anxiety through "behavior mechanism" (Katon et al., 1991). That is, the decreased enjoyment of previously pleasurable activities may contribute to withdrawal from social activities leading to lack of achievement of reinforcement. This may lead to feelings of hopelessness and helplessness, which may contribute to or initiate depressive illness.

Psychosocial impairment

The consequences of somatoform disorders are often profound. Somatoform disorders have been associated with functional impairment and suffering for the child, and may present a major problem for the health care system because patients with these disorders tend to overuse medical services and resources (Lipowski, 1987; Sartorius et al., 1990).

In the study by Essau and colleagues (1999), adolescents with pain disorder were the most impaired by the somatic symptoms. Those with undifferentiated somatoform disorder and conversion disorder were less impaired, with only 10.5 percent and 21.4 percent of them being bothered by the somatoform symptoms, respectively. Compared to adolescents with the other subtypes of somatoform disorders, most of those with pain disorder were severely to very severely impaired in their daily activities. Adolescents with pain disorder were also impaired, in the last four weeks before the interview in various life domains especially at work/schools and during leisure activities. About 28.7 percent of those with conversion disorder, 24.6 percent with undifferentiated somatoform disorder, and 11.1 percent with pain disorder had sought some professional help. More females than males also reported being unable to do their daily activities due to emotional problems; this was especially the case among those in the older than younger age groups. In another German study (Lieb et al., 2000), of all the somatoform disorders, conversion disorder, and the SS14.6 were associated with the highest level of impairment.

A number of reports have also described the level of functioning among patients with BDD. According to these reports, BDD is highly incapacitating, and almost all persons with this disorder have severe impairment in social and occupational activities. The types of impaired functioning experienced by children and adolescents with BDD include poor grades (Phillips et al., 1995), stopping sports and other activities (El-Khatib and Dickey, 1995), excessive school absences (Albertini et al., 1996), drop out from high school (Phillips et al., 1995), social withdrawal (El-Khatib and Dickey, 1995), and being housebound (Cotterill, 1996). BDD may also result in psychiatric hospitalization, suicidal ideation, and suicide attempts (Albertini and Phillips, 1999; Phillips et al., 1995). As shown by Albertini and Phillips (1999), 94 percent of the children and adolescents with BDD reported social impairment and 85 percent reported school or work impairment. About 11 percent of the patients reported extreme and disabling distress, 61 percent reported severe distress, and 25 percent reported moderate distress (Albertini and Phillips, 1999). Studies have also reported that adolescents and adults with BDD often seek help in dermatology and cosmetic surgery settings (Phillips and Diaz, 1997).

A high level of impairment has also been reported in studies among children and adolescents with different symptoms of somatoform disorders. For example, as reported by Abu-Arefeh and Russell (1994), up to 80 days of schooling has been lost a year by children and adolescents with migraine. Children with high physical symptoms were also rated by their parents as having greater academic difficulties and poorer grades, and missing more often from school than children in the control groups (Campo et al., 1999). Children and adolescents with high physical symptoms were also more likely to have a history of using mental health services sometimes in their life (Campo et al., 1999). In a study by Walker et al. (1995), former patients with recurrent abdominal pain were significantly more often absent from school or work in the past year compared to former well patients. Significantly more former patients with recurrent abdominal pain also made more mental health visits/and psychiatric hospitalization during the assessment period of five to six years than former well patients.

Course and outcome

Findings of community studies among adults have been very informative about the course and outcome of somatoform disorders (Canino et al., 1987; Wells et al., 1989; Wittchen et al., 1992). These studies indicated that most cases with somatoform disorders experienced their first somatic symptoms before 15 years of age; full remission was rare, and symptoms tended to be associated with long-term psychosocial impairment. However, such studies may be biased due to recall problems. Studies on the course and outcome of somatoform disorders in children and adolescents are limited to small sample size, or focus on specific types of somatoform disorders, or are limited to youths in clinical settings.

Among adults, the average duration of BDD was 18.3 years (Phillips et al., 1993). Furthermore, three patterns of course could be noted. The first pattern described BDD concerns as being persistent and unchanged, the second pattern involved an addition of new defects to the preexisting ones (Phillips et al., 1993). The third pattern consisted of complex additions of remission of symptoms, with frequent replacement of one symptom by the other. Regardless of these different patterns, the intensity of symptoms was described to wax and wane over time, with rare full remission of all symptoms. Among youngsters with BDD, the disorder has been described as generally a chronic condition, with a waxing and waning of intensity (Phillips et al., 1993). Veale and colleagues (1996) have regarded BDD as "a chronic handcapping disorder".

With respect to conversion disorder, a study by Pehlivantürk and Unal (2002) has shown that 85 percent of the youngsters with conversion disorder had recovered completely at the four-year follow-up investigation. Among patients with complete recovery, this occurred at an average of 7.2 months and frequently one month after the initial psychiatric interview; 7.5 percent of the patients who recovered in a short period following initial visit, relapsed 12–36 months later. One-third received a diagnosis of mood (major depression, dysthymic disorder) or anxiety disorder (generalized anxiety disorder, obsessive compulsive disorder) at follow-up. Factors that predicted poor outcome in conversion disorder included poly-symptomatic presentation, pseudoseizures, chronicity of the symptoms, comorbid psychiatric or medical disorders, poor capacity to gain insight, severe internal conflict and serious family dysfunction (Pehlivantürk and Unal, 2002). Favourable outcome was related to young age, early diagnosis, close liaison between pediatricians and child psychiatrists, good premorbid adjustment, the presence of an easily identifiable stressor, cooperation of the child and the family (Campo and Fritsch, 1994; Goodyer and Mitchell, 1989; Turgay, 1990; Wyllie et al., 1991). Adolescents with conversion disorder who were classified as polysymptomatic, compared to monosymptomatic, had significantly poorer prognosis (Murase et al., 2000). The poorer prognosis of patients who have been classified as polysymp-tomatic was explained in terms of the underlying psychological problems. That is, they had significantly more past psychiatric histories (e.g., recurrent psychosomatic complaints, violence) and family problems (e.g., live with a single parent, physically abusive father, have harsh, rejecting, verbally abusive parents) than patients who have been classified as monosymptomatic. In Wyllie et al.'s (1991) study early diagnosis and treatment was also found to be associated with good outcome in children and adolescents with psychogenic seizures. The outcome was significantly better for younger than for older patients (Wyllie et al., 1991). Goodyer and Mitchell (1989) showed that recovery rates for pseudoseizures (62.5 percent) were significantly lower than other conversion symptoms (90 percent). However, others reported high recovery rates for pseudoseizures ranging from 78 percent to 100 percent (Pehlivantürk and Unal, 2002; Turgay, 1990; Wyllie et al., 1991).

Information on the course of hypochondriasis and somatization disorder in children and adolescents are rare. Studies among adults have shown somatization disorder to be a chronic illness with fluctuation in the frequency and diversity of symptoms, and is rarely remit (Guze et al., 1986). Between 80 and 90 percent of patients diagnosed with somatization disorder retain the same diagnosis over many years (Cloninger, 1986). Among adults with hypochondriasis (Noyes et al., 1994), two-thirds of those with DSM-III-R defined hypochondriasis continued to meet criteria for the disorder one year later. While one-third of these patients no longer met the criteria, they had persisting hypochondriacal symptoms. In their prospective five-year study of DSM-III-R defined hypochondriasis, Barsky et al. (1998) found that 36.5 percent of the adults no longer met the criteria for hypochondriasis at follow up.

In the Ontario Child Health Study, adolescents with high somatic symptoms were found to have an increased risk of major depression four years later (Zwaigenbaum et al., 1999). It was argued that somatization is an alternative expression of emotional disorder. In fact, somatic complaints have been regarded as a presenting symptom of depression (Campo and Fritsch, 1994).

Risk factors

Data pertaining to the risk factors of somatoform disorders are weak and speculative. Additionally, most of the existing studies have focused on conversion disorder, and can be characterized as having a small sample size. The onset of conversion disorder was associated with psychosocial stressors such as relationship problems in the family (90 percent) and/or with peers (52.5 percent), medical problems in the family or close environment (25 percent) and school-related problems (12.5 percent) (Pehlivantürk and Unal, 2002). An early study by Siegel and Barthel (1986) also indicated that as many as 90 percent of the children with a conversion disorder have some family, peer, or school stress (Siegel and Barthel, 1986). Common stresses seen in the families of children with conversion disorders are parental discord, parental divorce (Volkmar et al., 1984), sexual abuse (Leslie, 1988; Volkmar et al., 1984), and psychiatric impairment of a parent (Lehmkuhl et al., 1989).

The study by Steinhausen et al. (1989) showed significant association between conversion disorder and socio-economic status. That is, two-thirds of conversion disorder patients were of lower socio-economic status or immigrants. Between 44 percent to 66 percent of the cases with conversion disorder reported the presence of illness models (Steinhausen et al., 1989; Thomson and Sills, 1988). Children with conversion disorder are also more likely to have a physically ill parent compared to children with other psychiatric disorders (Steinhausen et al., 1989). Family may be related to the onset or maintenance of conversion disorder through several ways (Seltzer, 1985). First, the family may be the source of the precipitating stressors such as family conflict, abuse or neglect. It has been suggested that a child or adolescent learns to transform overwhelming emotions and conflicts into an accepted scheme of expression (i.e., physical disease). Second, the illness behaviour may play an important role in organizing family life. Third, the illness of a family member may serve as a model for the child's disorder (Seltzer, 1985). As proposed by the social learning theory, people are more likely to engage in a behaviour if they observe another person receiving reinforcement for the behaviour. Hence, children who observe significant others engage in actual illness behaviour may be more prone to show similar behaviour themselves.

Barsky and colleagues (1994) examined the childhood histories of trauma, parental attitudes toward health, and physical illness in a group of hypochondriacal adults. Hypochondriacal compared to non-hypochondriacal patients reported traumatic sexual contact, physical violence, and major parental upheaval before the age of 17. Hypochondriacal patients also reported being sicker as children and missing more school. Traumatic experiences in childhood (e.g., childhood sexual and physical abuse) have been reported more frequently among patients with somatoform disorders, especially those with somatization disorder and chronic pain (Walker et al., 1995).

At the symptom level, children and adolescents with high level of medically unexplained physical symptoms tended to be girls, being a member of a minority group, have parents with low education level, and come from non-intact families (Campo et al., 1999). The physician may also influence the development or maintenance of somatization through their professional training (Fabrega et al., 1988), uncertainty of diagnosis (Walker and Greene, 1991), excessive reassurance (Warwick and Salkovskis, 1990), and through their clinical practices such as by conducting unnecessary medical tests. The latter could increase the conviction that the child is ill (Grattan-Smith et al., 1988).

Assessment

The main feature of somatoform disorders has been described as the presence of physical symptoms suggestive of a general medical condition, but which are not fully explained by a general medical condition (APA, 1994). As such, patients with somatoform disorders, present difficult diagnostic and management problems. That is, some somatoform disorders, such as BDD, are often under-recognized and misdiagnosed (Phillips, 1991; Zimmerman and Mattia, 1998). Some reasons why the BDD goes undiagnosed and untreated could be due to the fact that many patients are ashamed about the symptoms and reluctant to reveal them, their tendency to seek non-psychiatric treatment, and the fact that clinicians are not familiar with BDD (Phillips, 1991).

The first step in clinical assessment is to establish the diagnosis. A comprehensive medical investigation is needed to rule out the plausible physical causes, especially given the finding that between 27 and 46 percent of children diagnosed with a somatoform disorder (conversion disorder) had a physical disorder (Lehmkuhl et al., 1989). Information regarding any precipitating factors may give hint about the physical and the psychological stresses which may be involved at the outset of the disorders. Other important information includes earlier physical and developmental problems, the presence of functional symptoms and school adjustment. Towards the end of the interview, information about psychiatric history and information on family health, functioning, and relationships should be obtained.

The assessment of somatoform disorders or their symptoms is a difficult task. Due to the personal and subjective nature of physical symptom or pain, and the fact that children's ability to report their pain is limited, it is difficult to know what they feel. Nevertheless, careful assessment is the first step towards establishing a diagnosis of somatoform disorders in order to be able to intervene effectively.

The diagnostic process of somatoform disorder involves quantifying the children's pain. The most common assessment techniques include behavioral, physiological, and self-report. Behavioral assessment involves direct observation of the children's behavior (e.g., crying, facial expression) and can be completed by their parents or clinicians. Physiological approach includes measuring bodily responses to pain-inducing stimuli (e.g., heart rate, respiration). Self-report measures can be used to assess children's perception of their pain. Self-report measurement can be divided into visual and verbal scales. In visual pain scales, pictures are used to characterize pain such as pictures of faces (P.A. McGrath et al., 1985) and ladders (Jeans and Johnston, 1985). Visual pain scales are commonly used among children because they have limited ability to express their pain. Verbal scales involve verbal description of the pain, which are then anchored to a numerical value (P.J. McGrath and Unruh, 1987). Some of these scales include questions related to the temporal dimension of pain and pain descriptors (e.g., steady, up and down, increasing); the most commonly used scales under this category are the Children's Comprehensive Pain Questionnaire (P.A. McGrath, 1990) and the Varni Thompsons Pediatric Pain Questionnaire (Varni et al., 1987)

Additionally, a number of self-report questionnaires have been developed to measure symptoms of specific types of somatoform disorders (e.g., BDD). Some examples include the Body Dysmorphic Disorder Questionnaire (Phillips et al., 1995) and the Yale-Brown Obsessive-compulsive Scale Modified for Body Dysmorphic Disorder (BDD-YBOCS; Phillips, 1997).

Treatment

Most children and adolescents with somatoform disorders or symptoms of these disorders are seen in general medical services. In adult studies, patients with somatoform disorders account for a large number of visits to primary care settings, and of laboratory investigations and drug prescriptions (Sartorius et al., 1990). Consequently, the medical care expenditure for these patients is very high (Ford, 1983). Among children and adolescents, the somatoform disorders are often misdiagnosed and consequently mistreated. For example, in one study (Grant et al., 2001), none of the patients with BDD were given the diagnosis of a BDD by their treating physician during hospitalization. This finding was important because almost all of these patients reported their BDD preoccupation to have major problems or the biggest problems.

In order to gain the children's and their parents' compliance, the general practitioner needs, first, to show interest in the child's entire background, second, to carry out a comprehensive investigation to exclude organic disease confidently early on and helping parents in understanding the negative findings and the fact that organic disease has been ruled out, third, to encourage parents to explore emotional aspects of these problems, fourth, to help modify some aspects of the child's environment such as problems in peer relationships, or excessive academic pressure. Finally, in the presence of a school attendance problem, it should be helpful to get in contact with the school to facilitate attendance, and to help the child receive the necessary support (Garralda, 1999). In some cases, a psychiatric referral is needed. According to Garralda (1999), this is needed when there are some uncertainties about the relevance of psychological factors; when there are comorbid psychiatric disorders; when family problems are found to have the resolution of the symptoms; when the child fails to respond to pediatric treatment.

Youngsters with somatoform disorders are often treated with either medication (pharmacotherapy) or family therapy.

Pharmacotherapy

Based on several case reports, selective serotonin reuptake inhibitors (SSRIs) are effective in decreasing BDD symptoms and improving functioning in children and adolescents (Heimann, 1997). A 12- to 16-week trial of SSRI may be necessary for response to occur. However, these findings should be interpreted with caution because data are limited to a small number of cases. Furthermore, most treatment findings were obtained from uncontrolled studies and were obtained from self-report. For example, Phillips et al. (1995) reported four cases of adolescents with BDD, all of whom responded to a serotonin reuptake inhibitor (fluoxetine, clomipramine, fluvoxamine, paroxetine, and sertraline). The time to response could be up to 12 weeks, and high doses were required. In another study by Phillips et al. (1998), 63.3 percent of patients with BDD showed significant improvement and were considered responders to fluvoxamine. A high rate of side-effects was noted (i.e., sedation, fatigue, insomnia and agitation), although in most cases these adverse effects were well tolerated. In a study by Perugi et al. (1996), 10 of the 15 subjects with BDD responded to fluvoxamine. Side-effects were noted in 60 percent of the subjects, although they were generally mild, transcient, and well tolerated; only one subject dropped out of the study. The response of BDD symptoms to fluvoxamine could be attributed to the anti-obsessional qualities of the drug (Phillips, 1996).

Horowitz and colleagues (2002) presented a case report of a 16-year-old girl with BDD who has been found to respond to high doses of SSRIs. She was initiated on fluvoxamine 25 mg b.i.d., which has been titrated up over the course of her treatment to 400 mg. On this medication, her depression went into remission. After about six months of treatment with fluvoxamine, atypical antipsychotic was added to target her intense paranoia and psychotic episodes. Initially, quetiapine fumarate was added, with 25 mg once-daily dosing, and then risperidone up to a total of 1.5 mg/day was initiated. While on risperidone, she managed to leave her home and felt less paranoid outdoors, however, she developed a side-effect (hyperprolactinemia with galactorrhea), so risperidone was discontinued. She was then given an olazapine 2.5 mg at bedtime. Although she reported increased comfort outdoors and around peers at school, she gained 35 pounds over the course of about 2 months and this medication was discontinued.

Family therapy

The aim of a family therapy is to address the problems of families of youngsters with somatoform disorders and to increase family insight into interaction patterns (Seltzer, 1985). Further aims include the promotion of direct and honest communication between family members and the role of the child's illness in the family. Several techniques introduced by Minuchin (1974) to modify family structure have been applied to the family of a child with a conversion disorder. One technique involves moving family members to different places in the room to physically represent the boundaries which exist in the family system. The second technique involves forbidding family members to talk about each other; any comments about a family member have to be directed to that member, who then responds to the statement. This technique helps to interrupt enmeshed interaction patterns that family members think and feel for each other. The third technique involves the therapist pointing out and probing differences which the family tries to avoid. This technique allows processing of unstated issues that have an important impact on the system's interactions. The fourth technique involves the therapist joining a family member in a coalition. In this way, the position of that family member can be strengthened and can change his or her position in the family hierarchy.

Turgay (1990) examined the treatment outcome of children and adolescents with conversion disorder who were treated with an integrative child and family therapy approach. Each of the children was treated with individual and family therapy. The individual therapy was carried out two to three times per week with the child alone; the aims were to reduce anxiety symptoms, to gain insights into the meaning of symptoms, to resolve problems in their general functioning and behaviour, to decrease the need for primary and secondary gain through conversion symptoms and to strengthen the child's ego functioning. The family therapy was carried out once a week with all the family members. The aim was to unite the family, enhance their acceptance of the psychological nature of the symptoms, and to teach them about the nature and treatment of the disorder. The child participated, on the average, in 27 individual and 16 family sessions. Immediately after their discharge from the hospital, the patients were followed-up on a weekly, then biweekly, and monthly basis. Almost (99.9 percent) of the patients responded positively to the integrative treatment. About half of them (49.4 percent) recovered within the first two weeks of treatment, 47.1 percent responded within two to four weeks, and only 3.37 percent required more than four weeks to recover. Factors associated with positive treatment outcome (i.e., those who recovered less than two weeks after the initiation of the treatment) were younger age of patient, healthy personality characteristics, lack of psychopathology, insight and treatment compliance, healthy family functioning, acceptance by the family of the psychological nature of the illness, positive feelings towards the child and the family by the staff, lack of internal conflict and inflexible neurotic defences, and early therapeutic interventions.

Cognitive behaviour therapy

Case report by Phillips et al. (1995) showed cognitive behaviour therapy was effective in the treatment of BDD. The main components of the cognitive behaviour therapy used in that study included cognitive rehearsal, use of imagery, identification of cognitive distortions, graded exposure. Family involvement such as instructing parents not to respond to requests for reassurance and to help in hiding or covering mirrors has also been reported to be useful (Phillips et al., 1993). Cognitive-behavioral therapy that was combined with serotonin reuptake inhibitors had also been reported as helpful for children and adolescents with BDD (Albertini et al., 1996; Phillips et al., 1995).

Conclusion

Our knowledge about somatoform disorders in children and adolescents is still at an infancy stage. Epidemiological studies are needed to provide us with the prevalence and the associated features (e.g., comorbidity pattern, age of onset, impairment level) of somatoform disorders in various settings. However, such research should use standard assessment procedures in order to allow direct comparison across studies. Prospective longitudinal studies are also needed to determine the course of somatoform disorders, and to examine the relationship between childhood presentations and adult disorders.

Somatoform disorders are a difficult taxonomic challenge. As mentioned in an earlier section of this chapter, the same diagnostic criteria are used in children, adolescents, and adults. It is questionable whether the application of adult criteria is appropriate because they contain many symptoms that are not relevant to children (e.g., menstrual or genitourinary systems). Several other critics have been presented regarding disorders in general. First, it has been suggested that somatisation disorder and hypochondriasis cannot yet be conclusively regarded as psychiatric disorders, given their close association with anxiety and depressive disorders (Creed and Barsky, 2004; Gureje et al., 1997). Second, the validity of pain disorder has also been questioned, given its significant diagnostic overlap between somatoform pain disorder and conversion disorder (Birket-Smith and Mortensen, 2002). Third, the length in which the symptoms must be present (e.g., in DSM-IV, the duration of hypochondriasis has to be present for at least 6 months, or in the case of somatization disorder, it must be occurring over a period of several years) has also been criticized (Creed and Barsky, 2004). As argued by Creed and Barsky (2004), these criteria may be used to define only a limited group of people, specifically those with severe disorders. Fourth, in clinical practice, many categories of the somatoform disorders tend to exist as dimensions. Wise and Birket-Smith (2002) argued that the gradation of health anxiety to hypochondriasis is dependent on numerous factors such as the child's realistic health, his or her health-seeking behaviors, and the distress level experienced. Creed and Barsky (2004) have similarly argued that the number of somatic symptoms, the degree of worry about illness and the failure to be reassured by medical investigations be studied from a dimensional perspective. Finally, the "cutoff" points associated with marked impairment or increased use of health services need to be classified.

In addition to the classification issues discussed above, there is a need to integrate data from multiple informants, especially when disagreement among information sources occurs. There are real limitations to what children, parents and others (e.g., teachers) can know about children's experiences of pain.

Randomized controlled trials of psychological therapy for somatoform disorders in children and adolescents are lacking. The few existing studies have numerous methodological problems such as small sample size, lack of standardized measurement, and heterogenous samples. Therefore, there is an urgent need to conduct well-designed trials of psychological intervention for children and adolescents with somatoform disorders. Such intervention should aim to reduce or manage pain-associated disability and distress. Future studies should not focus on treatment among children alone, but also in combination with their parents. Additional studies are needed to examine the effectiveness of the different types and combinations of treatment interventions at different ages. The inclusion of a developmental perspective into this line of research could enhance our knowledge on how best to prevent and treat children and adolescents with somatoform disorders.

References

Abu-Arefeh, I. and Russell, G. (1994). Prevalence of headache and migraine in school children. *British Medical Journal, 309*, 765–769.

Albertini, R.S. and Phillips, K.A. (1999). Thirty-three cases of body dysmorphic disorder in children and adolescents. *Journal of the American Academy of Child and Adolescent Psychiatry, 38*, 453–459

Albertini, R., Phillips, K.A., and Guvremont, D. (1996). Body dysmorphic disorder in a young child (letter). *Journal of the American Academy of Child and Adolescent Psychiatry, 35*, 1425–1426.

American Psychiatric Association (1980). *Diagnostic and statistical manual of mental disorders*, 3rd edn. Washington, DC: APA.

American Psychiatric Association (1987). *Diagnostic and statistical manual of mental disorders*, 3rd edn revised. Washington, DC: APA.

American Psychiatric Association (1994). *Diagnostic and statistical manual of mental disorders*, 4th edn.Washington, DC: APA.

Aro, H., Paronen, O., and Aro, S. (1987). Psychosomatic symptoms among 14–16 year old Finnish adolescents. *Social Psychiatry, 22*, 171–176.

Barsky, A.J., Wyshak, G., and Klerman, G.L. (1992). Psychiatric comorbidity in DSM-III-R hypochondriasis. *Archives of General Psychiatry*, *49*, 101–108.

Barsky, A.J., Wool, C., Barnett, M.C., and Cleary, P.D. (1994). Histories of childhood trauma in adult hypochondriacal patients. *American Journal of Psychiatry*, *151*, 397–401.

Barsky, A.J., Fama, J.M., Bailey, E.D., and Ahern, D.K. (1998). A prospective 4- to 5-year study of DSM-III-R hypochondriasis. *Archives of General Psychiatry*, *55*, 737–744.

Bell, K.M., Cookfair, D., Bell, D.S., Reese, P., and Cooper, L. (1991). Risk factors associated with chronic fatigue syndrome in a cluster of pediatric cases. *Reviews of Infectious Diseases*, *13*, 32–38.

Benjamin, S. and Eminson, D. (1992). Abnormal illness behaviour: Childhood experiences and long-term consequences. *International Review of Psychiatry*, *4*, 55–70.

Biby, E.L. (1998). The relationship between body dysmorphic disorder and depression, self-esteem, somatization, and obsessive-compulsive disorder. *Journal of Clinical Psychology*, *54*, 489–499.

Birket-Smith, M. and Mortensen, E.L. (2002). Pain in somatoform disorders: Is somatoform pain disorder a valid diagnosis. *Acta Psychiatrica Scandinavica*, *106*, 103–108.

Bohne, A., Wilhelm, S., Keuthen, N.J., Florin, I., Baer, L., and Jenike, M.A. (2002). Prevalence of body dysmorphic disorder in a German college student sample. *Psychiatry Research*, *109*, 101–104.

Borge, A.I.H., Nordhagen, R., Botten, G., and Bakketeig, L.S. (1994). Prevalence and persistence of stomache ache and headache among children: Follow-up of a cohort of Norwegian children from 4 to 10 years of age. *Acta Paediatrica Scandinavica*, *83*, 433–437.

Bursch, B., Walco, G.A., and Zeltzer, L. (1998). Clinical assessment and management of chronic pain and pain-associated syndrome. *Journal of Developmental and Behavioral Pediatrics*, *19*, 45–53.

Campo, J.V. and Fritsch, S.L. (1994). Somatization in children and adolescents. *Journal of the American Academy of Child and Adolescent Psychiatry*, *33*, 1223–1235.

Campo, J.V., Jansen-McWilliams, L., Comer, D.M., and Kelleher, K.J. (1999). Somatization in pediatric primary care: Association with psychopathology, functional impairment, and use of services. *Journal of the American Academy of Child and Adolescent Psychiatry*, *38*, 1093–1101.

Canino, G.J., Bird, H.R., Shrout, P.E., Rubio-Stipec, M., Bravo, M., Martinez, R., et al. (1987). The prevalence of specific psychiatric disorders in Puerto Rico. *Archives of General Psychiatry*, *44*, 727–735.

Carroll, D.H., Scahill, L., and Phillips, K.A. (2002). Current concepts in body dysmorphic disorder. *Archives of Psychiatric Nursing*, *16*, 72–79.

Carter, B.D., Kronenberger, W.G., and Edwards, J.F. (1996). Differential diagnosis of chronic fatigue in children: Behavioral and emotional dimensions. *Journal of Developmental and Behavioral Pediatrics*, *17*, 16–21.

Cloninger, C.R. (1986). Somatoform and dissociative disorders. In G. Winokur and P. Clayton (Eds.), *The medical basis of psychiatry* (pp. 123–151). Philadelpha, PA: W.B. Saunders.

Cotterill, J.A. (1996). Body dysmorphic disorder. *Psychodermatology*, *14*, 457–463.

Creed, F. and Barsky, A. (2004). A systematic review of the epidemiology of somatisation disorder and hypochondriasis. *Journal of Psychosomatic Research*, *56*, 391–408.

El-Khatib, H.E. and Dickey, T.O. (1995). Sertaline for body dysmorphic disorder. *Journal of the American Academy of Child and Adolescent Psychiatry, 34*, 1404–1405.

Essau, C.A., Conradt, J., and Petermann, F. (1999). Frequency, comorbidity and psychosocial impairment of somatoform disorders in adolescents. *Psychology, Health, and Medicine, 4*, 169–180.

Fabrega, H., Mezzich, J., Jacob, R., and Ulrich, R. (1988). Somatoform disorder in a psychiatric setting: Systematic comparison with depression and anxiety disorders. *Journal of Nervous and Mental Disease, 176*, 431–439.

Feder, H., Dworkin, P., and Orkin, C. (1994). Outcome of 48 pediatric patients with chronic fatigue: A clinical experience. *Archives of Family Medicine, 3*, 1049–1055.

Ford, C. (1983). *The somatizing disorders: Illness as a way of life.* New York: Elsevier.

Fritz, G.K., Fritsch, S., and Hagino, O. (1997). Somatoform disorders in children and adolescents: A review of the past 10 years. *Journal of the American Academy of Child and Adolescent Psychiatry, 36*, 1329–1338.

Garber, J., Walker, L.S., and Zeman, J. (1991). Somatization symptoms in a community sample of children and adolescents: Further validation of the Children's Somatization Inventory. Psychological assessment. *Journal of Consulting and Clinical Psychology, 3*, 588–595.

Garralda, M.E. (1999). Practitioner review: Assessment and management of somatisation in childhood and adolescence: A practical perspective. *Journal of Child Psychology and Psychiatry, 40*, 1159–1167.

Garralda, M.E. and Rangel, L.A. (2001). Health attitudes in chronic fatigue syndrome of childhood [letter]. *American Journal of Psychiatry, 158*, 1161.

Garralda, M.E. and Rangel, L. (2002). Annotation: Chronic fatigue syndrome in children and adolescents. *Journal of Child Psychology and Psychiatry, 43*, 169–176.

Garralda, M.E. and Rangel, L. (2004). Impairment and coping in children and adolescents fatigue syndrome: A comparative study with other paediatric disorders. *Journal of Child Psychology and Psychiatry, 45*, 543–552.

Goodman, J.E. and McGrath, P.J. (1991). The epidemiology of pain in children and adolescents: A review. *Pain, 46*, 247–264.

Goodyer, I.M. (1981). Hysterical conversion reactions in childhood. *Journal of Child Psychology and Psychiatry, 22*, 179–188.

Goodyer, I.M. and Mitchell, C. (1989). Somatic emotional disorders in childhood and adolescence. *Journal of Psychosomatic Research, 33*, 681–688.

Grant, J.E., Kim, S.W., and Crow, S.J. (2001). Prevalence and clinical features of body dysmorphic disorder in adolescent and adult psychiatric inpatient. *Journal of Clinical Psychiatry, 62*, 517–522.

Grattan-Smith, P., Fairley, M., and Procopis, P. (1988). Clinical features of conversion disorder. *Archives of Disease in Childhood, 63*, 408–414.

Gureje, O., Simon, G.E., Ustun, T.B., and Goldberg, D.P. (1997). Somatization in cross-cultural perspective: A World Health Organization study in primary care. *American Journal of Psychiatry, 154*, 989–995.

Guze, S.B., Cloninger, C.R., Martin, R.L., and Clayton, P.J. (1986). A follow-up and family study of Briquet's syndrome. *British Journal of Psychiatry, 149*, 17–23.

Heimann, S.W. (1997). SSRI for body dysmorphic disorder [letter]. *Journal of the American Academy of Child and Adolescent Psychiatry, 36*, 868.

Horowitz, K., Gorfinkle, K., Lewis, O., and Phillips, K.A. (2002). Body dysmorphic disorder in an adolescent girl. *Journal of the American Academy of Child and Adolescent Psychiatry, 41*, 1503–1509.

Jeans, M.E. and Johnston, C.C. (1985). Pain in children: Assessment and management. In S. Lipton and J. Miles (Eds.), *Persistent pain: Modern methods of treatment* (pp. 111–127). London: Grune and Stratton.

Jordan, K.M., Ayers, P.M., Jahn, S.C., Taylor, K.K., Huang, C.F., Richman, J., et al. (2000). Prevalence of fatigue and chronic fatigue syndrome-like illness in children and adolescents. *Journal of Chronic Fatigue Syndrome, 6,* 3–21.

Katon, W., Lin, E., Von Korff, M., Russo, J., Lipscomb, P., and Bush, T. (1991). Somatization: A spectrum of severity. *American Journal of Psychiatry, 148,* 34–40.

Krilov, L.R., Fisher, M., Friedman, S.B., Reitman, D., and Mandel, F.S. (1998). Course and outcome of chronic fatigue in children and adolescents. *Pediatrics, 102,* 360–366.

Larsson, B. (1991). Somatic complaints and their relationship to depressive symptoms in Swedish adolescents. *Journal of Child Psychology and Psychiatry, 32,* 821–832.

Lehmkuhl, G., Blanz, B., Lehmkuhl, U., and Braun-Scharm, H. (1989). Conversion disorder: Symptomatology and course in childhood and adolescence. *European Archives of Psychiatry and Clinical Neuroscience, 238,* 155–160.

Leslie, S.A. (1988). Diagnosis and treatment of hysterical conversion reactions. *Archives of Disease in Childhood, 63,* 506–511.

Lieb, R., Pfister, H., Mastaler, M., and Wittchen, H.U. (2000). Somatoform sndromes and disorders in a representative population sample of adolescents and young adults: Prevalence, comorbidity and impairment. *Acta Psychiatrica Scandinavica, 101,* 194–206.

Lipowski, Z.J. (1987). Somatization: The experience and communication of psychological distress as somatic symptoms. *Psychotherapy and Psychosomatics, 47,* 160–167.

McGrath, P.A. (1990). Pain in children: Nature, assessment, and treatment. *Psychosomatics, 28,* 294–295.

McGrath, P.A., DeVeber, L.L., and Hearn, M.T. (1985). Multidimensional pain assessment in children. In H.L. Fields, R. Dubner, and F. Cervero (Eds.), *Advances in pain research and therapy* (pp. 387–393). New York: Raven Press.

McGrath, P.J. and Larsson, B. (1997). Headache in children and adolescents. *Child and Adolescent Psychiatric Clinics of North America, 6,* 843–859.

McGrath, P.J. and Unruh, A.M. (1987). *Pain in children and adolescents.* New York: Elsevier.

Martin, R.L. and Yutzy, S.H. (1994). Somatoform disorders. In R.E. Hales, S.C. Yudofsky, and J.A. Talbott (Eds.), *The American Psychiatric Press Textbook of Psychiatry* (pp. 591–622). Washington, DC: American Psychiatric Press.

Mayville, S., Katz, R.C., Gipson, M.T., and Cabral, K. (1999). Assessing the prevalence of body dysmorphic disorder in an ethnically diverse group of adolescents. *Journal of Child and Family Studies, 8,* 357–362

Minuchin, S. (1974). The McGill Pain Questionnaire: Major properties and scoring methods. *Pain, 1,* 277–299.

Murase, S., Sugiyama, T., Ishii, T., Wakako, R., and Ohta, T. (2000). Polysymptomatic conversion disorder in childhood and adolescence in Japan: Early manifestation or incomplete form of somatization disorder? *Psychotherapy and Psychosomatics, 69,* 132–136.

Noyes, J. Jr., Kathol, R.G., Fisher, M.M., Phillips, B.M., Suelzer, M.T., and Woodman, C.L. (1994). One-year follow-up of medical outpatients with hypochondriasis. *Psychosomatics, 35,* 533–545.

Offord, D.R., Boyle, M.H., Szatmari, P., Rae-Grant, N.L., Links, P.S., Cadman, D.T., et al. (1987). Ontario Child Health Study. II. Six-month prevalence of disorder and rates of service utilization. *Archives of General Psychiatry, 44*, 833–836.

Pehlivantürk, B. and Unal, F. (2002). Conversion disorder in children and adolescents: A 4-year follow-up study. *Journal of Psychosomatic Research, 52*, 187–191.

Perquin, C.W., Hazebroek-Kampschreur, A.A.J.M., Hunfeld, J.A.M., Bohnen, A.M., van Suijlekom-Smit, L.W.A., Passchier, J., et al. (2000). Pain in children and adolescents: A common experience. *Pain, 87*, 51–58.

Perugi, G., Giannotti, D., Di Vaio, S., Frare, F., Saettoni, M., and Cassano, G.B. (1996). Fluvoxamine in the treatment of body dysmorphic disorder (dysmorphophobia). *International Clinical Psychopharmacology, 11*, 247–254.

Phillips, K.A. (1991). Body dysmorphic disorder: The distress of imagined ugliness. *American Journal of Psychiatry, 148*, 1138–1149.

Phillips, K.A. (1996). *The broken mirror: Understanding and treating body dysmorphic disorder.* New York: Oxford University Press.

Phillips, K.A. (1997). A severity rating scale for body dysmorphic disorder: Development, reliability, and validity of a modified version of the Yale-Brown Obsessive Compulsive Scale. *Psychopharmacological Bulletin, 33*, 17–22.

Phillips, K.A. and Diaz, S. (1997). Gender differences in body dysmorphic disorder. *Journal of Nervous and Mental Disease, 185*, 570–577

Phillips, K.A., McElroy, S.L., Keck, P.E., Pope, H.G., and Hudson, J.I. (1993). Body dysmorphic disorder: 30 cases of imagined ugliness. *American Journal of Psychiatry, 150*, 302–308.

Phillips, K.A., Atala, K.D., and Pope, H.G. Jr. (1995). Diagnostic instruments for body dysmorphic disorder. *New research program and abstracts: American Psychiatric Association Annual Meeting* (p. 157). Miami, FL: American Psychiatric Association.

Phillips, K.A., Dwight, M.M., and McElroy, S.L. (1998). Efficacy and safety of fluvoxamine in body dysmorphic disorder. *Journal of Clinical Psychiatry, 59*, 165–171.

Rangel, L.A., Garralda, M.E., Levin, M., and Roberts, H. (2000). The course of chronic fatigue syndrome. *Journal of the Royal Society of Medicine, 93*, 129–134.

Sartorius, N., Goldberg, D., de Girolamo, G., Costa e Silva, J.A., Lebrubier, Y., and Wittchen, H-U. (1990). *Psychological disorders in general medical settings.* Bern: Hogrefe and Huber.

Sarwer, D.B., Wadden, T.A., Pertschuk, M.J., and Whitaker, L.A. (1998a). Body image dissatisfaction and body dysmorphic disorder in 100 cosmetic surgery patients. *Plastic and Reconstructive Surgery, 101*, 1644–1649.

Sarwer, D.B., Whitaker, L.A., Pertschuk, M.J., and Wadden, T.A. (1998b). Reconstructive surgery patients: An underrecognized problem. *Annals of Plastic Surgery, 40*, 403–407.

Seltzer, W.J. (1985). Conversion disorder in childhood and adolescence: A familial/cultural approach. Part I. *Family Systems Medicine, 3*, 261–280.

Siegel, M. and Barthel, R.P. (1986). Conversion disorders on a child psychiatry consultation service. *Psychosomatics, 27*, 201–204.

Steinhausen, H.C., Aster, M., Pfeiffer, E., and Göbel, D. (1989). Comparative studies of conversion disorders in childhood and adolescence. *Journal of Child Psychology and Psychiatry, 30*, 615–621.

Taylor, D.C., Szatmari, P., Boyle, M.H., and Offord, D.R. (1996). Somatization and the vocabulary of everyday bodily experiences and concern: A community study of adolescents. *Journal of the American Academy of Child and Adolescent Psychiatry, 35*, 491–499.

Thomson, A.P. and Sills, J.A. (1988). Diagnosis of functional illness presenting with gait disorder. *Archives of Disease in Childhood, 63*, 148–153.

Turgay, A. (1990). Treatment outcome for children and adolescents with conversion disorder. *Canadian Journal of Psychiatry, 35*, 585–588.

Varni, J.W., Thompson, K.L., and Hanson, V. (1987). The Varni-Thompson pediatric pain questionnaire: chronic musculoskeletal pain in juvenile rheumatoid arthritis. *Pain, 28*, 27–38.

Veale, D. (2000). Outcome of cosmetic surgery and "DIY" surgery in patients with body dysmorphic disorder. *Psychiatric Bulletin, 24*, 218–221.

Veale, D., Gournay, K., Dryden, W., and Boocock, A. (1996), Body dysmorphic disorder: A cognitive behavioral model and pilot randomized controlled trial. *Behaviour Research and Therapy, 34*, 717–729.

Volkmar, F.R., Poll, J., and Lewis M. (1984). Conversion reactions in childhood and adolescents. *Journal of the American Academy of Child and Adolescent Psychiatry, 23*, 424–430.

Walker, L.S. and Greene, J.W. (1991). Negative life events and symptom resolution in pediatric abdominal pain patients. *Journal of Pediatric Psychology, 14*, 231–243.

Walker, L.S., Garber, J., van Slyke, D.A., and Greene, J.W. (1995). Long-term health outcomes in patients with recurrent abdominal pain. *Journal of Pediatric Psychology, 20*, 233–245.

Warwick, H. and Salkovskis, P.M. (1990). Hypochondriasis. *Behaviour Research and Therapy, 28*, 105–117.

Wells, J.E., Bushnell, J.A., Hornblow, A.R., Joyce, P.R., and Oakley-Browne, M.A. (1989). Christchurch epidemiology study: Part I. Methodology and lifetime prevalence for specific psychiatric disorders. *Australian and New Zealand Journal of Psychiatry, 23*, 315–326.

Wise, T.N. and Birket-Smith, M. (2002). The somatoform disorders for DSMV: The need for changes in process and content. *Psychosomatics, 43*, 437–440.

Wittchen, H-U., Essau, C.A., von Zerssen, D., Krieg, C., and Zaudig, M. (1992). Lifetime and six-month prevalence of mental disorders in the Munich Follow-up Study. *European Archives of Psychiatry and Clinical Neuroscience, 241*, 247–258.

World Health Organization (WHO) (1992). *International classification of diseases: Tenth revision*. Chapter V. Mental and behavioural disorders: Diagnostic criteria for research. Geneva: WHO.

Wyllie, E., Friedman, D., Lüders, H., Morris, H., Rothner, D., and Turnbull, J. (1991). Outcome of psychogenic seizures in children and adolescents compared with adults. *Neurology, 41*, 742–744.

Zimmerman, M. and Mattia, J. I. (1998). Body dysmorphic disorder in psychiatric outpatients: Recognition, prevalence, comorbidity, demographic, and clinical correlates. *Comprehensive Psychiatry, 39*, 265–270.

Zwaigenbaum, L., Szatmari, P., Boyle, M.H., and Offord, D.R. (1999). Highly somatizing young adolescents and the risk of depression. *Pediatrics, 103*, 1203–1209.

10

AUTISM

A psychological perspective

Hanna Kovshoff, Corinna F. Grindle, and Richard P. Hastings

First identified in 1943 by Leo Kanner, autism affects an individual's ability to communicate verbally and non-verbally, interact socially, play imaginatively, and relate to those around them. Autism is a spectrum disorder such that it affects individuals differently, and with varying degrees of severity. It is estimated that between 3.3 and 16 children per 10,000 are affected with autism, taking into account differing diagnostic criteria, genetic factors, environmental influences, and/or case finding methods of a range of epidemiological studies. The latest incidence rates of persons living with autism spectrum disorders in the United Kingdom, according to the National Autistic Society, are 91 per 10,000, and 1 in 1000 (Bryson, 1997) in the United States. Autism is three to five times more likely to affect boys than girls (American Psychiatric Association 1994; Klinger and Dawson, 1996).

Autism is not a behavioural disorder; however, diagnosis relies on the presence, as well as the absence, of various key behaviours. It is a lifelong, complex neurodevelopmental disability, which affects central nervous system and brain functioning. Behaviours commonly associated with autism may become apparent by the time the child reaches the age of 18 months, and are usually present by 3 years of age. As described in the DSM-IV (APA, 1994) and the ICD-10 (WHO, 1992) diagnostic manuals, autism is characterized by a pattern of deficits in social behaviour, communication, and imagination, and is associated with repetitive and/or stereotypical patterns of behaviours or interests. Autism forms part of a subcategory of Pervasive Developmental Disorders (DSM-IV; APA, 1994) which are characterized by severe and lifelong impairment in multiple areas of development. These areas of impairment are relative to the individual's developmental level or mental age (DSM-IV; APA, 1994). Apart from autism spectrum disorder, pervasive developmental disorders include Rett's disorder, child disintegrative disorder, Asperger's disorder, and pervasive developmental disorder – not otherwise specified (PDD-NOS). All of these conditions have in common that they are evident in the first year of life, and most are associated with some level of intellectual disability. Autism occurs at all intelligence levels, although it is widely believed that approximately 75 percent of persons with autism also have associated learning difficulties and a below average intelligence quotient (IQ), while approximately 25 percent of individuals with autism have average or above average intelligence (Newsom, 1998; Sigman, 1998). It is noteworthy to say that tests of intelligence and cognitive potential find a different pattern of performance than other children with intellectual disabilities. Autism is associated with a pattern of strengths and weaknesses characterized by deficits in abstract and conceptual thinking, receptive and expressive language, and socially related tasks. Conversely, non-verbal performance, and visual spatial and motor skill areas are often better developed (Happé, 1994; Shah and Frith, 1993; Volkmar et al., 1997).

Although a large body of research has been conducted as to its nature, the aetiology of autism is still unknown. While autism is widely believed to be a neuro-logical disorder with a strong genetic component, exact brain-location or biological markers remain unidentified, and diagnosis of autism continues to rely solely on the presence and absence of particular behavioural patterns. Epidemiological studies reveal that autism is associated with several known genetic disorders including Fragile X syndrome which is found in approximately 2.5 percent of cases of autism (Rutter et al., 1997). Other conditions have also been linked to autism including tuberous sclerosis (Dykens and Volkmar, 1997) and seizure disorders. Inheritance studies have found that between 36 percent (Folstein and Rutter, 1978) and 91 percent (Bailey et al., 1995) of monozygotic twins are concordant for autism. The rate of autism in siblings of children with autism is between 3 and 7 percent, and approximately 8 percent of extended families have a member with autism (Bailey et al., 1996; Newsom, 1998). Additionally, family studies of genetics indicate that non-autistic siblings and parents of children with autism have subtle cognitive, linguistic, or social abnormalities (Fombonne et al., 1997; Hughes et al., 1999; Piven and Palmer, 1997; Rutter et al., 1993; Tsai and Ghaziuddin, 1991). The mode of genetic transmission remains unknown; however, the case is strong for several interacting genes (Simonoff et al., 1996), perhaps triggered by an environmental insult either in the womb or within the first two years of life.

The triad of impairments in autism

In 1979 Lorna Wing and Judith Gould examined the prevalence of autism amongst a group of children with special needs in the former London borough of Camberwell. They found a prevalence of 5 out of 10,000 in children with IQ levels below 70. However, 15 out of 10,000 children in this group were identified as having deficits in communication, social interaction, and in imagination skills (along with repetitive or stereotyped patterns of behaviour), which they referred to as the "Triad of Impairments". This work formed the basis of the DSM-IV (APA, 1994) and ICD-10 (WHO, 1992) diagnostic criteria, which requires deficits in each of these three areas in order to diagnose autism. This work led to the understanding of autism as a "spectrum disorder" with varying cognitive profiles, behavioural patterns, and adaptive skills.

Deficits in social interaction

Persons with autism are mistakenly believed to be entirely non-social. While this is not the case, and sociability levels differ from individual to individual, qualitative impairments are present in the area of social interaction. This may involve lack of, or abnormal use of eye contact and eye gaze. Some persons with autism find eye contact difficult to make, and/or use their peripheral vision to look at objects or persons in their environment. Additionally, use of gestures while speaking, body posture and proximity, as well as facial expression may be impaired. Difficulties range from indifference and aloofness of other persons, to wanting to interact with others socially, but not having a good enough command of social norms and rules in order to do this effectively and as a result, they experience social rejection.

Deficits in social communication

While autism is associated with both a developmental delay and deviance in the production of language, many individuals with autism do learn to use language to communicate. The form and function of these communications are often impaired such that the social rules of give and take in conversations with others are not learned or understood. Thus, a person with autism may talk "at" another, rather than with them. Additionally, they may not be able to read social cues of when it is time to let another have their turn to speak, recognize when their conversational partner is no longer interested in what they are saying, or fail to produce an appropriate emotional response to other people's verbal or non-verbal behaviour. There may also be impairments in the tone of speech, such that the voice may remain in monotone, be high-pitched, or disfluid.

Deficits in imagination

People with autism have impaired make-believe and pretend play skills. Most children with autism are unable to play pretend or imagination games with toys or objects, either alone or with other children or adults. When pretend play is modelled for children, it may be learned, however there is the risk of this becoming a scripted play routine, rather than an inherent ability to build on and change the play sequence. There is also an impairment in the ability to imitate others spontaneously. This has effects in both the ability to learn as well as to fit in with society. As many children learn by watching others around them in order to find out how things are done, children with autism may need to be explicitly shown and taught how to perform certain activities.

Repetitive and/or stereotyped behaviours

In addition to impairments in social interaction, communication, and imagination, persons with autism also display repetitive and stereotyped qualities in their activities or behaviour. This is manifest in a tendency to play with parts, rather than wholes of objects, lining objects up, spinning parts of objects, an intense desire for "sameness" and routine, over or undersensitivities to sensory information including sound, taste, touch, and sight, and repeated looking at books or watching videos. In addition, poor motor coordination, disturbances in sleep and eating patterns, and problems of attention may also be present.

Theoretical accounts of the nature of autism

Several attempts have been made to identify the core or pivotal skill deficit of autism. Researchers have compared the development of children with autism with their typically developing peers, as well as with children with other developmental disorders, in order to identify some fundamental deficit that might underlie and account for the features of autism. What follows is a brief description of four of the most prominent and well researched theories to date which attempt to explain the cause of autism spectrum disorders: executive dysfunction, central coherence, theory of mind, and social orienting theory.

Executive dysfunction

The term "executive functioning" is used to describe a frontally mediated behaviour of the brain whose purpose is to organize, plan, manage, and strategize thoughts and behaviour. Children and adults with autism perform more poorly than their typically developing peers on tests of executive functions (McEvoy et al., 1993; Ozonoff, 1997). A typical example lies in the Tower of Hanoi task, which requires planning and forethought in order to rearrange rings on a pegboard such that they are ordered according to certain rules. Bailey et al. (1996), among others, find that persons with autism have difficulty in planning ahead, switching rules, and in disregarding irrelevant information that leads to an increased number of errors on this test. However, while performance on executive functioning tasks points to deficits in this area, it is difficult to control for attentional issues which may be at the root of poor performance (e.g. Burack et al., 1997). Additionally, while this theory can account for the inflexibility of thought, as well as the stereotypical and repetitive patterns of behaviour that are seen in this population, it cannot comprehensively explain the social or linguistic deficits that are also associated with autism.

Central coherence

Central coherence refers to the ability to integrate incoming information in context, or view both the parts and the wholes of visual scenes to view a complete picture. Persons with autism are reported to have a heightened ability to view the parts of visual stimuli, often at the expense of being able to interpret the global whole, thus having weak central coherence (Happé, 1994). For example, when shown pictures of either a face or parts of a face and asked to identify the person, typically developing children are better able to recognize the whole face, rather than parts of it. Conversely, children with autism are equally able to identify a face from only seeing parts of the face, as they are when seeing the whole face (Baron-Cohen and Swettenham, 1997). Thus, having weak central coherence can be advantageous when attention to the detail or parts of a picture are important. Consequently, persons with autism are often better than their typically developing peers at tasks that involve using smaller parts in order to build a whole, such as jigsaw puzzles. In addition, they perform better than normally developing matched comparison groups on the Block Design task on the Wechsler Intelligence Scales for Children (WISC; Shah and Frith, 1993). This is likely due to the fact that children with autism are able to break down pictures, and the locally viewed segments are as or more salient than the whole picture. Furthermore, in an embedded figures task which involves finding a shape that is hidden within and helps make up a larger picture, children with autism also outperform their peers (Jolliffe and Baron-Cohen, 1997).

Finally, children with autism seem to be able to resist visual illusions, for example being able to tell that two lines are of the same size when arrows are pointed both outwards and inwards (Happé, 1996). While these studies have helped to show that weak central coherence is a cognitive style of persons with autism, it is not a likely cause of autism as children with autism perform in line with mental age on a variety of tasks that involve integrating information, including transitive inference tests and analogical reasoning tests (Scott and Baron-Cohen, 1996), as well as counter-factual syllogistic reasoning tests (Scott et al., 1999).

Theory of mind

The study of theory of mind in persons with autism has led to conclusions regarding the way in which this population are able to infer the mental states of others, represent the world in the mind (metarepresentation), as well as understand that other people have thoughts and feelings that can differ from their own. Children and adults with autism have difficulty using the above points to "read others' minds" (Baron-Cohen, 1994, 1995). The prototypical theory of mind task is the Sally-Ann test, which tests the understanding that others can hold beliefs that are false. In this task, Sally puts a marble into a cup and leaves the room. Ann enters the room and puts the marble into a box. The child is then asked where they think that Sally will look for the marble upon return. Between 3 and 4 years of age, typically developing children are able to understand that Sally will look in the cup for the marble, as she will hold the false belief that it is still there, not knowing that Ann has moved it, and this belief will guide her action. Baron-Cohen et al. (1985) found that 80 percent of preschool children with autism failed the Sally-Ann task by saying that Sally would look into the box for the marble. Lending support to a lack of theory of mind, deficits also exist in pretend or symbolic play (Baron-Cohen, 1987), in recognizing mental state words (e.g. anxious, depressed) (Baron-Cohen et al., 1994), in using a range of mental state words (Tager-Flüsberg, 1993), and in understanding complex causes of emotion (Baron-Cohen, 1991). These impairments highlight major difficulties in the ability to attribute or comprehend the mental states to others, and proponents of this theory argue that a lack of theory of mind is central to the major social and communication deficits seen in persons with autism.

Social orienting theory

Peter Mundy suggested that the primary deficit in autism revolves around an impairment in social orienting, specifically joint attention behaviours. Joint attention refers to the ability to respond to, initiate or maintain a communicative channel with a partner (Adamson and McArthur, 1995) and involves the ability to coordinate visual attention with others regarding objects and events (Mundy and Gomes, 1998). In typical development, joint attention develops between the ages of 6 and 12 months. Deviances in the development of joint attention skills are evident early in life in children with autism. For example, Osterling and Dawson (1994) conducted an analysis of first year birthday party video tape data. They found at 12 months, compared to their normally developing peers, children with autism were less likely to look at others, to show an object or point out an object, and to respond by orienting to their name.

While developing his theory, Mundy and colleagues worked for many years on the Early Social Communication Scales (ESCS; Mundy et al., 1996), a semi-structured video-taped observation measure in which an experimenter attempts to elicit joint attention, requesting, and social interaction behaviours through toy play, turn taking attempts, commands to follow instructions, and bids to engage in play. They have, through this paradigm, been able to identify deficits in the ability to initiate joint attention bids with a social partner, as well as in the ability to point out items of interest for the sake of sharing the experience (Mundy et al., 1990). Conversely, responding to the joint attention bids from others, as well as pointing in order to attain an item is less impaired.

Mundy and colleagues believe that a frontally mediated neuroaffective motivation system whose purpose is to prioritize social information is impaired in children with autism (Mundy, 1995; Mundy and Neal, 2001). This leads to a negative feedback loop where social information is continually not prioritized in the brain, and thus social information becomes even less salient or motivating to attend to. While it is clear that a deficit in higher order cognitive processes plays an important role in the manifestation of the social and communication deficits in autism, a clear neurological pathway leading to the disorder remains unidentified. These neuro-logical links remain important goals for autism researchers.

Treatment for children with autism

We have already noted that autism is a chronic, severely handicapping medical condition with onset in early childhood. Conventional long-term studies of people with autism have suggested that, without treatment, most will continue to have serious deficits in communication and social skills throughout their lives (DeMyer et al., 1973; Rutter, 1970). Thus, treatment is a crucial issue. In a major review of autism, Rapin (1997) concluded: "The most important intervention in autism is early and intensive remedial education that addresses both behavioural and communication disorders. The effective approaches use a highly structured environment with intensive individual instruction and a high teacher-to-student ratio" (Rapin, 1997, p. 104). Similarly, McGee et al. (1999) concluded that "The issue is not whether to intervene, but how to provide information when it will help the most . . . Strong consensus exists on this one point: early intervention is a critical factor in [the] effective treatment [of autism]" (McGee et al., 1999, p. 133).

Dozens of treatments for autism are currently being promoted, many of which are said to benefit most, if not all, children with autism. In the following sections, we review the claims and evidence about some of these treatments and evaluate whether or not proposed treatment outcomes are supported by sound scientific evidence which rules out alternative explanations for apparent effects. Our focus is on intervention that has been used with children with autism and often with young children, constituting an interest in early intervention as opposed to long-term support methods. The terms *intervention therapy* and *treatment* will be used interchangeably to describe anything that is done to or with a child with the intention of changing their behaviour or symptomatology.

Sensory integration therapy

A popular view about children with autism is that they have a dysfunctional sensory system and that they may be over or under reactive to normal levels of sensory stimulation. Consequently, the child may try to moderate their arousal levels by engaging in such self-stimulatory behaviours as rocking or hand flapping. Sensory integration therapy (SIT) was developed in a series of studies by Ayres (1972, 1979) to overcome these problems by improving the sensory processing capabilities of the brain. Typically, SIT is delivered in one-to-one treatment sessions by occupational therapists who stimulate the child's skin, vestibular, and proprioceptive systems. This stimulation might consist of activities such as playing on a rocking horse or engaging in activities which require balance. Success on the programme is usually inferred from observing improvements in areas such as eye contact, learning, communication, motor skills, and so on.

Although SIT is clearly enjoyed by many children with autism, there have been no published, methodologically sound documentations that SIT alone actually produces significant lasting changes in reducing autistic behaviours or enhancing skills in areas like language and communication (see Hoehn and Baumeister, 1994, for a critique of the literature). Most studies have not ruled out the possibility that something other than SIT (e.g., maturation, adult attention, possible reinforcing effects of sensory stimulation) could be responsible (e.g., Ayres and Maillouz, 1981).

Auditory integration training

Advocates of auditory integration training (AIT) believe that children with autism are hypersensitive to certain frequencies of sound and that these distortions in hearing significantly contribute to many of the symptoms commonly associated with autism (e.g., aggression, inability to follow instructions, poor social interaction skills). The main aim of AIT, therefore, is to reduce the child's hypersensitivity to sound, subsequently alleviating deficits in these areas (Rimland and Edelson, 1995; Stehli, 1991).

Training begins with an assessment (audiogram) to discover the frequencies at which the child's hearing is too sensitive. The child then spends two thirty-minute sessions daily for ten consecutive days, listening to music played through a specialized electronic device. The device randomizes and filters out the frequencies identified by the audiogram and sends these sounds to the child's ears through a set of headphones. The randomized frequencies are said to mobilize and exercise the inner ear and brain. After twenty sessions the child's hearing should show significant improvement with all or most frequencies being perceived at or near equal level. Behavioural changes and benefits are said to eventually follow, although they may take up to one year to become apparent.

Although some studies claim substantial improvements in behaviour due to AIT (e.g., Rimland and Edelson, 1995; Stelhi, 1991), it is difficult to draw definite conclusions from this research. The audiogram, for example, has actually never been shown to be a valid measure of hypersensitive hearing. Furthermore, inherent in the philosophy of AIT is the claim that hypersensitivity causes the problems displayed by children with autism. This has never been demonstrated in a scientific way, so even if AIT did reduce hypersensitivity, there should be no reason to expect that it could produce improvements in behaviour.

There is also much contradictory evidence against the efficacy of AIT (e.g., Gillberg et al., 1999; Link, 1997; Mudford et al., 2000). For example, Mudford et al. (2000), using a variety of objective assessment and control procedures, found that not one child benefited clinically or educationally from AIT. Evidence such as this should raise concerns as to the validity or utility of AIT as a treatment of choice for children with autism.

Facilitated communication

The essence of the facilitated communication (FC) approach is that a child with autism is taught to communicate by "facilitators" physically prompting him or her to point to letters or words on a communication board or to type using a word processor. Typically the child is non-verbal or has severe language delay. The intention is not to teach independent pointing or typing but to release the hidden thoughts and desires of the child through the facilitator. This technique has been claimed to be remarkably effective; many children have been said to reveal fluent literacy, cognitive, and communication skills (Crossley, 1992; Sabin and Donnellan,

1993). These claims, however, have been backed up only by using anecdotal or subjective evidence. For example, published research supporting the efficacy of FC usually failed to control for the possibility that it was, in fact, the facilitators who were doing the spelling (e.g., Biklen, 1993). However, when these controls were implemented (e.g., by having facilitators look away from the spelling device), the vast majority of "facilitated" communications come from the facilitators, not from the people with disabilities (e.g., Jacobsen et al., 1995; Smith and Belcher, 1994).

Not only has FC failed to "release" hidden language skills, but also it has caused serious errors of judgment. For example, under the misconception that their child possessed highly developed language skills, parents have been known to stop other interventions aimed at improving their child's skills, instead putting their child into mainstream classes to follow an age-appropriate curriculum with the help of their facilitator.

Diets

The dietary approach supports the view that some of the symptoms of autism (e.g., aggression, hyperactivity, deficits in attending skills) may be linked to certain food products, particularly those containing casein (milk and dairy produce) or gluten (wheat and other cereal products). Consequently, advocates of this approach advise the removal of casein and/or gluten from the diet to help reduce symptoms commonly associated with autism (e.g., Reichelt et al., 1990; Shattock and Lowdon, 1991). Specifically, casein free diets are often recommended for those children whose autism appears at or around the time of birth (neonatal onset), whereas a gluten free diet may be recommended for those children whose autism becomes apparent at about 2 years of age (when a wheat based diet is more likely to be introduced).

To date, most of the evidence supporting the efficacy of dietary intervention is anecdotal, with many parents reporting their child's successful reactions to an exclusion diet. Unfortunately, however, the effectiveness of dietary intervention has yet to be demonstrated in a scientifically rigorous way. For example, studies which have attributed positive changes in symptomatology to an exclusion diet (e.g., Knivsberg et al., 1990; Reichelt et al., 1990, 1997) did not include a control group of children who were not put on the diet. Thus, it was not possible to see whether it was the dietary intervention or another variable, like maturation effects, that was the critical variable.

A major drawback to this approach is that shopping and cooking can become extremely arduous. Several foods (e.g., bread, pasta) have to be either cooked from scratch or bought at inflated prices. Furthermore, whoever does the cooking may find themselves cooking separate meals for different family members. Birthday parties can also be a problem for the child with autism, who is restricted from eating much of the party food. Despite these drawbacks, however, parents often claim that the positive changes they see in their child are worth the pitfalls of implementing the diet.

Son-Rise

The Son-Rise approach (Options) was developed in the 1970s by two parents, to teach their own son with autism and severe mental retardation (e.g., Kaufman, 1995). The essence of this approach is that the adult should show total non-judgmental acceptance of the child and their actions. The adult follows the child's lead and although the child is invited to join in interactive activities, the adult always accepts when the child refuses. The child is also never made to either stop or undertake any activity. Importantly, this programme does not aim to provide the child with any information, or to teach the child to master predetermined skills. The child's current level of performance is viewed as being the best the child can do.

It has been claimed that this process helps to resolve unhappiness and discard self-limiting beliefs (The Option Institute and Fellowship, 1997), in some cases effecting a "cure". For example, Kaufman (1995) explained how his son acquired a near genius IQ with few traces of his original condition. There are, however, no peer-reviewed, published studies of the Son-Rise Programme's effectiveness or any outcome statistics, so these claims should be viewed with the utmost caution.

Project TEACCH

Project TEACCH (The Treatment and Education of Autistic and related Communication handicapped Children) was developed in the 1970s by Eric Schopler at the University of North Carolina and has become one of the most influential and widely used teaching approaches for children with autism. One of the defining characteristics of the TEACCH approach is its emphasis on designing structured classroom environments for the child, rather than focusing on integrating the child into more "typical" settings (Lord and Schopler, 1994). Thus, it is based on the idea that the environment should be adapted to the child with autism, not the child to the environment.

Most children with autism on a TEACCH programme are taught in classrooms arranged in such a way to minimize distractions, usually working alone at "work stations", separated by screens from the rest of the class. Another central feature of this approach is that the teacher chooses a work programme for each child based on the skills they already have, rather than trying to teach any new skills or behaviours. Thus, class work often involves repetitive visual-motor activities such as sorting objects by size or colour. Materials are often clearly marked and arranged to help children carry out these tasks independently (e.g., trays of different colours for colour sorting). Teaching strategies generally emphasize visual rather than verbally mediated strategies. As such, children may be taught to follow picture schedules which depict a series of activities to be completed in one sitting. Pictures or photographs are also commonly used to communicate with others.

Although TEACCH is one of the most widely used programmes for children with autism, there has been surprisingly little done in the way of scientifically rigorous research. Several studies purportedly show that children on the TEACCH programme show a significant increase in appropriate behaviours as a result of being on the programme (e.g., Panerai et al. 1997; Schopler et al., 1982; Short, 1984; Venter et al., 1992). However, none of these studies had any control groups, so it is unclear whether it was the TEACCH programme that produced gains. For example, Schopler et al. (1982) showed that the individuals with autism in their study had a lower rate of institutionalization than did individuals in studies conducted in the 1960s, and inferred that this finding was proof of the efficacy of TEACCH. Without a control group, however, it was not possible to see if changes in national policy may have made institutionalization less likely anyway, regardless of treatment. Furthermore, much of the evidence offered to demonstrate the effectiveness of TEACCH comes only from parent satisfaction surveys, rather than any objective measures like IQ.

With its emphasis on developing a programme around a child's existing skills and interests, and keeping the child independently and usefully occupied, TEACCH has become the treatment of choice for many teachers and parents. However, many argue that with its emphasis on structure and special environments, children with autism can miss out on the opportunity to become more like typically developing children by being integrated into mainstream settings. Scientifically rigorous evaluations of TEACCH are also needed to assess its long term effectiveness.

Applied behaviour analysis

A long-running research programme at UCLA (see, e.g., Lovaas, 1993) has developed a practical method of early intervention for children with autism based on applied behaviour analysis (ABA), a scientific approach derived from psychological learning theory (see, e.g., *Journal of Applied Behavior Analysis*, 1968 to present). Applied behaviour analysts adopt the view that the symptoms of autism have a biological basis but can nonetheless be changed through intensive, structured teaching. The main aim of ABA is to build socially useful repertoires of behaviours at the same time as reducing problematic ones. This is achieved by using principles based on Skinnerian operant conditioning from the 1960s, namely that the probability of appropriate behaviours will increase if they are reinforced immediately, but that problematic behaviours will decrease if they are not reinforced. The ABA treatment approach focuses on the development of many different types of skills, including attention, imitation, communication, social skills, reading, writing and self-help skills.

ABA for children with autism also focuses on breaking down these skills into very small steps and teaching only one of these steps at a time. Using a one-to-one therapist–child ratio, teaching begins with the therapist presenting a specific cue or instruction to the child. If the child needs help to respond correctly the teacher provides a prompt such as physical guidance or a verbal reminder. Then, either with or without a prompt, the child responds to the instruction. If the child responds incorrectly they are corrected or given another chance. If correct, the teacher gives a reward or praise to encourage them. This single cycle of the behaviourally based instruction routine (e.g., antecedent-behaviour-consequence) is known as a discrete-trial. A particular trial may be repeated several times in succession, several times a day, over several days (or even longer) until the child can perform the response readily without any help from the teacher.

One of the most thorough of studies of the effectiveness of ABA on children with autism was published by Lovaas (1987), who assessed the effect of beginning ABA intervention with children during the pre-school period (aged 3–4 years), working intensively, and continuing therapy for at least two years. He compared the progress of 19 children who received intensive intervention (40 hours a week) with those who were either treated only 10 hours a week (the minimal-treatment control group) or who were treated in programmes other than the UCLA project. After two years of treatment, the IQ of the intensive-treatment experimental group increased by an average of 30 points compared to the controls, and 47 percent of the treated children improved sufficiently to be enrolled in mainstream schools, where their behaviour was indistinguishable from their peers on blind tests of IQ and adaptive functioning. In contrast, only 2 percent of the children in the control conditions showed a similar level of improvement.

The nine best-outcome children from the intensive treatment group, who had achieved normal functioning, participated in a long-term follow-up study (McEachin et al., 1993). These children were re-evaluated when they were about 13 years old. "Blind" examiners could not distinguish eight out of the nine children from typically developing children of the same age on measures of cognitive, academic, social or adaptive skills. Thus, the results of the follow-up study showed that the gains made by these children persisted.

Given the potentially profound implications of Lovaas's treatment, with its apparent capacity to transform the lives of children suffering from autism, replication of these results has been of the utmost importance. Several studies have now shown that ABA can result in improvements in many children with autism, including the development of an effective skills repertoire, the control of challenging behaviour (e.g., self-injury), successful integration in mainstream schools and apparently normal levels of functioning for some (e.g., Anderson et al., 1987; Birnbrauer and Leach, 1993; Fenske et al., 1985). Although the original study (Lovaas, 1987) has been criticized for the relatively small number of children in the study and the procedures used for measuring improvement (Gresham and MacMillan, 1997), Lovaas's work has attracted strong support from the research community (e.g. Green, 1996). There is also scientific evidence that older children can develop a wide range of skills on the programme. For example, Eikeseth and his colleagues demonstrated that some 4–7 year olds can make clinically valuable gains with intensive behavioural intervention (Eikeseth et al., 2002).

Autism and the family

We have seen in previous sections of this chapter that autism is often a disorder that has serious consequences for children in terms of social development and long term outcomes. Children with autism, despite their lack of interest generally in the social world, still live within family environments. Thus, parents, siblings, and other family members have to develop ways of coping with the unusual social and behavioural characteristics of the child with autism who lives with them. There has been considerable research attention given to adjustment in family members of children with autism, especially parents and siblings. There is also the question of how the well-being of other family members might affect the development of the child with autism, whether clinicians can intervene to alleviate any negative impact on the family, and whether the impact on the family is always negative.

In the following sections, we review the research literature relating to the issues raised above. However, there is a further question about autism and the family that we will not address in detail but may be important to consider when trying to understand the interactions between children with autism and their family members. Autism is likely to have an underlying genetic component, and so there has been research interest in whether the broad autism phenotype is found in family members of children with autism (see earlier). Thus, it may be important to consider how we might disentangle any measures of the impact of a child with autism on the psychological well-being of family members from the presence of psychological characteristics resulting from the impact of shared genes rather than the impact of the child with autism per se.

Parental adaptation in families of children with autism

In the research literature on parents of children with autism, adaptation is a general phrase applied to studies that measure the psychological well-being of parents using constructs such as depression, anxiety, and parenting stress. We will use the general term "stress" to describe the results of these studies. Three conclusions in particular are significant in the research literature concerning the adaptation of parents to the presence of a child with autism in the family:

- Parents of children with autism report more stress than other parents.
- Mothers typically report more stress than fathers.
- It is the behaviour problems of the child with autism in particular that are the most predictive of parental stress.

Almost without exception, research studies comparing stress in parents of children with autism and stress in parents of children without disabilities, parents of children with intellectual disabilities, physical disabilities or chronic illnesses, have found that parents of children with autism report more stress (Bouma and Schweitzer, 1990; Dumas et al., 1991; Kasari and Sigman, 1997; Koegel et al., 1992; Konstantareas et al., 1992; Rodrigue et al., 1990, 1992; Sanders and Morgan, 1997; Wolf et al., 1989). The stressful impact of the child with autism can be quantified from studies where measures of mental health have been used and clinical caseness can be established by considering whether parents meet cut-off scores. For example, in a study of parents of school age children with autism, Hastings and Brown (2002) found that one-half of mothers and one-quarter of fathers scored in the borderline or clinical range for anxiety, 40 percent of mothers and 15 percent of fathers scored within clinical range for depression.

An obvious question to ask is why parents of children with autism report these high levels of stress compared to other parents. As indicated above, it may be that some increased psychological problems are due to shared genetic factors within the family but this is unlikely to account fully for these findings. What does seem to be clear is that the increase in stress results mainly from the level of behaviour problems in children with autism. Autism is a risk factor for the presence of significant behaviour problems in many studies of children with developmental disabilities (e.g., Hastings and Mount, 2001). Furthermore, the child characteristics most strongly predictive of stress in parents of children with autism are their behaviour problems and not adaptive skills (cf. severity of cognitive impairment, and level of dependence) (see Hastings, 2002, for a review).

Research findings on the differential impact of children with autism on mothers and fathers are more varied and also reflect a general pattern in research on parents of children with other disabilities. Many studies suggest that mothers are more affected by their child with autism in that they typically report more stress than fathers (e.g., Bristol et al., 1988; Gray and Holden, 1992; Hastings, 2003b; Hastings and Brown, 2002; Konstantareas et al., 1992; Moes et al., 1992). However, these differences are not always found. Some studies have reported no differences in maternal and paternal stress (e.g., Bebko et al., 1987; Factor et al., 1990; Wolf et al., 1989) but, as far as we are aware, no researchers have yet reported data from a sample where fathers report more stress than mothers.

The most obvious explanation for higher levels of stress in mothers compared with fathers of children with autism is that in many families, fathers may still be less involved with their children (e.g., Bristol et al., 1988). Thus, fathers may not be exposed to as much of the child's behaviour problems on a day-to-day basis. However, the picture is unlikely to be this simple. In particular, fathers are also more likely to be employed outside of the home and thus have ready access to social support from colleagues. Social support, and also coping styles, are predictive of stress in parents of children with autism (e.g., Hastings and Johnson, 2001). Mothers may have very different social support and may adopt different coping strategies than fathers and this may underscore some of the differences found in reported stress. Very few research studies have considered potential differences in social support and coping for mothers and fathers in families of children with autism. Thus, it is difficult to comment any further on these questions at present.

A further issue worth considering at this point is that the discussion so far on parental adaptation has focused on negative outcomes such as stress and mental health problems. Recent research (see Hastings and Taunt, 2002, for a review) has shown that parents of children with autism, in common with parents of children with other disabilities, also report that their child has a positive impact on themselves (e.g., increased sensitivity) and their family (e.g., bringing the family closer together). As with any family, parents of children with autism experience not only stresses (perhaps in the extreme), but also a number of positive effects. It is important to remember this point and perhaps to encourage parents specifically to recognise these positive effects when they may be feeling overly negative.

Sibling adjustment

Research seems to suggest that siblings of children with autism may be at increased risk of negative outcomes such as depression when compared to control groups but also to siblings of children with other disabilities (Bågenholm and Gillberg, 1991; Fisman et al., 1996, 2000; Gold, 1993; Hastings, 2003a; Rodrigue et al., 1993; Roeyers and Mycke, 1995). However, not every study has found negative effects. Some of the variation in findings may well be due to the influence of a number of moderating factors. In particular, variables such as the age of the sibling, whether the sibling is younger or older than the child with autism, and the gender match between the siblings have been identified in several studies (e.g., Gold, 1993; Hastings, 2003a; Mates, 1990; McHale et al., 1986; Roeyers and Mycke, 1995).

It is difficult to draw firm conclusions from the research literature on the adjustment of siblings of children with autism. A meta-analysis of research with siblings of children with mental retardation suggested that there was evidence of a small negative effect on siblings (Rossiter and Sharpe, 2001). There is no real reason to suppose that such a review of autism-specific studies would find any different. The effects of potential moderating variables are also mixed. For example, some studies have suggested that a child younger than their sibling with autism is more at risk of adjustment problems and some studies find that it is those older than their sibling with autism that are at most risk.

Clinical implications

There is some argument as to the nature of the increase in prevalence of newly diagnosed cases of autism since the 1970s. There is evidence to suggest that changes in case definition and improved awareness explain much of the upward trend of rates since the 1970s (Fombonne, 2003). In addition, since the 1990s we have heard much about the possible link between the combined MMR vaccine and autism. After reviewing 32 published epidemiological surveys published between 1966 and 2001, Fombonne (2003) concedes that the available studies do not provide an adequate picture to fully explain why the incidence of autism and other pervasive developmental disorders (e.g., Asperger's Disorder) have increased. While the cause of autism remains unidentified, and the number of new cases continues to rise, autism spectrum disorders will undoubtedly require a greater amount of financial, educational, and clinical resources over the next few years.

While the major theories outlined in this chapter have gone a long way towards outlining possible sources of the deficits seen in autism, no one theory can account for all of the features of autism. While theory of mind or social orienting deficits can explain the social and communication impairments seen in autism, they cannot account for the repetitive or stereotyped behaviours that are also a feature of this disorder. Similarly, whilst executive functioning deficits and weak central coherence theory are able to explain many of the cognitive and visual characteristics of autism, they do not provide straightforward account of autism's social and communication deficits. Furthermore, few links between theoretical accounts of autism and intervention techniques exist. Most interventions that are used with the autistic population do not seem to be based on key psychological theories. Where attempts have been made to develop therapeutic approaches based on theory (e.g., Teaching Children with Autism how to Mindread, Hadwin et al., 1997), there is not strong evidence of success. Similarly, while the TEACCH approach is often said to be loosely based on executive functioning theory, little research evidence exists to support this link. One theory that does highlight the importance of intervention is social orienting theory. Mundy and colleagues (Mundy, 1995; Mundy and Neal, 2001) believe that early intervention increases the tendency of young children with autism to process social information within a critical period. Thus, the earlier that therapeutic intervention can begin with these children, the better the chance of increasing the saliency of social communication skills. This should in turn lessen the degree of social and communication deficit (Mundy and Crowson, 1997) and if proven correct, would help explain accounts of why early intervention works better than later intervention and why more is better than less. Mundy does not however link his theory to any intervention in particular, except to say that many of the current therapies are provided within the context of a social interaction, and should thus have the desired effects.

As mentioned previously, dozens of treatments have been proposed for the treatment of autism. Choosing between them can be a daunting and overwhelming experience for most families. To help families make informed decisions about what is best for their child, clinicians should recommend only those treatments whose effectiveness has been established by sound scientific evidence. This research should be based upon objective observation and measurement of behavioural changes and also rule out alternative explanations for apparent effects. In addition, there should be repeated replications of the treatment's effectiveness by researchers working independently of one another. Treatments which are not evidence based in this way ought not to be recommended.

At present, only one treatment approach for autism – early intensive intervention using the methods of applied behaviour analysis – has produced satisfactory scientific evidence to support its claims of effectiveness. No other treatment for autism offers comparable scientific evidence (e.g., Lovaas and Smith, 1989). Thus, because treatments derived from ABA have such a strong evidence base, they are often regarded as the treatment of choice for children with autism (New York State Department of Health, 1999; US Department of Health and Human Services, 1999). However, it is also important to consider the possibility that other treatments may well be effective but lack the scientific evidence to back them up. For example, many parents report beneficial changes in their child's behaviour when they are put on a casein or gluten free diet, but unfortunately these claims have yet to be supported by scientifically rigorous research. Thus, a key priority in autism research must be to design more robust evaluations of these treatment outcomes.

Worryingly, out of the dozens of treatments currently available for children with autism, most have little or no sound scientific evidence to support their effectiveness. In some cases, scientific evidence exists to show that treatment claims are completely unsubstantiated and that treatment may even be harmful to the child. Despite this, many of these treatments are still being used routinely in services around the world. Clinicians should keep up-to-date with the research literature and take on board the ethical responsibility of advising parents about the negative evidence of such treatments.

The research literature on parental adaptation reviewed above suggests that the needs of many families of children with autism might be addressed via direct stress management intervention from clinicians. Parents are clearly experiencing significant levels of stress and mental health problems and stress interventions could potentially alleviate their psychological distress. There is also a further reason why clinicians should consider direct stress management interventions with parents. Especially with respect to children's behaviour problems, there is evidence from prospective research designs with families of children with developmental disabilities that parental stress is predictive of changes in children's behaviour problems over time (Baker et al., 2003; Orsmond et al., 2003). Thus, children whose behaviour problems deteriorate over time tend to have parents who are experiencing higher levels of stress. The mechanism for this effect may well be that parents under stress respond differently to their child's behaviour problems and one important difference in behaviour may be that they are more likely to reinforce problem behaviour (Hastings, 2002).

Parental stress has also been identified as a variable that predicts lack of success or less significant change in the context of interventions for children with disabilities. For example, a number of researchers have shown that high parental stress predicts less beneficial outcomes for children in early intervention programmes (e.g., Brinker et al., 1994; Robbins et al., 1991). Furthermore, high parental stress predicts fewer gains in parenting skills in behavioural parenting training interventions (e.g., Baker et al., 1991).

Although the evidence base is small, there are some controlled studies that support the use of cognitive behavioural group interventions for parents of children with developmental disabilities including parents of children with autism (Gammon and Rose, 1991; Greaves, 1997; Nixon and Singer, 1993; Singer et al., 1988, 1989). We could find only two studies reporting the impact of a stress intervention specifically for parents of children with autism. Bitsika and Sharpley (2000) described outcomes of a stress management group intervention for parents of children with autism, and Bristol et al. (1993) reported the results of a psycho-educational intervention. Despite the lack of research relating to parents of children with autism specifically, the results of the more general literature on interventions for parents of children with developmental disabilities can probably be used to guide clinical practice.

262

In addition to working with parents, the literature on sibling adjustment suggests that at least a proportion of siblings might benefit from support from clinical services. A more detailed assessment of the family system, perhaps also including extended family members and their role in supporting the family, is probably needed in order to consider how best to provide treatment for families of children with autism (Harris, 1984). The difficulties faced by children with autism themselves are clearly very significant, but it is important to remember that the child's family also has to adapt to these difficulties. Thus, clinical services must be aware of the needs of family members.

References

Adamson, L. and McArthur, D. (1995). Joint attention, affect and culture. In C.P. Moore and P. Dunham (Eds.), *Joint attention: Its origins and role in development*. Hillsdale, NJ: Lawrence Erlbaum.

American Psychiatric Association (1994). *Diagnostic and statistical manual of mental disorders*, 4th edn. Washington, DC: APA.

Anderson, S.R., Avery, D.L., DiPietro, E.K., Edwards, G.L., and Christian, W.P. (1987). Intensive home based early intervention with autistic children. *Education and Treatment of Children*, *10*, 352–366.

Ayres, A.J. (1972). *Sensory integration and learning disorders*. Los Angeles, CA: Western Psychological Association.

Ayres, A.J. (1979). *Sensory integration and the child*. Los Angeles, CA: Western Psychological Association.

Ayres, A.J. and Mailloux, Z. (1981). Influence of sensory integration procedures on language development. *American Journal of Occupational Therapy*, *35*, 383–390.

Bågenholm, A. and Gillberg, C. (1991). Psychosocial effects on siblings of children with autism and mental retardation: A population-based study. *Journal of Mental Deficiency Research*, *35*, 291–307.

Bailey, A., Le Couteur, A., Gottesman, I., Bolton, P., Simonoff, E., Yuzda, E., et al. (1995). Autism as a strongly genetic disorder: Evidence from a British twin study. *Psychological Medicine*, *25*, 63–78.

Bailey, A., Phillips, W., and Rutter, M. (1996). Autism: Towards an integration of clinical, genetic, neuropsychological, and neurobiological perspectives. *Journal of Child Psychology and Psychiatry*, *37*, 89–126.

Baker, B.L., Landen, S.J., and Kashima, K.J. (1991). Effects of parent training on families of children with mental retardation: Increased burden or generalized benefit? *American Journal on Mental Retardation*, *96*, 127–136.

Baker, B.L., McIntyre, L.L., Blacher, J., Crnic, K., Edelbrock, C., and Low, C. (2003). Preschool children with and without developmental delay: Behaviour problems and parenting stress over time. *Journal of Intellectual Disability Research*, *47*, 217–230.

Baron-Cohen, S. (1987). Autism and symbolic play. *British Journal of Developmental Psychology*, *5*, 139–148.

Baron-Cohen, S. (1991). Do people with autism understand what causes emotion? *Child Development*, *62*, 385–395.

Baron-Cohen, S. (1994). Development of a theory of mind: Where would we be without the intentional stance? In M. Rutter and D. Hay (Eds.), *Development through life: A handbook for clinicians*. Oxford: Blackwell Scientific.

Baron-Cohen, S. (1995). *Mindblindness: An essay on autism and theory of mind.* Cambridge, MA: Bradford, MIT Press.

Baron-Cohen, S. and Swettenham, J. (1997). Theory of mind in autism: Its relationship to executive functions and central coherence. In D.J. Cohen and F.R. Volkmar (Eds.), *Handbook of autism and pervasive developmental disorders.* New York: Wiley.

Baron-Cohen, S., Leslie, A.M., and Frith, U. (1985). Does the autistic child have a "Theory of mind"? *Cognition, 21,* 37–46.

Baron-Cohen, S., Ring, H., Moriarty, J., Schmitz, B., Costa, D., and Ell, P. (1994). Recognition of mental state terms: Clinical findings in children with autism and a functional neuroimaging study of normal adults. *British Journal of Psychiatry, 165,* 640–649.

Bebko, J.M., Konstantareas, M.M., and Springer, J. (1987). Parent and professional evaluations of family stress associated with characteristics of autism. *Journal of Autism and Developmental Disorders, 17,* 565–576.

Biklen, D. (1993). *Communication unbound: How facilitated communication is challenging traditional views of ability/disability.* New York: Teacher's College.

Birnbrauer, J.S. and Leach, D.J. (1993). The Murdoch Early Intervention Program after 2 years. *Behaviour Change, 10,* 63–74.

Bitsika, V. and Sharpley, C. (2000). Development and testing of the effects of support groups on the well-being of parents of children with autism, II: Specific stress management techniques. *Journal of Applied Health Behaviour, 2,* 8–15.

Bouma, R. and Schweitzer, R. (1990). The impact of chronic childhood illness on family stress: A comparison between autism and cystic fibrosis. *Journal of Clinical Psychology, 46,* 722–730.

Brinker, R.P., Seifer, R., and Sameroff, A.J. (1994). Relations among maternal stress, cognitive development, and early intervention in middle- and low-SES infants with developmental disabilities. *American Journal on Mental Retardation, 98,* 463–480.

Bristol, M.M., Gallagher, J.J., and Schopler, E. (1988). Mothers and fathers of young developmentally disabled and nondisabled boys: Adaptation and spousal support. *Developmental Psychology, 24,* 441–451.

Bristol, M.M., Gallagher, J.J., and Holt, K.D. (1993). Maternal depressive symptoms in autism: Response to psychoeducational intervention. *Rehabilitation Psychology, 38,* 3–10.

Bryson, S.E. (1997). Epidemiology of autism: Overview and issues outstanding. In D.J. Cohen and F.R. Volkmar (Eds.), *Handbook of autism and pervasive developmental disorders.* New York: Wiley.

Burack, J.A., Enns, J.T., Stauder, J.E.A., Mottron, L., and Randolph, B. (1997). In D.J. Cohen and F. R. Volkmar (Eds.), *Handbook of autism and pervasive developmental disorders.* New York: Wiley.

Crossley, R. (1992). Getting the words out: Case studies on facilitated communication training. *Topics in Language Disorders, 12,* 46–59.

DeMeyer, M.K., Barton, S., DeMeyer, W.E., Norton, J.A., Allen, J., and Steele, R. (1973). Prognosis in autism: A follow-up study. *Journal of Autism and Childhood Schizophrenia, 3,* 199–246.

Dumas, J.E., Wolf, L.C., Fisman, S.N., and Culligan, A. (1991). Parenting stress, child behavior problems, and dysphoria in parents of children with autism, Down syndrome, behavior disorders, and normal development. *Exceptionality, 2,* 97–110.

Dykens, E.M. and Volkmar, F.R. (1997). Medical conditions associated with autism. In D.J. Cohen and F.R. Volkmar (Eds.), *Handbook of autism and pervasive developmental disorders.* New York: Wiley.

Eikeseth, S., Smith, T., Jahr, E., and Eldevik, S. (2002). Intensive behavioral treatment at school for 4- to 7-year-old children with autism: A 1-year comparison controlled study. *Behavior Modification, 26,* 49–68.

Factor, D.C., Perry, A., and Freeman, N. (1990). Stress, social support, and respite care use in families with autistic children. *Journal of Autism and Developmental Disorders, 20,* 139–146.

Fenske, E.C., Zalenski, S., Krantz, P.J., and McClannahan, L.E. (1985). Age at intervention and treatment outcome for autistic children in a comprehensive intervention program. *Analysis and Intervention in Developmental Disabilities, 5,* 49–58.

Fisman, S., Wolf, L., Ellison, D., Gillis, B., Freeman, T., and Szatmari, P. (1996). Risk and protective factors affecting the adjustment of siblings of children with chronic disabilities. *Journal of the American Academy of Child and Adolescent Psychiatry, 35,* 1532–1541.

Fisman, S., Wolf, L., Ellison, D., and Freeman, T. (2000). A longitudinal study of siblings of children with chronic disabilities. *Canadian Journal of Psychiatry, 45,* 369–375.

Folstein, S. and Rutter, M. (1978). A twin study of individuals with infantile autism. In M. Rutter and E. Schopler (Eds.), *Autism: A reappraisal of concepts and treatment.* New York: Plenum.

Fombonne, E. (2003). Epidemiological surveys of autism and other pervasive developmental disorders: An update. *Journal of Autism and Developmental Disorders, 33,* 365–382.

Fombonne, E., Bolton, P., Prior, J., Jordan, H., and Rutter, M. (1997). A family study of autism: Cognitive patterns and levels in parents and siblings. *Journal of Child Psychology and Psychiatry, 38,* 667–683.

Gammon, E.A. and Rose, S.D. (1991). The Coping Skills Training Program for parents of children with developmental disabilities: An experimental evaluation. *Research on Social Work Practice, 1,* 244–256.

Gillberg, C., Johansson, M., Steffenburg, S., and Berlin, O. (1997). Auditory integration training in children with autism. *Autism, 1,* 97–100.

Gold, N. (1993). Depression and social adjustment in siblings of boys with autism. *Journal of Autism and Developmental Disorders, 23,* 147–163.

Gray, D.E. and Holden, W.J. (1992). Psycho-social well-being among parents of children with autism. *Australia and New Zealand Journal of Developmental Disabilities, 18,* 83–93.

Greaves, D. (1997). The effect of rational-emotive parent education on the stress of mothers of young children with Down syndrome. *Journal of Rational-Emotive and Cognitive-Behavior Therapy, 15,* 249–267.

Green, G. (1996). Early intervention for autism: What does research tell us? In C. Maurice, G. Green, and S.C. Luce (Eds.), *Behavioral intervention for young children with autism: A manual for parents and professionals.* Austin, TX: Pro-Ed.

Gresham, F.M. and MacMillan, D.L. (1997). Autistic recovery? An analysis and critique of the empirical evidence on the early intervention project. *Behavioral Disorders, 22,* 185–201.

Hadwin, J., Baron-Cohen, S., Howlin, P., and Hill, K. (1997). Does teaching theory of mind have an effect on the ability to develop conversation in children with autism? *Journal of Autism and Developmental Disorders, 27,* 519–537.

Happé, F.G.E. (1994). Wechsler IQ profile and theory of mind in autism: A research note. *Journal of Child Psychology and Psychiatry, 37,* 873–878.

Happé, F.G.E. (1996). Studying weak central coherence at low levels: Children with autism do not succumb to visual illusions. *Journal of Child Psychology and Psychiatry*, *37*, 873–878.

Harris, S.L. (1984). The family of the autistic child: A behavioral-systems view. *Clinical Psychology Review*, *4*, 227–239.

Hastings, R.P. (2002). Parental stress and behaviour problems of children with developmental disability. *Journal of Intellectual and Developmental Disability*, *27*, 149–160.

Hastings, R.P. (2003a). Behavioural adjustment of siblings of children with autism. *Journal of Autism and Developmental Disorders*, *33*, 99–104.

Hastings, R.P. (2003b). Child behaviour problems and partner mental health as correlates of stress in mothers and fathers of children with autism. *Journal of Intellectual Disability Research*, *47*, 231–237.

Hastings, R.P. and Brown, T. (2002). Behavior problems of autistic children, parental self-efficacy and mental health. *American Journal on Mental Retardation*, *107*, 222–232.

Hastings, R.P. and Johnson, E. (2001). Stress in UK families conducting intensive home-based behavioral intervention for their young child with autism. *Journal of Autism and Developmental Disorders*, *31*, 327–336.

Hastings, R.P. and Mount, R.H. (2001). Early correlates of behavioural and emotional problems in children and adolescents with severe learning disabilities. *Journal of Applied Research in Intellectual Disabilities*, *14*, 381–391.

Hastings, R.P. and Taunt, H.M. (2002). Positive perceptions in families of children with developmental disabilities. *American Journal on Mental Retardation*, *107*, 116–127.

Hoehn, T.P. and Baumeister, A.A. (1994). A critique of the application of sensory integration therapy to children with learning disabilities. *Journal of Learning Disabilities*, *27*, 338–350.

Hughes, C., Plumet, M.H., and Leboyer, M. (1999). Towards a cognitive phenotype for autism: Increased prevalence of executive dysfunction and superior spatial span amongst siblings of children with autism. *Journal of Child Psychology and Psychiatry*, *40*, 705–718.

Jacobson, J.W., Mulick, J.A., and Schwartz, A.A. (1995). A history of facilitated communication: Science, pseudoscience, and antiscience. *American Psychologist*, *50*, 750–765.

Jolliffe, T. and Baron-Cohen, S. (1997). Are people with autism and Asperger syndrome faster than normal on the Embedded Figures Test? *Journal of Child Psychology and Psychiatry*, *38*, 527–534.

Journal of Applied Behavior Analysis (1968–). Lawrence, KS: Society for the Experimental Analysis of Behavior. Online. Available http://www.envmed.rochester. edu/wwwrap/behavior/jaba/jabahome.htm (accessed 26 Jan. 2004).

Kasari, C. and Sigman, M. (1997). Linking parental perceptions to interactions in young children with autism. *Journal of Autism and Developmental Disorders*, *27*, 39–57.

Kaufman, B.N. (1995). *Son-Rise: The miracle continues*. New York: Kramer.

Klinger, L.G. and Dawson, G. (1996). Autistic disorder. In E.J. Mash and R.A. Barkley (Eds.), *Child psychopathology*. New York: Guilford.

Knivsberg, A.M., Wiig, A., Lind, G., Nodland, M., and Reichelt, K. L (1990). Dietary intervention in autistic syndromes. *Brain Dysfunction*, *3*, 315–327.

Koegel, R.L., Schreibman, L., Loos, L.M., Dirlich-Wilheim, H., Dunlap, G., Robbins, F.R., et al. (1992). Consistent stress profiles in mothers of children with autism. *Journal of Autism and Developmental Disorders*, *22*, 205–216.

Konstantareas, M.M., Homatidis, S., and Plowright, C.M.S. (1992). Assessing resources and stress in parents of severely dysfunctional children through the Clarke modification of Holroyd's Questionnaire on Resources and Stress. *Journal of Autism and Developmental Disorders*, 22, 217–234.

Link, H.M. (1997). Auditory Integration Training (AIT): Sound therapy? Case studies of three boys with autism who received AIT. *British Journal of Learning Disabilities*, 25, 106–110.

Lord, C. and Schopler, E. (1994). TEACCH services for preschool children. In S. Harris and J. Handleman (Eds.), *Preschool programs for children with autism*. Austin, TX: Pro-Ed.

Lovaas, O.I. (1987). Behavioural treatment and normal educational and intellectual functioning in young autistic children. *Journal of Consulting and Clinical Psychology*, 55, 3–9.

Lovaas, O.I. (1993). The development of a treatment-research project for developmentally disabled and autistic children. *Journal of Applied Behavior Analysis*, 26, 617–630.

Lovaas, O.I. and Smith, T. (1989). A comprehensive behavioral theory of autistic children: Paradigm for research and treatment. *Journal of Behavior Therapy and Experimental Psychiatry*, 20, 17–29.

McEachin, J.J., Smith, T., and Lovaas, O.I. (1993). Long-term outcome for children with autism who received early intensive behavioural treatment. *American Journal on Mental Retardation*, 97, 359–372.

McEvoy, R.E., Rogers, S.J., and Pennington, B.F. (1993). Executive functions and social communication deficits in young autistic children. *Journal of Child Psychology and Psychiatry*, 34, 563–578.

McGee, G.G., Morrier, M.J., and Daly, T. (1999). An incidental teaching approach to early intervention for toddlers with autism. *Journal of the Association for Persons with Severe Handicaps*, 24, 133–146.

McHale, S.M., Sloan, J., and Simeonsson, R.J. (1986). Sibling relationships of children with autistic, mentally retarded, and nonhandicapped brothers and sisters. *Journal of Autism and Developmental Disorders*, 16, 399–413.

Mates, T.E. (1990). Siblings of autistic children: Their adjustment and performance at home and in school. *Journal of Autism and Developmental Disorders*, 20, 545–553.

Moes, D., Koegel, R.L., Schreibman, L., and Loos, L.M. (1992). Stress profiles for mothers and fathers of children with autism. *Psychological Reports*, 71, 1272–1274.

Mudford, O.C., Cross, B.A., Breen, S., Cullen, C., Reeves, D., Gould, J., et al. (2000). Auditory integration training for children with autism: No behavioral benefits detected. *American Journal on Mental Retardation*, 105, 118–129.

Mundy, P. (1995). Joint attention and social-emotional approach behavior in children with autism. *Development and Psychopathology*, 7, 63–82.

Mundy, P. and Crowson, M. (1997). Joint attention and early social communication: Implications for research on intervention with autism. *Journal of Autism and Developmental Disorders*, 27, 653–676.

Mundy, P. and Gomes, A. (1998). Individual differences in joint attention skill development in the second year. *Infant Behavior and Development*, 21, 469–482.

Mundy, P. and Neal, R. (2001). Neural plasticity, joint attention and autistic developmental pathology. In L.M. Glidden (Ed.), *International Review of Research in Mental Retardation*, 23. New York: Academic Press.

Mundy, P., Kasari, C., and Sigman, M. (1990). A longitudinal study of joint attention and language development in autistic children. *Journal of Autism and Developmental Disorders*, *20*, 115–128.

Mundy, P., Hogan, A., and Doehring, P. (1996). *A preliminary manual for the Abridged Early Social Communication Scales (ESCS)*. Online. Available http:/www.psy.miami. edu/child.pmundy (accessed 26 Jan. 2004).

Newsom, C. (1998). Autistic disorder. In E.J. Mash and R.A. Barkley (Eds.), *Treatment of childhood disorders*. New York: Guilford.

New York State Department of Health (1999). *Report of the Recommendations: Autism/ Pervasive Developmental Disorders*. Publication no. 4215. New York: State Department of Health.

Nixon, C.D. and Singer, G.H.S. (1993). Group cognitive-behavioral treatment for excessive parental self-blame and guilt. *American Journal on Mental Retardation*, *97*, 665–672.

Orsmond, G.I., Seltzer, M.M., Krauss, M.W., and Hong, J. (2003). Behavior problems in adults with mental retardation and maternal well-being: Examination of the direction of effects. *American Journal on Mental Retardation*, *108*, 257–271.

Osterling, J. and Dawson, G. (1994). Early recognition of children with autism: A study of first birthday home videotapes. *Journal of Autism and Developmental Disorders*, *24*, 247–257.

Ozonoff, S. (1997). Casual mechanisms of autism: Unifying perspectives from an information-processing framework. In D.J. Cohen and F.R. Volkmar (Eds.), *Handbook of autism and pervasive developmental disorders*. New York: Wiley.

Panerai, S., Ferrante, L., and Caputo, V. (1997). The TEACCH strategy in mentally retarded children with autism. A multidimensional assessment: Pilot study. *Journal of Autism and Developmental Disorders*, *27*, 345–347.

Piven, J. and Palmer, P. (1997). Cognitive deficits in parents from multiple-incidence autism families. *Journal of Child Psychology and Psychiatry*, *38*, 1011–1022.

Rapin, I. (1997). Current concepts: Autism. *New England Journal of Medicine*, *337*, 97–104.

Reichelt, K.L., Ekrem, J., and Scott, H. (1990). Gluten, milk proteins and autism: Dietary intervention effects on behaviour and peptide secretion. *Journal of Applied Nutrition*, *42*, 1–9.

Reichelt, W.H., Knivsberg, A.M., Nodland, M., Stensrud, M., and Reichelt, K.L. (1997). Urinary peptide levels and patterns in autistic children from seven countries, and the effect of dietary intervention after 4 years, *Developmental Brain Dysfunction*, *10*, 44–55.

Rimland, B. and Edelson, S.M. (1995). Auditory integration training in autism: A pilot study. *Journal of Autism and Developmental Disorders*, *25*, 61–70.

Robbins, F.R., Dunlap, G., and Plienis, A.J. (1991). Family characteristics, family training, and the progress of young children with autism. *Journal of Early Intervention*, *15*, 173–184.

Rodrigue, J.R., Morgan, S.B., and Geffken, G. (1990). Families of autistic children: Psychological functioning of mothers. *Journal of Clinical Child Psychology*, *19*, 371–379.

Rodrigue, J.R., Morgan, S.B., and Geffken, G.R. (1992). Psychosocial adaptation of fathers of children with autism, Down syndrome, and normal development. *Journal of Autism and Developmental Disorders*, *22*, 249–263.

Rodrigue, J.R., Geffken, G.R., and Morgan, S.B. (1993). Perceived competence and behavioral adjustment of siblings of children with autism. *Journal of Autism and Developmental Disorders, 23,* 665–674.

Roeyers, H. and Mycke, K. (1995). Siblings of children with autism, with mental retardation and with a normal development. *Child: Care, Health and Development, 21,* 305–319.

Rossiter, L. and Sharpe, D. (2001). The siblings of individuals with mental retardation: A quantitative integration of the literature. *Journal of Child and Family Studies, 10,* 65–84.

Rutter, M. (1970). Autistic children: Infancy to adulthood. *Seminars in Pychiatry, 2,* 435–450.

Rutter, M., Bailey, A., Bolton, P., and Le Couteur, A. (1993). Autism: Syndrome definition and possible genetic mechanisms. In R. Plomin and G.E. McClearn (Eds.), *Nature, nuture and psychology.* Washington, DC: American Psychological Association.

Rutter, M., Bailey, A., Simonoff, E., and Pickles, A. (1997). Genetic influences and autism. In D.J. Cohen and F.R. Volkmar (Eds.), *Handbook of autism and pervasive developmental disorders.* New York: Wiley.

Sabin, L.A. and Donnellan, A.M. (1993). A qualitative study of the process of Facilitated Communication. *Journal of the Association for the Severely Handicapped, 18,* 200–211.

Sanders, J.L. and Morgan, S.B. (1997). Family stress and adjustment as perceived by parents of children with autism or Down syndrome: Implications for intervention. *Child and Family Behavior Therapy, 19,* 15–32.

Schopler, E., Mesibov, G., and Baker, A. (1982). Evaluation of treatment for autistic children and their parents. *Journal of the American Academy of Child Psychiatry, 21,* 262–267.

Scott, F.J. & Baron-Cohen, S. (1996a). Imagining real and unreal things: Evidence of a dissociation in autism. *Journal of Cognitive Neuroscience, 8,* 371–382.

Scott, F.J., Baron-Cohen, S., and Leslie, A. (1999). "If pigs could fly": A test of counterfactual reasoning and pretence in children with autism. *British Journal of Developmental Psychology, 17,* 349–362.

Shah, A. and Frith, U. (1993). Why do autistic individuals show superior performance on the block design task? *Journal of Child Psychology and Psychiatry, 34,* 1351–1364.

Shattock, P. and Lowdon, G. (1991). Proteins, peptides and autism. Part 2: Implications for the education and care of people with autism. *Brain Dysfunction, 4,* 323–334.

Short, A.B. (1984). Short-term treatment outcome using parents as co-therapists for their own autistic children. *Journal of Child Psychology and Psychiatry and Allied Disciplines, 25,* 443–458.

Sigman, M. (1998). Change and continuity in the development of children with autism. *Journal of Child Psychology and Psychiatry, 39,* 817–828.

Simonoff, E., Bolton, P., and Rutter, M. (1996). Mental retardation: Genetic findings, clinical implications and research agenda. *Journal of Child Psychology and Psychiatry, 37,* 259–280.

Singer, G.H.S., Irvin, L.K., and Hawkins, N. (1988). Stress management training for parents of children with severe handicaps. *Mental Retardation, 26,* 269–277.

Singer, G.H.S., Irvin, L.K., Irvine, B., Hawkins, N., and Cooley, E. (1989). Evaluation of community-based support services for families of persons with developmental disabilities. *Journal of the Association for Persons with Severe Handicaps, 14,* 312–323.

Smith, M.D. and Belcher, R.G. (1994). Facilitated communication and autism: Separating fact from fiction. *Journal of Vocational Rehabilitation, 4,* 66–74.

Stehli, A. (1991). *The sound of a miracle: A child's triumph over autism*. New York: Doubleday.

Tager-Flüsberg, H. (1993). What language reveals about the understanding of minds in children with autism. In S. Baron-Cohen, H. Tager-Flüsberg, and D.J. Cohen (Eds.), *Understanding other minds*. New York: Oxford University Press.

The Option Institute and Fellowship (1997). *The Option Institute: The worldwide teaching centre for the option process*. 1998 programs catalogue. Sheffield, MA: Option Institute and Fellowship.

Tsai, L.Y. and Ghaziuddin, M. (1991). Autistic disorder. In J.M. Wiener (Ed.), *Textbook of child and adolescent psychiatry*. Washington, DC: American Psychiatric Press.

US Department of Health and Human Services (1999). Children and mental health. In *Mental health: A report of the surgeon general*. Online. Available http://www.surgeongeneral.gov/library/mentalhealth/toc.html#chapter3 (accessed 2 Dec. 2003).

Venter, A., Lord, C., and Schopler, E. (1992). A follow-up study of high-functioning autistic children. *Journal of Child Psychology and Psychiatry and Allied Disciplines*, *33*, 489–507.

Volkmar, F.R., Klin, A., and Cohen, D.J. (1997). Diagnosis and classification of autism and related conditions: Consensus and issues. In D.J. Cohen and F.R. Volkmar (Eds.), *Handbook of autism and pervasive developmental disorders*. New York: Wiley.

Wolf, L.C., Noh, S., Fisman, S.N., and Speechley, M. (1989). Psychological effects of parenting stress on parents of autistic children. *Journal of Autism and Developmental Disorders*, *19*, 157–166.

World Health Organization (1992). *International classification of diseases: Tenth revision*. Chapter V. Mental and behavioural disorders: Diagnostic criteria for research. Geneva: WHO.

11

LEARNING DISORDERS

Maureen Samms-Vaughan

Children and adolescents may fail to learn and/or perform at school because of intrinsic or external causes. Intrinsic causes imply some impairment to the learning pathways of the central nervous system. External causes impairing school performance include a wide range of factors, such as family dysfunction (e.g. divorce, domestic violence, poor parent–child interaction); sensory (visual or auditory) impairment or disability; acute or chronic physical illnesses; nutritional deficiencies, behavioral or emotional disorders; socio-economic disadvantage and environmental and cultural differences.

The term *learning disorder* has been used broadly to refer to all factors affecting school performance, but has also been used in a very narrow sense to include only those learning difficulties attributable to central nervous system dysfunction. The term *learning disability* has been used interchangeably with learning disorders in its broadest sense and has sometimes included mental retardation (Gillberg and Soderstrom, 2003). Conversely, the term learning disability has been used to refer specifically to the intrinsic learning disorders. The lack of consensus as to the use of the terms *learning disorder* and *learning disability* is well demonstrated by the terms and definitions used by the legal, educational and professional bodies in the United States.

The Individuals with Disabilities Education Act of 1999 (IDEA) in the United States, which is used to identify children in need of special education services, defines a *learning disability* as

> a disorder in one or more of the basic psychological processes involved
> in understanding or in using language, spoken or written, that may
> manifest itself in an imperfect ability to listen, think, speak, read, write,
> spell or to do mathematical calculations, including conditions such
> as perceptual disabilities, brain injury, minimal brain dysfunction,
> dyslexia and developmental aphasia.

This definition excludes children whose learning difficulties are primarily due to visual, hearing or motor disabilities; mental retardation; emotional difficulties and environmental, cultural or economic disadvantage. The identification of learning disabled children in the IDEA also requires that having been provided with appropriate learning experiences, the child's performance is below age and ability levels and there is a severe discrepancy between achievement and intellectual ability.

The DSM-IV (American Psychiatric Association, 1994) uses the term *learning disorder* in its restricted sense, and states that this condition is diagnosed when an individual's achievement on standardized tests in reading, mathematics or written expression is substantially below that expected for age, schooling and level of intelligence. The learning disorder must also significantly impair academic achievement or activities of daily living.

The IDEA definition of a *learning disability* and the DSM-IV definition of a *learning disorder* are clearly defining the same entity using different terms. There are, however, some minor differences in the definitions. The DSM-IV is more specific in its description of the discrepancy between achievement and level of intelligence. While acknowledging that a variety of statistical approaches can be used to determine what "substantially below" means, the DSM-IV suggests clearly that more than two standard deviations between IQ and achievement is an acceptable difference. Additionally, this definition takes some account of individual differences in intellectual ability as determined by intelligence tests. As a result, a discrepancy of between one and two standard deviations is acceptable, where the intelligence of a child may have been compromised by associated cognitive processing deficits, mental disorder, medical disorder or the child's ethnic or cultural background.

The requirement of a two standard deviation ability-achievement difference has been challenged. Lyon and colleagues (2001) have recommended that academic under-achievement, the common presenting characteristic, be the main factor used to identify learning disability, that external factors should not be used to exclude children from a diagnosis of learning disability and that the student's response to intervention should be considered in the identification process. Lyon's recommendations would lead to a greater proportion of under-achieving children being diagnosed with learning disabilities or disorders. However, Shaywitz has suggested that there is some merit in the ability-achievement definition, particularly for children of high ability, whose learning disability would be undiagnosed by comparing their performance with age-appropriate standards (Shaywitz, 1998). These newer concepts have not yet been universally accepted by educators and policy makers and have not been reflected in the recognized reference texts, such as the DSM-IV.

The use of the terms learning disorder and learning disability and their respective definitions remain controversial at this time. In this chapter, the term learning disorder is used in the restricted sense and includes those learning difficulties attributable to intrinsic central nervous system dysfunction, where there is a significant discrepancy between ability or potential and school achievement or performance.

Classification

There are four main types of learning disorders: reading disorder, mathematics disorder, disorder of written expression and non-verbal learning disorder. Reading disorder, the commonest of the learning disorders, was the first to be identified and consequently, has been the most studied. While reading disorder was earlier thought to account for approximately 80 per cent of all learning disorders (Aaron, 1997), more recent reports suggest that the prevalence of the other disorders may be considerably higher than previously thought, with reading disorder accounting for approximately 50 per cent of all learning disorders (Kronenberger and Dunn, 2003).

Epidemiology

The differences in definition and diagnostic criteria have led to wide variation in the reported prevalence of learning disorders. Prevalence rates of 5–15 percent for all learning disorders have been reported by early investigators (Silver, 1991). However, the prevalence rate for the commonest form of reading disorder, dyslexia, has been reported to be as high as 17.5 per cent (Shaywitz et al., 1994). The DSM-IV reports dyscalculia, the commonest of the mathematics disorders, to be a rare disorder with a prevalence of 1 per cent in the population (American Psychiatric Association, 1994). However, more recent prevalence studies have yielded rates of dyscalculia of between 3 and 6.5 per cent (Gross-Tsur et al., 1996; Lewis et al., 1994). Disorders of written expression are relatively common, reported to occur in 8–15 per cent of children at school age (Lyon, 1996). Non-verbal learning disorders are more rare, accounting for only 0.1 to 1 per cent of all learning disorders (Pennington, 1991)

An increase in prevalence over time has been particularly noticeable in the school system. In a period spanning less than 20 years, between 1977 and 1995, the number of children participating in special educational programmes in the United States increased by 47 per cent, with almost a half of children in these programmes diagnosed with learning disabilities (MacMillan et al., 1998; US Department of Education, 1997). The prevalence of learning disabilities in the United States is reported to have tripled since the 1960s, due to a combination of changes in assessment methods and criteria for eligibility for special educational services (Kidder-Ashley et al., 2000). Educational laws in the United States now mandate the use of more accurate and more sensitive diagnostic measures and require mandatory reporting. While improved diagnosis and reporting is largely thought to be responsible for the increase in identified cases, some have also considered the possibility of a true increase in prevalence due to environmental and other contextual risk factors (Margai and Henry, 2003).

Early studies of learning disorders, particularly dyslexia, suggested a male predominance (Finnuci and Childs, 1981). More recent studies report no gender differences (Shaywitz et al., 1990; Wadsworth et al., 1992). There are also no gender differences in dyscalculia or disorders of written expression (Gross-Tsur et al.,

1996; Lyon, 1996). Earlier gender differences may have reflected a greater likelihood for boys to be identified as having learning disorders.

Reading disorder

A reading disorder occurs when reading achievement, as measured by standardized tests of reading accuracy, fluency or speed and comprehension, is substantially below that expected for age, education and intelligence and interferes significantly with academic achievement or activities of daily living requiring reading. Reading disorder, also known as dyslexia, may be of two types – developmental dyslexia or acquired dyslexia. Developmental dyslexia refers to an innate and unexpected difficulty in reading, while acquired dyslexia refers to a loss of previously acquired reading ability consequent on brain dysfunction as a result of trauma, infection or other causes. This chapter confines itself to developmental dyslexia.

Reading disorder is a spectrum disorder with children having varying degrees of impairment along a normal distribution. Children with poor reading ability are at one end of the normal distribution curve. Reading, the process of converting printed symbols to their appropriate meaning, involves two main processes: decoding or word recognition and comprehension. Decoding occurs before comprehension, with children typically able to read words before fully understanding their meaning. Decoding involves a number of processes: phonologic awareness, orthographic awareness, semantic and pragmatic awareness. Phonologic awareness refers to the ability to recognize that words can be broken down into smaller units, such as syllables and phonemes. Phonemes, of which there are approximately forty in the English language, are the smallest discernible units of speech. Orthographic awareness is the ability to recognize how words look and discern unlikely letter combinations. For example, a series of letters without an intervening vowel is unlikely to be a true word. While phonemic and orthographic awareness can be considered the building blocks necessary for the development of early reading skills, semantic and pragmatic awareness, which refer to grammatical rules and structure and the abstract use of words, are skills required at a more advanced stage of reading. Comprehension requires higher order functioning such as general intelligence and reasoning.

A deficit in phonologic awareness has been identified as the core abnormality in reading disorder. Children who have a reading disorder are unable to segment the words they see into syllables and phonemes. Because words are either not recognized or take great effort and time to be recognized, their meaning is not able to be appreciated. Phonologic deficits do not affect higher-order reading processes, so children with reading disorder, who are of normal intelligence and reasoning, quickly grasp meaning and comprehend expressed concepts when words are read to them.

The phonologic deficit theory explains the common clinical presentation of an ability-achievement discrepancy in children with reading disorders. Additionally, phonologic awareness predicts later reading achievement; phonologic deficits readily identify children with reading disorder from those without and specific instruction in phonologic awareness improves reading ability (Shaywitz, 1998). Probably, the most definitive support for the phonologic deficit theory is the recent evidence of a change in brain functioning by functional magnetic resonance imaging techniques (fMRI) when poor readers were exposed to an intensive reading programme based on phonemic awareness (Shaywitz et al., 2004). At the end of the one-year period of intervention, there was an increase in activation in the left hemisphere inferior frontal gyrus and middle temporal gyrus, areas known to have deficient functioning in children with reading disorders. Further, the effects persisted a year after the intervention ended, with children showing further activation in inferior frontal gyri bilaterally and in the left superior temporal and occipital brain regions. The patterns of activation were matched by an increase in reading accuracy, fluency and comprehension.

Reading disorders are diagnosed most frequently at school age, when children are exposed to the art of reading and expected to attain reading skills. Additionally, the testing processes and materials used to identify an ability–achievement discrepancy are more accurate for children at school age. In the pre-school years, children with reading disorder may have difficulty naming letters and associating sounds with letters. This would precede the reading and spelling difficulties typically identified in the school years.

Mathematics disorder

Mathematics disorder occurs when mathematical ability, as measured by calculation or reasoning, is substantially below that expected for an individual's age, intelligence and education and significantly interferes with academic achievement or activities of daily living requiring mathematics (APA, 1994). There are a number of similarities between reading disorder and mathematics disorder. Mathematics disorder is believed to be on a continuum, with children with poor mathematical ability at one end of the normal distribution. There are two main types of mathematics disorder, developmental dyscalculia and acquired dyscalculia. This chapter confines itself to developmental dyscalculia. There are, however, notable differences between the learning of reading and the learning of mathematics. While reading must be taught, there is an innate ability to acquire mathematical skills, such as counting, adding and comparing size and quantity, existing from as early as infancy (Ginsburg, 1997; Wynn, 1992, 1998). Children of 3 to 4 years count to 4 and by 5 years count to 15 or 20. Higher order mathematical function, such as the interpretation of mathematical symbols and the ability to perform addition, subtraction, multiplication and division are usually learnt at school.

The neuro-anatomic and physiological theories for the learning of mathematics and the development of mathematics disorder have not been as well studied as those for reading disorder, but important information has emerged throughout the last few decades, with the latest theories receiving support from neuro-imaging studies. Shalev and Gross-Tsur traced the development of the theories, showing that each step built on the foundation of the previous theories (Shalev and Gross-Tsur,

275

2000). The early scientists of the 1920s correctly suggested then that difficulties in mathematics were due to a specific cognitive defect (Henschen, 1925), but were unable to identify the cognitive functions necessary for learning or those specifically affected in mathematics disorder. By the 1980s, McCloskey identified three possible mathematical cognitive function skills: comprehension of number concept, production of numbers and calculation (McCloskey et al., 1985). Rourke then suggested that dyscalculia was secondary to visuo-spatial or verbal or auditory-perceptual dysfunction (Rourke, 1993). Dehaene and Cohen in 1995 proposed that the understanding of mathematics had three components: verbal, visual and magnitude representation (Dehaene and Cohen, 1995). Simple arithmetic operations were processed by the verbal system in the left hemisphere, while more complex procedures, such as those requiring visual representation and those of magnitude estimation, were processed bilaterally.

Functional magnetic resonance imaging (fMRI) in normal individuals support Dehaene and Cohen's theory. When performing language-dependent mathematical processes, normal individuals activate the left frontal lobe, but when performing complex calculations, both parietal lobes become activated. Dehaene and Cohen further proposed that two neural circuits are necessary for the understanding of mathematics: lingusitic and visuo-spatial (Dehaene et al., 1999). Linguistic skills are necessary for naming mathematical terms and decoding written problems; perceptual skills allow the understanding of numerical symbols and signs and facilitate their manipulation.

Children with mathematics disorder have difficulty with counting and grasping numerical concepts during pre-school. While doing so later than their peers, they eventually grasp counting, recognize and write numerals and compare numbers by the age of 10 years, successfully completing the verbal tasks. However, they are unable to handle the more complex tasks. They are unable to retrieve learned information rapidly and have difficulty solving mathematical problems. Their errors include failure to link the appropriate operation to the sign (e.g. adding when a subtraction sign is present), putting digits in the wrong place and failing to manipulate numbers across value lines (e.g. hundreds, tens and units).

Similar to reading disorder, children with mathematics disorder are not usually identified until the early primary grades, when mathematical concepts are expected to be learnt.

Disorder of written expression

A disorder of written expression occurs when writing skills fall substantially below that expected for an individual's age, intelligence and education experience. The difficulty in written expression should also significantly interfere with academic achievement or with activities of daily living that require writing skills (APA, 1994). Unlike reading disorder, the underlying deficit for disorders of written expression has not yet been identified. However, the characteristics of children with disorders of written expression have been determined.

Writing is the conversion of thoughts and/or auditory information to an under-standable visual form. In the earliest stages of learning to write, children are required to produce visual representations of the building blocks of words (e.g. the English alphabet, Japanese characters). This requires memory, fine-motor coordination, visual-spatial and visual-motor integration skills. In the later stages, children are required to produce words, sentences and paragraphs that express their ideas, feelings and/or knowledge in an organized, accurate and efficient manner. These later writing skills require the development of ideas, the correct use of grammar, spelling and punctuation and organizational skills as well as the efficient fine motor, visual-motor and visual-spatial co-ordination skills mentioned earlier.

Children with a disorder of written expression may manifest their difficulty in a variety of ways. Some may be unable to plan, generate or organize their thoughts for the writing process. These children will produce simple and brief written work after a prolonged period of time, but will be able to express their thoughts extremely well verbally. Other children will produce written work, that is difficult for others to understand, as multiple spelling errors will be made and the rules of punctuation and grammar will not be followed. Children with handwriting difficulties or dysgraphia will produce written work that only they can decipher. Typically, a child with a disorder of written expression will have a combination of difficulties. The diagnosis is not usually made when there are only spelling errors, when a reading disorder may be more likely, or when there is only dysgraphia. Dysgraphia as a single entity is more likely due to an underlying motor co-ordination impairment.

Unlike reading and mathematics skills, copying of written work, dictation, spontaneous and expressive writing skills are not usually required until grade three level, at 8 to 9 years of age. Disorders of written expression are therefore not often detected prior to this stage.

Non-verbal learning disorder

Non-verbal learning disorder (NVLD) describes a specific pattern of cognitive strengths and weaknesses. There are strengths in memory, rote learning, factual knowledge and basic verbal skills. The core deficits in NVLD are visual perceptual organization, motor skills, novel and non-verbal problem solving and integration and organization of information (Rourke, 1995). Additional deficits include psycho-motor coordination, tactile perception, visual memory, reading comprehension, concept formation, and social relations. The deficits not only result in academic achievement falling below that expected for age, intelligence and educational experience, but manifest in deficient social skills.

NVLD typically presents first with mathematical underachievement. In the early years, when mathematical aptitude is dependent on rote learning and mathematical facts, children with NVLD are able to function well. At about grade three or four, equivalent to ages 8 or 9 years, when the learning of mathematics requires an understanding of concepts and non-verbal problem solving skills, the deficits of children with NVLD become apparent. NVLD may also manifest at these higher grade levels as difficulties with reading comprehension or a slow writing speed. Written expression deficits reflect difficulty producing and organizing novel information and poor psycho-motor coordination (Kronenberger and Dunn, 2003). Children with NVLD are therefore likely to be misdiagnosed as having reading disorder, mathematics disorder or disorder of written expression. Additionally, as social skills require the learning and understanding of non-verbal cues, children with NVLD may display impairment in their social interactions and may be mis-diagnosed as having primary behavior difficulties.

There is some evidence to suggest that the deficit in NVLD may be due to deficiencies in white matter functioning in the brain (Rourke, 1995). Children who have neurologic disorders affecting white matter manifest many of the cognitive deficits that children with NVLD have.

Aetiology

The aetiology of learning disorders is multi-factorial. While the underlying problem is believed to be central nervous system dysfunction, both genetic and biological factors have been implicated as contributors.

Genetic

The genetic basis of learning disorders has been suggested for decades by the recognition that learning disorders were more common in children with a family history of learning difficulties. Accurate determinations since the mid 1990s identified 23 to 65 percent of children with a dyslexic parent and 40 percent of children with a dyslexic sibling to have this disorder (Pennington and Gilger, 1996; Scarborough, 1998). More recently, molecular genetics has implicated specific chromosomes for reading disorder. Both linkage analysis and association analysis have been performed and found useful. Linkage analysis detects genes that have large effects, while association analysis detects genes with much smaller effects. These analyses have identified loci for reading disability on chromosomes 6, 15 and 18 and more recently chromosomes 16 and 19 have been associated with language impairment (Grigorenko et al., 1997; Plomin and Walker, 2003). Though scientific evidence is available primarily for dyslexia, this suggests that genetic associations with other learning disorders may be discovered in the future.

Biological

A neurobiological basis for learning disorders was first suggested by changes in central nervous system morphology on examination of post-mortem brain specimens. Enlarged cerebral ventricles, reversed cerebral asymmetry and cortical anomalies, particularly in the tempero-parieto-occipital regions and particularly in the left hemisphere, were found in some persons with dyslexia (Denckla et al., 1985; Galaburda et al., 1985; Lyon, 1996; Rosenberger and Hier, 1980; Thatcher,

1996). Many CT and MRI studies later showed that persons with dyslexia had atypical cerebral symmetry, particularly in the posterior regions of the brain (Dalby et al., 1998; Leisman and Ashkenazi, 1980). However, some studies have failed to find abnormal asymmetry (Best and Demb, 1999; Rumsey et al., 1997). Differences in findings are believed to be due to differences in definition, variation in sample size and study methodology.

EEG studies identified electrophysiological differences, particularly in latency and amplitude, in the brains of learning disabled children when compared with their non learning disabled peers (Ackerman et al., 1994, 1998; Mattson et al., 1992). Unlike the morphological studies, the electrophysiological studies do not show differences confined to one hemisphere.

Functional brain imaging studies, such as regional cerebral blood flow, positron emission tomography (PET), and functional MRI support functional differences in persons with dyslexia. PET studies show reduced or absent activity in the left hemisphere, particularly in the angular gyrus area; fMRI studies show reduced or absent activity in the left temporal and frontal regions during language related tasks (Collins and Rourke, 2003).

Collins and Rourke (2003) reviewed the literature on the brain findings of persons with learning disability and concluded that dyslexic brains have subtle but important differences when compared with others and that the neuroanatomical evidence is suggestive of abnormal neurodevelopment (Collins and Rourke, 2003).

Emerging associations between prenatal and postnatal biological insults, minor neurological abnormalities and learning disorders support a neuro-biological basis for learning disorders. Children with severe growth retardation have a higher prevalence of learning difficulties (O'Keefe et al., 2003; Rooney et al., 2003). Communities with clusters of children with learning disabilities are also those with historically significant levels of lead toxicity and air pollution (Margai and Henry, 2003). Children with minor neurological abnormalities on physical examination have poorer academic and cognitive performance than their peers.

Experimental induction of prenatal and postnatal insults in laboratory animals also support a neuro-biological aetiology for learning disorders. Induction of hyperglycaemia in female rats, simulating diabetes mellitus in humans, led to gender-dependent deficits in learning and memory of offspring, suggesting that diabetes mellitus in pregnancy may be associated with learning and memory disorders in children (Kinney et al., 2003). Exposure of laboratory animals to common anaesthetic agents used in paediatric practice during the period of formation of synapses in the brain resulted in persistent learning deficits (Jevtovic-Todorovic et al., 2003).

Despite the advances being made in the aetiology of learning disorders, our current knowledge is limited by the small sample size in many of the studies. Additionally, for the majority of children with learning disorders, the aetiology is unknown.

Early identification

Children with learning disorders are most commonly identified in the third grade (Lyon et al., 1997). Yet, research has suggested that classroom and reading instruction interventions should occur early, preferably from kindergarten through to grade two, to be most effective (Foorman et al., 2003). Early identification allows programmes of sufficient intensity, duration and support to be introduced. Improved understanding of the deficits associated with learning disorders now allow earlier identification.

In the case of reading disorder, historically significant features are a family history of reading difficulties, a history of delayed expressive language development in the child, difficulty playing rhyming games and confusion of words with similar sounds (Scarborough, 1998). School readiness reading tests have also been shown to be predictive of later reading difficulties and can be used to identify children at risk for dyslexia at school entry. Children who have difficulty with naming letters of the alphabet, identifying words beginning with the same sound from a word list, identifying the word that would remain when the first letter is removed from a word, rapidly naming a series of familiar objects, poor story or sentence recall or naming objects presented as a single picture should be identified as being at risk for reading disorder at school entry (Shaywitz, 1998).

School age children read slowly and with difficulty, particularly when faced with unfamiliar words, and will make spelling errors. They also have a relatively poor performance on tests requiring them to name items, but will perform well on tests requiring them to point out objects named by someone else (Shaywitz, 1998). They will also perform well on oral comprehension tests. At adolescence, reading is slow and labored and lacks fluency.

At the end of pre-school, children at risk for mathematics disorder may not be able to count as well as their peers. They rely heavily on the use of aids such as fingers or drawing of circles for simple arithmetic functions in which their peers would use memory. At school age, errors in mathematical operations become apparent. The features of disorders of written expression and non-verbal learning disorder are not usually amenable to early identification.

In instances where readiness tests are either not available or not routinely used, children's early learning difficulties are often apparent during normal classroom activities at kindergarten. Teacher's subjective ratings of performance at kindergarten are sensitive enough to identify children who had poor achievement on standardized tests, and are predictive of later learning difficulties (Taylor et al., 2000; Teisl et al., 2001.)

Comorbidity

Learning disorders

There is a high degree of comorbidity among the learning disorders. For example, 17 percent of children with dyscalculia also had reading disorder (Shalev and Gross-Tsur, 2001).

Behavior and emotional disorders

Children with different types of disability have been identified as being at greater risk for emotional and behavioral disorders (Witt et al., 2003). In keeping with this, children with learning disorders have been found to have a higher prevalence of psychopathology. There are two possible explanations for this association. Children who experience persistent failure may recognize themselves to have functional academic limitations, a situation comparable to children with physical disabilities who recognize themselves to have functional activity limitations in comparison to their peers. Low self-esteem and a sense of hopelessness may develop, which can manifest as externalizing disorders, such as aggressive and disruptive behavior or as internalizing disorders, such as anxiety, depression or withdrawn behavior. Alternatively, the central nervous system dysfunction associated with the development of a learning disorder may predispose children to the development of behavior disorders. Both factors may also operate simultaneously.

Behavioral and emotional disorders are often not recognized by educational professionals working with children with learning disorders (Morgan and Hastings, 1998). However, they are major concerns for parents. Some 40 per cent of parents were dissatisfied with the community learning disability services their children received. Psychological and behavioral services were particularly identified as either unmet or inadequately provided (McKenzie et al., 2001)

Though other behavioral and emotional disorders, such as aggression and depression have been reported in children with learning disorders (Howard and Tryon, 2002; Jahoda et al., 2001), the most consistently identified behavioral and emotional disorders are social skills deficits and attention deficit hyperactivity disorder (ADHD).

Poor social skills have been associated with the deficient information processing, self monitoring and self regulation skills that may accompany learning disorders. Using a meta-analytical approach, Kavale demonstrated that approximately 75 per cent of children with learning disabilities have social skill deficits (Kavale and Forness, 1996). Social skills deficits manifest prominently in the friendship patterns of children. In comparison with children without learning disorders, children with learning disorders have fewer friends without a disorder, more friends with learning disorders and more friends below the age of their peer group (Wiener and Schneider, 2002). They also have less stable relationships, more conflicts and more difficulties with relationship repair following conflict. Some social skill deficits, such as loneliness and a poor sense of coherence, can be identified in pre-school children at high risk of developing a learning disorder, prior to the recognition of academic difficulties (Margalit, 1998). This supports the theory that central nervous system dysfunction may be responsible for at least some of the emotional and behavioral manifestations associated with learning disorders.

Behavioral and emotional disorders are not limited to children with learning disorders. As with children with other forms of disability, family members are at higher risk for emotional distress. Additionally, family stressors and family adjustment impact significantly on the child with learning disability (Witt et al., 2003).

ADHD, with its core behavior manifestations of hyperactivity, impulsivity and inattention, is a behavior disorder believed to be due to deficient neuro-transmitters in specific regions of the brain. Approximately 50 per cent of children with learning disorders have ADHD and up to 70 per cent of children diagnosed with ADHD have a learning disability (Mayes et al., 2000). A learning disability of written expression was twice as common as learning disabilities in reading, spelling or mathematics. In this study, the existence of attention difficulties in children with learning disabilities, but without ADHD, and the existence of learning problems in children with ADHD, but without learning disability, led the authors to theorize that learning and attention problems are on a continuum, are interrelated and usually coexist. The coexistence of ADHD and learning disability is associated with more severe learning and attentional difficulties.

Clinical implications

Diagnosis

Educators and parents or other care givers are the persons most likely to suspect a learning disorder in a child. Such suspicion warrants a complete multidisciplinary evaluation based on the immediate and long term consequences of a diagnosis of learning disorder for children, their families and the local educational authority. The evaluation process should be sensitive enough to correctly identify a learning disorder if present and specific enough to exclude other disorders that may manifest in a similar manner. Common mental and physical disorders that need to be excluded are mental retardation, behavior disorders, hearing and visual impairment. Environmental factors such as inadequate schooling and cultural factors will also need to be excluded. In some situations, mental and physical disorders and environmental factors may coexist with a learning disorder.

The multidisciplinary team should include a pediatrician, an educational psychologist, and a specialist in child mental health. Child mental health services may be provided by a clinical psychologist, developmental and behavioral pediatrician or a child and adolescent psychiatrist.

A detailed medical, developmental and behavioral, social, family and educational history will obtain information on the child's past and current academic achievement status, identify possible risk factors (e.g. family history, perinatal injury) and complications (e.g. behavioral disorders), determine the degree of family support and the child and family's coping strategies and the effectiveness of any previous interventions. A complete medical examination, with a focus on neuro-developmental examination, and hearing and visual evaluations will identify any physical medical conditions that are associated with learning disorders and/or are known to impair learning. Behavioral evaluation will identify specific behavior disorders that are present and determine their cause.

The educational evaluation has as its objectives a determination of the child's general intelligence, academic performance and neuropsychological functioning. General intelligence is determined by the use of standardized tests of intelligence which include verbal and non-verbal measures, such as the Weschler Preschool and Primary Scale of Intelligence (WPPSI), Weschler Intelligence Scale for Children (WISC), Stanford-Binet Intelligence Scales and Woodcock Johnson Test of Cognitive Abilities. Tests of academic achievement include general tests which evaluate performance in a range of academic subjects such as the Weschler Individual Achievement Test (WIAT), Wide Range Achievement Test (WRAT) and the Woodcock Johnson Tests of Achievement, or specific tests of achievement in which only a single academic area is tested, such as the Gray Diagnostic Reading Tests and the Test of Written Language (TOWL). Neuropsychological functioning determines how a child processes information and may include tests of visual-motor perception and integration, visual perception, auditory perception and motor proficiency, as in the Bender Gestalt Test.

The comprehensive evaluation process allows an accurate diagnosis of a learning disorder to be made based on a difference between general intellectual ability and achievement, identifies possible causes and complications and allows for the planning of an appropriate intervention programme.

Educational intervention

Educational intervention for reading disorder has been the most well documented. For young children, remedial education is most important, with particular emphasis on phonemic awareness, such as teaching rhyming and non-rhyming words, teaching word blends and syllabication. The success of a phonologically based reading intervention in activating neural pathways and improving reading fluency has been documented (Shaywitz et al., 2004). For older children, interventions depend on accommodation of the environment. Older children with reading disorder have similar word recognition skills as their peers, but the phonologic deficit makes reading slow and labored. These students require extra time to decode the words that they can and to use their higher order cognitive and linguistic skills to assist in determining the meaning of the words they cannot decode (Shaywitz et al., 1999). Other recommended accommodations for older children include the use of note takers, tape recording of lectures, using recordings for blind people for texts that they find difficult to read and the opportunity to take tests in an alternative format, such as short answers or oral tests (Shaywitz, 1998).

For children with mathematics disorder, disorders of written expression and non-verbal learning disorders, where there are a variety of presentations, interventions are directed at addressing the child's specific weaknesses using existing strengths. Children with disorders of written expression are encouraged to write at leisure, such as keeping a journal; write outlines and make jottings in draft format before compiling final written work and record ideas on tape, later playing the recorded information while writing (Kronenberger and Dunn, 2003). The verbal and rote learning strengths of children with NVLD are used to memorize academic algorithms and to teach social and non-verbal material using extensive practice and examples, such as role play. Children are also encouraged to engage in supervised and structured peer activities.

Behavioral intervention

Children with behavior disorders may require counseling or specific therapy such as Cognitive Behavior Therapy. Families may also benefit from Family Therapy. Children diagnosed with ADHD may require pharmaco-therapeutic agents such as methylphenidate. Other pharmaco-therapeutic agents such as anti-histamines and motion sickness medication are unsubstantiated.

Other interventions

Many publicized therapies for learning disorders, such as elimination of food additives, use of antioxidants and megavitamins have not been proven to be beneficial. Other interventions, such as auditory and optometric training are either unproven or controversial.

Course and outcome

Learning disorders are lifelong conditions with significant social and academic consequences. Young adults with learning disorders have lower graduation rates, are less likely to be enrolled in post-secondary education and are more likely to aspire to low-prestige occupations than their peers (Rojewski, 1999). The school dropout rate for children and adolescents with learning disorders is one and a half times the average rate (DSM-IV; APA, 1994). At work, even in part-time, unskilled jobs, young adults with learning disorders report high levels of stress in learning job tasks and the need to develop coping strategies to overcome difficulties in the work environment (Stacey, 2001). Students recommended practice and real life experiences prior to entering the workforce.

Recent studies of adolescents are suggesting more positive outcomes. Students who received an inclusive education with periods of specific instruction had similar social and academic outcomes as their peers when they made the transition from elementary school to middle school in the early adolescent years (Forgan and Vaughan, 2000). A study of adolescents with reading disorder, followed to the age of 14 years, found that their non-academic outcomes, as measured by trouble with the law, use of alcohol or tobacco and teacher behavior reports were similar to that of their peers (Shaywitz et al., 1999). Their reading disorder, as manifested by rate of reading and spelling errors, persisted, showing no evidence of remission or catch up with the skills of their peers.

Where students' learning disorders are identified and appropriate intervention provided, their academic and social outcomes improve, though their specific deficits persist.

Conclusion

Much new information on learning disorders has been obtained over the last few decades that has challenged previous knowledge and has also suggested areas requiring further investigation. Most important for future research is the determination of an accurate and internationally acceptable definition, allowing consistency across studies of prevalence, aetiology, intervention and outcome. Based on current knowledge, learning disorders have been shown to occur with a relatively high prevalence rate in the populations studied, affecting both genders equally. There is little information on learning disorders from non-English-speaking countries and developing countries. Similarities in cross-cultural findings strengthen existing theories and differences suggest new theories.

Aetiological studies have elicited genetic and biological associations. Genetic associations have suggested a possible role for genetic intervention and counseling in reducing the prevalence of dyslexia. Biological neuro-imaging studies have contributed to the understanding and management of dyslexia by the identification of phonemic awareness as the specific deficit and by showing conclusively that phonological interventions lead to alteration in brain structure and improved reading skills. The benefits of years of research in reading disorders are evident. Similar attention needs to be paid to the other learning disorders.

Learning disorders are lifelong conditions. Long term social, educational, behavioral and emotional consequences for children and their families occur, particularly if learning disorders are unrecognized and adequate services are not provided. As early identification and appropriate intervention improve outcome, teacher training curricula for the early childhood and primary years, should place emphasis on the development of competencies in this area. Curricula will need ongoing revision as new information emerges from the scientific literature. Additionally, public education programmes will improve general education and reduce the stigma and emotional disorders associated with this condition.

Early identification and better diagnostic techniques have implications for service provision. Educational authorities will need to provide the comprehensive services necessary to improve the outcome for children identified with learning disorders. Cost–benefit analysis is an area for future research.

References

Aaron, P.G. (1997). The impending demise of the discrepancy formula. *Review of Educational Research, 67*, 461–502

Ackerman, P.T., Dykman, R.A., and Oglesby, D.M. (1994). Visual event-related potentials of dyslexic children to rhyming and non-rhyming stimuli. *Clinical and Experimental Neuropsychology, 16*, 136–154.

Ackerman, P.T., McPherson, B.D., Oglesby, D.M., and Dykman, R.A. (1998). EEG power spectra of adolescent poor readers. *Journal of Learning Disabilities, 31*, 83–90.

American Psychiatric Association (1994). *Diagnostic and statistical manual of mental disorders*, 4th edn. Washington, DC: APA.

Bastra, L., Neeleman, J., and Hadders-Algra, M. (2003). The neurology of learning and behaviour problems in pre-adolescent children. *Acta Psychiatrica Scandinavica, 108*, 92–100.

Best, M. and Demb, J.B. (1999). Normal planum temporale asymmetry in dyslexics with a magnocellular pathway deficit. *Neuroreport, 10*, 607–612.

Collins, D.W. and Rourke, B.P. (2003). Learning disabled brains: A review of the literature. *Journal of Clinical and Experimental Neuropsychology, 25*, 1011–1034.

Dalby, M.A., Elbro, C., and Stodilke-Jorgensen, H. (1998). Temporal lobe asymmetry and dyslexia: An in vivo study using MRI. *Brain and Language, 62*, 51–69.

Dehaene, S. and Cohen, L. (1995). Towards an anatomical and functional model of number processing. *Math Cognition, 1*, 83–120.

Dehaene, S., Spelke, E., Pinel, P., Stanescu, R., and Tsivkin, S. (1999). Sources of mathematical thinking: Behavioral and brain-imaging evidence. *Science, 284*, 970–974.

Denckla, M.B., LeMay, M., and Chapman, C.A. (1985). Few CT scan abnormalities found even in neurologically impaired learning disabled children. *Journal of Learning Disabilities, 18*, 13–135.

Finnuci, J.M. and Childs, B. (1981). Are there really more dyslexic boys than girls? In A. Ansara, N. Geschwind, M. Albert, and N. Gartrell (Eds.), *Sex differences in dyslexia* (pp. 1–9). Towson, MD: Orton Dyslexic Society.

Foorman, B.R., Breier, J.I., and Fletcher, J.M. (2003). Interventions aimed at improving reading success: an evidence based approach. *Developmental Neuropsychology, 24*, 613–639.

Forgan, J.W. and Vaughn, S. (2000). Adolescents with and without LD make the transition to middle school. *Journal of Learning Disabilities, 33*, 33–43.

Galaburda, A.M., Sherman, G.F., Rosen, G.D., Aboitz, F., and Geschwind, N. (1985). Developmental dyslexia: Four consecutive patients with cortical anomalies. *Annals of Neurology, 18*, 222–233.

Gillberg, C. and Soderstrom, H. (2003). Learning disability. *The Lancet, 362*, 811–821.

Ginsburg, H.P. (1997). Mathematics learning disabilities: A view from developmental psychology. *Journal of Learning Disabilities, 30*, 20–33.

Grigorenko, E.L., Wood, F.B., Meyers, M.S., Hart, L.A., Speed, W.C., Shuster, A., et al. (1997). Susceptibility loci for distinct components of developmental dyslexia on chromosomes 6 and 15. *American Journal of Human Genetics, 60*, 27–39.

Gross-Tsur, V., Manor, O., and Shalev, R.S. (1996). Developmental dyscalculia: Prevalence and demographic features. *Developmental Medicine and Child Neurology, 38*, 25–33.

Henschen, S.E. (1925). Clinical and anatomical contributions in brain pathology. *Archives of Neurology and Psychiatry, 13*, 226–249.

Howard, K.A. and Tryon, G.S. (2002). Depressive symptoms in and type of classroom placement for adolescents with LD. *Journal of Learning Disabilities, 35,* 185–190.

Jahoda, A., Trower, P., Pert, C., and Finn, D. (2001). Contingent re-inforcement or defending the self? A review of evolving models of aggression in people with mild learning disabilities. *British Journal of Medical Psychology, 74,* 305–321.

Jevtovic-Todorovic, V., Hartman, R.E., Izumi, Y., Benshoff, N.D., Dikranian, K., Zorumski, C.F., et al. (2003). Early exposure to common anesthetic agents causes widespread neurodegeneration in the developing rat brain and persistent learning deficits. *Journal of Neuroscience, 23,* 876–882.

Kavale, K.A. and Forness, S.R. (1996). Social skills deficits and learning disabilities: A meta-analysis. *Journal of Learning Disabilities, 3,* 226–237.

Kidder-Ashley, P., Deni, J.R., and Anderton, J.B. (2000). Learning disabilities eligibility in the 1990s: An analysis of state practices. *Education, 121,* 65–72.

Kinney, B.A., Rabe, M.B., Jensen, R.A., and Steiger R.W. (2003). Maternal hyperglycemia leads to gender-dependent deficits in learning and memory in offspring. *Experimental Biology and Medicine* (Maywood), *228,* 152–159.

Kronenberger, W.G. and Dunn, D.W. (2003). Learning disorders. *Neurological Clinics of North America, 21,* 941–952.

Leisman, G. and Ashkenazi, M. (1980). Aetiological factors in dyslexia: IV. Cerebral hemispheres are functionally equivalent. *International Journal of Neuroscience, 11,* 157–164.

Lewis, C., Hitch, J., and Walker, P. (1994). The prevalence of specific arithmetic difficulties and specific reading difficulties in 9 to 10 year old boys and girls. *Journal of Child Psychology and Psychiatry, 35,* 283–292.

Lyon, G.R. (1996). Learning disabilities. *Future of Children, 6,* 54–76.

Lyon, G.R., Alexander, D., and Yaffee, S. (1997). Progress and promise in research in learning disabilities. *Learn Disabilities, 8,* 1–6.

Lyon, G.R., Fletcher, J.M., Shaywitz, S.E., Shaywitz, B.A., Torgesen, J.K., Wood, F.B., et al. (2001). Rethinking learning disabilities. In C.E. Finn, Jr., A.J. Rotherham, and C.R. Hokanson, Jr. (Eds.), *Rethinking special education for a new century* (pp. 259–287). Washington, DC: Thomas B. Fordham Foundation and the Progressive Policy Institute.

McCloskey, M., Caramazza, A., and Basili, A. (1985). Cognitive mechanisms in number processing and calculation: Evidence from dyscalculia. *Brain Cognition, 4,* 171–196.

McKenzie, K., Paxton, D., and Murray, G.C. (2001). An evaluation of community learning disability services for children with a learning disability. *Health Bulletin, Scottish Office Department of Health, 59,* 91–96.

MacMillan, D.L., Gresham, F.M., and Bocian, M. (1998). Discrepancy between definitions of learning disabilities and school practices: An empirical investigation. *Journal of Learning Disabilities, 31,* 314–326.

Margai, F. and Henry, N. (2003). A community based assessment of learning disabilities using environmental and contextual risk factors. *Social Sciences in Medicine, 56,* 1073–1085.

Margalit, M. (1998). Loneliness and coherence among preschool children with learning disabilities. *Journal of Learning Disabilities, 31,* 173–180.

Mattson, A.J., Sheer, D.E., and Fletcher, J.M. (1992). Electrophysiological evidence of lateralized disturbances in children with learning disabilities. *Journal of Clinical and Experimental Neuropsychology, 14,* 707–716.

Mayes, S.D., Calhoun, S.L., and Crowell, E.W. (2000). Learning disabilities and ADHD: overlapping spectrum disorders. *Journal of Learning Disabilities, 33*, 417–424.

Morgan, G.M. and Hastings, R.P. (1998). Special educators' understanding of challenging behaviour in children with learning disabilities: Sensitivity to information about behavioral function. *Behavioral and Cognitive Psychotherapy, 26*, 43–52.

O'Keefe, M.J., O'Callaghan, M., Williams, G.M., Najman, J.M., and Bor, W. (2003). Learning, cognitive and attentional problems in adolescents born small for gestational age. *Pediatrics, 112*, 301–307.

Pennington, B.F. (1991). *Diagnosing learning disorders: A neuropsychological framework*. New York: Guilford.

Pennington, B.F. and Gilger, J.W. (1996). How is dyslexia transmitted? In C.H. Chase, G.D. Rosen, and G.F. Sherman (Eds.), *Developmental dyslexia: Neural, cognitive and genetic mechanisms* (pp. 41–61). Baltimore, MD: York Press.

Plomin, R. and Walker, S.O. (2003). Genetics and educational psychology. *British Journal of Educational Psychology, 73*, 3–14.

Rojewski, J.W. (1999). Occupational and educational aspirations and attainment of young adults with and without LD 2 years after High School completion. *Journal of Learning Disabilities, 32*, 533–552.

Rooney, R., Hay, D., and Levy, F. (2003). Small for gestational age as a predictor of behavioural and learning problems in twins. *Twin Research, 6*, 46–54.

Rosenberger, P.B. and Hier, D.B. (1980). Cerebral asymmetry and verbal intellectual deficits. *Annals of Neurology, 8*, 300–304.

Rourke, B.P. (1993). Arithmetic disabilities, specific and otherwise: A neuropsychological perspective. *Journal of Learning Disabilities, 26*, 214–226.

Rourke, B.P. (1995). Introduction: The NLD Syndrome and the white matter model. In B.P. Rourke (Ed.), *Syndrome of non-verbal learning disabilities* (pp. 1– 26). New York: Guilford.

Rumsey, J.M., Nace, K., Donohue, B., Wise, D., Maisog, J.M., and Andreason, P. (1997). A positron emission study of impaired word recognition and phonological processing in dyslexic men. *Archives of Neurology, 54*, 562–573.

Scarborough, H.S. (1998). Early identification of children at risk for reading disabilities: phonologic awareness and some other promising predictors. In B. Shapiro, P. Accardo, and A. Capute (Eds.), *Specific reading disability*. Baltimore, MD: York Press.

Shalev, R.S. and Gross-Tsur, V. (2001). Developmental dyscalculia. *Pediatric Neurology, 24*, 337–342.

Shaywitz, S.E. (1998). Dyslexia. *New England Journal of Medicine, 338*, 307–312.

Shaywitz, S.E., Shaywitz, B.A., Fletcher, J.M., and Escobar, M.D. (1990). Prevalence of reading disability in boys and girls: Results of the Connecticut Longitudinal Study. *Journal of the American Medical Association, 264*, 998–1002.

Shaywitz, S.E., Fletcher, J.M., and Shaywitz, B.A. (1994). Issues in the definition and classification of attention deficit disorder. *Topics in Language Disorders, 14*, 1–25.

Shaywitz, S.E., Fletcher, J.M., Holahan, J.M., Shneider, A.E., Marchione, K.E., Stuebing, K.K., et al. (1999). Persistence of dyslexia: The Connecticut Longitudinal Study at Adolescence. *Pediatrics, 104*, 1351–1359.

Shaywitz, B.A., Shaywitz, S.E., Blachman, B.A., Pugh, K.R., Fulbright, R.K., Skudlarski, P., et al. (2004). Development of left occipitotemporal systems for skilled reading in children after a phonologically based intervention. *Biological Psychiatry, 55*, 926–933.

Silver, L.B. (1991). Developmental learning disorders. In M. Lewis (Ed.), *Child and adolescent psychiatry: A comprehensive textbook* (pp. 522–528). Baltimore, MD: Williams and Wilkins.

Stacey, W.A. (2001). The stress of progression from school to work for adolescents with learning disabilities: What about life progress? *Work, 17*, 175–181.

Taylor, H.G., Anselmo, M., Foreman, A.L., Schatschneider, C., and Angelopoulos, J. (2000). Utility of kindergarten judgements in identifying early learning problems. *Journal of Learning Disabilities, 33*, 200–210.

Thatcher, R.W. (1996). Neuroimaging of cyclical cortical reorganization during human development. In R.W. Thatcher, G.R. Lyon, J. Rumsey, and N. Krasgenor (Eds.), *Developmental neuroimaging: Mapping the development of brain and behaviour* (pp. 91–106). San Diego, CA: Academic Press.

Teisl, J.T., Mazzocco, M.M., and Myers, G.F. (2001). The utility of kindergarten teacher ratings for predicting low academic achievement in first grade. *Journal of Learning Disabilities, 34*, 286–293.

US Department of Education (National Center for Education Statistics) (1997). *The condition of education 1997: Supplemental and standard error tables NCES97–988*. Washington, DC: US Government Printing Office.

Wadsworth, S.J., DeFries, J.C., Stevenson, J., Gilger, J.W., and Pennington, B.F. (1992). Gender ratios among reading-disabled children and their siblings as a function of parental impairment. *Journal of Child Psychology and Psychiatry, 33*, 1229–1339.

Wiener, J. and Schneider, B.H. (2002). A multisource exploration of the friendship patterns of children with and without learning disabilities. *Journal of Abnormal Child Psychology, 30*, 127–141.

Witt, W.P., Riley, A.W., and Coiro, M.J. (2003). Childhood functional status, family stressors, and psychosocial adjustment among school-aged children with disabilities in the United States. *Archives of Pediatric and Adolescent Medicine, 157*, 687–695.

Wynn, K. (1992). Addition and subtraction by human infants. *Nature, 358*, 749–750.

Wynn, K. (1998). Psychological foundations of number: Numerical competence in human infants. *Trends in Cognitive Science, 2*, 296–303.

INDEX

Academic problems, 54
Academic performance, 62
Accommodation, 4
Acute stress disorder, 79
Adjustment disorder, 149
Adolescent-onset, 31, 36, 41
Affective consequences model, 205
Affective disorders, 166
Aggressive, 39; behaviours, 31
Agoraphobia, 79, 81, 83
Alcohol, 60, 184–185; consumption, 195; abuse/dependence, 230; dexoxification, 206; use, 193; use disorders, 186, 193, 195–196
Alcoholism, 16, 193, 197–198
Alpha-adrenrgic blockers, 101
Amphetamines, 194–195, 202
Amphetamine abuse/dependence, 230
Amygdala, 94–96, 98; -hippocampal, 97
Amygdalar: abnormalities, 95; activation, 96–97; damage, 96; dysfunction, 98; volumes, 97
Annenberg Eating Disorder Commission, 162
Anorexia nervosa, 160–166, 168–169, 174
Anorexia Nervosa Treatment Work Group, 173
Antidepressants, 173–175
Antidepressant medication, 125, 175
Antisocial behaviour, 35, 43, 151, 204, 207
Antisocial outcomes, 61
Antisocial personality disorder, 197, 198
Anxiety, 16, 29, 30, 79, 82, 86, 94, 121, 258; disorders, 55, 78, 80, 82–84, 86, 100, 166, 175, 197–198, 205, 230–231; -related traits, 84; pathogenesis of, 95; severity of, 97; symptoms, 97

Anxiolytics, 174
Applied behaviour analysis, 256
Asperger's disorder, 260
Assessment, 202, 235–236, 253
Assimilation, 4
Attention, 16, 96
Attention-deficits, 53
Attention-deficit/Hyperactivity disorder (ADHD), 39, 52, 54–55, 57–59, 60–61, 65, 67, 101, 115, 198
Attention studies, 88
Attentional: biases, 91; dysfunction, 91; processes, 8; problems, 145
Attributional style, 144–145, 147–148
Auditory integration training, 253
Autism, 246–247, 249, 251–254, 257–262

Behavior: problem, 27–28, 259; therapy, 66, 68
Behavioral inhibition (BI), 83–84
Behavioral: data, 94; disruptions, 145; fluctuations, 146
Benzodiazepines, 100
Binge eating, 161, 168, 175
Binge-purge, 167
Biological: factors, 147, 199; processes, 147
Bipolar disorder, 124, 197
Birth cohort, 170
Body dysmorphic disorder, 224
Body satisfaction, 171–172
Borderline symptoms, 150–151, 156
Bottom-up study, 83
Bulimia nervosa, 160–166, 168–169, 175–176

Cannabis, 184; abuse, 191; dependence, 191; use disorders, 186

Case-control, 87, 170
Central coherence, 249
Child Behavior Checklist, 12
Childhood adversities, 120
Childhood-limited disorder, 62
Childhood-onset, 30–31, 36, 41, 43
Chronic abdominal pain, 227; disability, 226; fatigue syndrome (CFS), 222; illness, 258; pain, 226
Circular reaction, 4
Classification, 113, 240, 273; system, 114, 197
Clomipraimine, 237
Cocaine, 202; dependence, 187
Cognitive: ability, 6, 13; abnormalities, 86; capacity, 174; dysfunction, 227; factors, 198–199; function, 86; impairment, 259; paradigms, 86; patterns, 126; potential, 247; processes, 86, 251; processing, 86, 101, 174; tests, 65; theory, 4; style, 250; vulnerabilities, 145
Cognitive-behavioral: approach, 38; therapy, 99, 175, 239; treatment, 126; treatment studies, 81
Color-naming delay, 87
Color-word stroop test, 87
Communication deficits, 261
Communication skills, 251, 253
Community-based studies, 184
Community samples, 27, 36, 81, 113, 229
Comorbid, 29, 78, 81, 196, 204; anxiety disorder, 29; associations, 197; concomitants, 116; conditions, 115; depression, 29–30; disorders, 123, 165, 188, 231; disruptive behavior disorders, 82; pattern, 231; psychiatric condition, 124; psychiatric disorders, 205; psychopathology, 101, 165; substance use disorders, 167
Comorbidity, 29, 55, 67, 81–82, 115, 127, 140, 167, 175, 184, 195–196, 203, 205, 225, 228, 230; patterns, 206
Conduct disorder, 196, 198
Conduct problems, 26–30, 32, 36–37, 41, 43, 61, 67
Constructivist view, 18
Contingency management, 37; programs, 37; system, 40
Conversion disorder, 221–223, 228–229, 230, 233–234, 238–239
Co-occurring, 56, 61

Coping, 121, 156; skills, 155, 207; strategies, 259
Correlational studies, 168
Course, 82, 184; chronic, 122; fluctuating, 82; of depression, 113; of disorder, 122–123; of illness, 113; longitudinal, 186; protracted, 122
Course and outcome, 30, 165–166, 232, 284
Cross-sectional, 169
Culture, 7

Daily hassles, 144
Definition, 113
Depression, 15, 29, 56–57, 82–83, 101, 119, 121–122, 127, 146–147, 149, 151–152, 155, 165, 197, 205, 258; adolescent, 113, 116, 120, 125, 127, 129; childhood 118, 124; chronic form of, 114; increase of, 116; maternal, 15–16, 20; pediatric, 95; recurrence of, 155, 157; recurrent, 123
Depressive: cycle, 155; disorders, 115–116, 123–124, 128, 198, 230; episode, 113, 122–123, 125, 127, 140, 142, 144, 146, 148–149; symptoms, 113, 120, 126–127, 129, 142–143, 156; symptomatology, 118; rumination, 156
Development, 1, 2, 4, 6, 11, 14, 20, 42, 67; abnormal, 3, 20; abnormal and normal, 10; child's, 11; cognitive, 4–5, 8; critical periods of, 11; differences, 117; emotional, 17; intellectual, 13; human, 4, 6 11; normal and abnomal, 20; of a chronic course, 113; of effective intervention, 113; of conduct problems, 34–35; of cognition, 4; of depression, 143; of depressive symptoms, 121; of disorders, 128; of disordered eating, 169; of eating disorders, 172; of neurotic symptoms, 84; of reasoning in childhood, 4; psychosexual, 3; psychosocial, 3; social and emotional, 17–19; social and intellectual, 2; social cognitive, 8; theories of, 1; transitions, 78
Developmental, 42, 128, 282; challenges, 140; changes, 20, 85; course, 52, 60; difficulties, 19–20; disabilities, 262; dyscalculia, 275; epidemiology, 116; functioning, 3; human, 1; impact, 125;

lifespan, 9; level, 10, 86; mechanisms, 44; other aspects of, 3; outcomes, 13, 62; pathways, 11, 35, 113; pattern, 116; psychopathology, 1, 9–10, 78, 85, 116, 129, 160; problems, 2, 18, 175; processes, 12, 32, 122; progression, 162, 186; psychosocial, 3; research, 14; questions, 10; stages, 2; tasks, 123; trajectory, 17, 30, 62

Diagnostic: criteria, 64, 160, 163, 186, 229, 247, 273; levels, 184; measures, 184; strategies, 115; symptoms, 193; system, 202

Diathesis-stress model, 121

Dissociative symptom, 223

Disruptive behaviour disorders, 55, 196

Dizygotic, 59

Dot probe task, 90

Double-depression, 114

Drug use disorders, 195, 196

Drug experimentation, 200

Dyscalculia, 273

Dysfunction family environments, 40

Dysfunctional: body image, 174; mechanisms, 85; parenting practices, 34; families, 38; thinking, 156; sensory system, 252

Dyslexia, 273, 278

Dysmorphic disorder, 221–222

Dysmorphophobia, 224

Dysphoria, 146, 151, 153

Dysphoric mood, 148, 150

Dysthymia, 122, 124

Dysthymic disorder, 113–114, 230, 233

Early adulthood, 120

Early childhood, 120

Eating disorders, 16, 162–171, 197

Eating syndromes, 164

Ecological perspective, 7

Ecological theory, 5

Emotional: arousal, 9, 34; dependence, 121; development, 19; difficulties, 271; dispositions, 9; disorders, 95, 234, 281; events, 153; learning, 92; memory, 92, 98; problems, 10, 12–13; processing, 154; regulation, 34–35; reliance, 123, 148, 150–151, 156; stroop task, 87; stroop test, 87; salience, 87; well-being, 19

Emotionally valent stimuli, 87

Emotionally valent words, 87

Empirically based treatment, 206

Endrocrine influences, 147

Environment, 6–8, 15, 18; prenatal, 20; cultural context of the, 7

Environmental: contributions, 11, 14, 59, 84; cultural context, 7; effects, 20, 33; events, 7; factors, 12, 59–60, 84; influences, 20, 148, 246; origins, 11; systems, 6; variables, 65, 151

Epidemiologic Catchment Area study, 193, 198

Epidemiologic studies, 118, 122, 185, 187, 246, 247

Epidemiological: data, 80, 169; studies, 80, 171

Epidemiology, 27, 80, 115, 140, 184, 206, 273

Episode severity, 122

Ethnicity, 13, 118

Ethnic groups, 27, 80, 118

Etiology, 59, 67, 127, 168, 206–207

Eurocentric meanings, 7

Executive dysfunction, 249

Executive functioning, 249

Exosystem, 7

Experimental treatment, 174

Explicit memory, 93

Externalizing behaviour, 18

Facilitated communication, 253

Family: adjustment, 282; factors, 119, 199; interaction patterns, 204; history, 92, 280; therapy, 42, 175, 238–284; stressors, 282; studies, 83, 170; system, 263

Familial: transmission, 119; rejection, 121; relationships, 121

First-degree relatives, 123

Fluoxetine, 100, 125, 237

Functional: analysis, 64; deficits, 64; neuroimaging data, 96; polymorphisms, 119

Functional Family Therapy, 204

Functional magnetic resonance imaging (fMRI), 276

Functioning, 15; abnormal, 14; cognitive, 18; emotional, 34; family, 13, 56–57; impaired psychosocial, 30; maladaptive, 15; neuropsychological; parental, 15; peer, 57; poor adaptive, 13; psychological, 9; psychosocial, 125, 200; social, 57, 123; school, 53; social and emotional, 17; occupational, 200

Gastrointestinal complaints, 226
Gastrointestinal symptoms, 223
Gene-environment interactions, 119
Genes, 14, 258, 278
Generalized anxiety disorder, 78–80, 90, 224, 233
Genetic factors, 199
Genetic predispositions, 119
Genetic transmission, 247
Genetics, 59
Genotypic, 14
Growth hormone, 120

Hallucinogen abuse/dependence, 23
Hallucinogen disorders, 195
Hallucinogens, 185,
Hard drug use abuse/dependence, 187
Hard drug use disorders, 186, 195–196
Hyperactive, 52
Hyperactivity, 62, 254
Hypersensitivity, 92
Hypochondiasis, 221, 224, 228, 233–234, 239
Hypothalamic-endocrine-adrenal (HPA) axis, 120

Imipramine, 125
Immunity factors, 141, 248, 261
Impairment, 53, 80, 114, 123, 125, 128, 185, 205, 221, 224, 231–232, 234, 246, 247, 248, 261
Impulsive behaviour, 58
Impulsivity, 52, 62, 65
Inattention, 52, 58, 62, 65
Inattentive symptoms, 58
Incidence, 115; rates, 116, 194
Independent factors, 206
Information-processing biases, 88
Insomnia, 114
Integrative theory of depression, 141, 143, 152–153, 155–157
Intergenerational transmission, 207
Internalizing behaviour problems, 144, 146
Internalizing disorders, 55
Interpersonal 94; communication skills, 128; difficulties, 123; problems, 185
Interpersonal relationships, 126, 141
Interpersonal therapy, 126
Intervention, 66
Interviews, 64; semi-structured clinical, 64; structured, 64; unstructured, 64
Intrapersonal factors, 141
Irritability, 56

Juvenile antisocial behaviour, 26
Juvenile crime, 26

Learning disability, 271–273, 280, 282
Learning disorders, 271–273, 279, 280–282, 284–285
Life events, 120, 142, 144, 146, 154, 157
Life experiences, 141, 153
Life Skills Training Program, 203
Lifetime prevalence, 116
Linguistic skills, 276
Longitudinal: period, 153; study, 82, 116, 165–166; research, 146

Macroparadigm, 9
Macrosystem, 7
Major depression, 120, 122, 124, 156, 230, 233
Major depressive disorder, 100, 113–114, 117, 140, 146
Major depressive episode, 122
Major life stress, 144, 148, 153, 155
Major stressful life events, 153
Marijuana, 185, 202; abuse/dependence, 186, 194; smoking, 201; use, 201; use disorders, 186–187, 194, 196
Mathematics disorder, 273–274, 276, 280
Memory bias, 93
Mental disorder, 79
Mental retardation, 12, 271
Mesosystem, 6–7
Metarepresentation, 250
Methods for the Epidemiology of Child and Adolescent Mental Disorders (MECA), 80
Methylphenidate, 66
Microsystem, 6
Minor hassles, 120
Monozygotic, 59
Monozygotic twins, 247
Monitoring the Future Study, 185
Mood disorders, 223
Mood dysregulation, 101
Mortality rate, 165
Motivational Enhancement Therapy, 173
Multi-Family Psychoeducaional Groups (MFPG), 126
Multi-modal treatment, 66
Multi-Systemic Therapy (MST), 42
Multisystemic family therapy, 204
Multiple causal pathways, 31
Multiple pathways, 128

National Survey on Drug Use and Health, 185
Natural course, 164
Negative affectivity, 170
Negative experiences, 142
Neural: data, 99; studies, 95
Neuroaffective motivation system, 251
Neurobehavioral functions, 94
Neurochemistry, 120
Neurodevelopmental conditions, 95
Neurodevelopmental examination, 283
Neuroimaging studies, 95, 275
Neuroleptics, 100
Neurological disorder, 223
Neurological tests, 65
Neurophysiological changes, 85
Neuropsychological functioning, 283
Neurophysiological responses, 95
Neurotransmitter systems, 173
Nicotine dependence, 186, 192, 195–196
Non-verbal learning disorder, 277, 280
Nosology, 79
Nutritional therapy, 174

Observational: learning, 8; studies, 100
Obsessive-compulsive disorder, 79–80, 87, 167, 224, 233
Oedipus complex, 2
Oestrogen levels, 120
Offspring, 83
Onset, 113; adolescent, 119, 165; late adolescent, 168; of depression, 120, 153–154; of eating disorders, 163, 171; of bulimia nervosa, 166
Oppositional behaviour, 145
Oppositional defiant disorder, 27, 196
Orbital frontal cortex, 94
Oregon Adolescent Depression Project, 184
Oregon Youth Substance Use Project, 184, 191
Orthographic awareness, 274
Outcomes, 13; developmental, 13; emotional, 13; for children, 15; poor academic, 13

Pain disorder, 221–222, 224–226, 230–231
Panic disorder, 79, 81, 87
Parent-child interactions, 119
Parental: attachment, 122; history, 119; obesity, 170; psychopathology, 15
Parenting, 56; attitudes, 56; stress, 258; styles, 57, 262

Parent Management Training, 38
Paroxetine, 125–126
Partial syndrome, 164
Pathophysiology, 78–79, 84, 97, 101
Pathophysiologic theories, 140
Peer factors, 199; rejection, 121; relationship, 58
Perception studies, 89
Personality disorders, 166–167, 197
Pervasive Developmental Disorders, 246, 260
Pharmacotherapy, 99, 125
Phenotypic, 14
Phonologic awareness, 274
Phonologic deficit theory, 274–275
Physical complaints, 221
Physical symptoms, 79, 221, 223, 226
Pituitary gland, 120
Play therapy, 66
Point prevalence estimates, 116
Polymorphism, 97
Postmenarcheal females, 161
Post-scan memory test, 98
Posttraumatic stress disorder, 79–80, 90, 231
Pragmatic awareness, 274
Precursor, 55
Predisposing characteristics, 143
Pre-pubertal, 124; onset, 124
Prevalence, 27, 80, 185, 187, 194, 227, 229, 247, 273; estimates, 27, 116; of major depression, 117; of substance use disorder, 167; rates, 27–28, 163
Problems: behavior, 27–28; behavior and emotional, 13; behavioral and emotional, 14, 20; conduct and social, 13; emotional developmental, 17; learning, 29; rates of behavioural, 28; social and emotional, 17
Problem Behavior Theory, 207
Problem-solving, 38, 148, 150, 156
Process, 9; of modelling, 9
Prognosis, 115, 168, 233
Prospective study, 170–171
Prospective cohort, 170
Protective factors, 128, 147–148, 151, 156
Pseudoneurological symptom, 223
Pseudoseizures, 227, 233
Psychiatric: conditions, 196; diagnoses, 127 ; disorders, 99, 160, 166, 198, 203–204, 221, 227, 231, 234; medications, 18
Psychoanalytic theory, 1

Psychometric properties, 63
Psychopathology, 2, 14, 26, 127, 170, 198, 201, 228; adult, 82, 86; child, 16; childhood, 29; competing models of, 14; fathers', 16; maternal, 16; mothers', 16; parental, 15, 83, 118, 170; paternal, 16; risk of, 16
Psychopharmacological agents, 126
Psychosocial, 184; factors, 121, 141; functioning, 162, 164–166; influences, 128, 140, 147; morbidity, 160; understanding, 141; variables, 156
Psychotherapy, 126
Purging behaviours, 175
Purging type, 161

Randomized control trials, 100, 173
Rating scales, 63, 64
Reading disorder, 273–275, 280, 283, 285
Reciprocal relations, 206
Recovery, 184
Recovery rates, 166
Recurrent abdominal pain, 232
Recurrent: episodes, 118, 123; substance-related legal problems, 185; psychopathology, 204
Reinforcement, 143, 146, 153, 156–157; patterns, 145
Relapse, 176, 184; rates, 165
Relaxation training, 65
Response rate, 125
Retrospectively, 168
Retrospective reporting, 168
Rett's disorder, 246
Risk factors, 83, 113, 117, 121, 128, 168–169, 171–172, 198–199, 201, 234
Risk-taking behaviours, 201
Risperidone, 238
Ritalin, 40

School-based programs, 203
School drop-out, 124
Self-analyze, 142
Self-awareness, 142, 155, 157
Self-consciousness, 144
Self-efficacy, 155
Self-esteem, 114, 121, 141, 147–148, 166, 170, 172–173, 225
Self-evaluation, 161, 169
Self-injurious acts, 167
Self-medication model, 205
Self-monitor, 142, 146
Self-mutilation, 225

Self-perceptions, 121
Self-rated, 147
Self-rated social competence, 147–148
Self regulation, 9
Self-report, 146, 236
Self-worth, 161
Sensory integration therapy, 252
Sensory stimulation, 252
Separation anxiety disorder, 78–79
Serotonin-norepinephrine reuptake inhibitors, 100
Serotonin-reuptake inhibitors (SSRI), 100–101, 125, 175, 237
Serotonin transporter promoter gene, 97
Sertraline, 125, 237
Service utilization, 12
Simple animal phobia, 87
Social: anxiety disorder, 83; cognitive theory, 8; communication, 248 ; information, 251; interaction, 248; interaction behaviours, 251; phobia, 78–80; self-disturbance, 170; skills, 256; support, 121; support system, 141
Socialization, 9, 32, 37
Sociocultural factors, 13, 118
Sociocultural variables, 13
Sociodemographic factors, 118
Socioeconomic, 80; status, 13, 118, 170, 228–229, 234
Socioethnic group, 7
Sociohistorical events, 7
Somatic symptoms, 232
Somatization disorder, 221–223, 225, 228, 234, 239
Somatoform disorders, 221–224, 225, 228–232, 235–237, 240
Son-Rise approach, 255
Specific phobia, 79
Spectrum disorder, 246
Stability, 35; of conduct problems, 35; in diagnoses of CD, 35
Stereotypical patterns, 246
Stimulant, 39; medication, 39, 66, 68
Stressful events, 146
Stressful environment, 147
Stressful life experiences, 145
Stressors, 120–121
Structural equation modelling, 14
Structural-strategic family therapy, 204
Substance, 185, 191; abuse, 19, 30, 78, 148, 184–185, 198, 201–202, 206–207; dependence, 185; disorder, 119; use, 30, 172, 184–186, 191, 198, 200,

202–203, 206–207; use disorders, 145, 166, 184–185, 230
Subsyndromal depression, 197
Subthreshold eating disorders, 169
Subthreshold syndromes, 164
Suicidal: ideation, 29, 124, 225, 232; behaviours, 124; thoughts, 126
Suicide attempts, 78, 150, 167, 225, 232
Supportive interventions, 128
Supportive therapy, 127, 175

Taxonomy, 115
Temperament, 33–34
Temperamental style, 33
Theory of mind, 250
Tobacco use, 195
Top-up study, 83
Traits of impairment, 247
Tranquilizers, 185

Trauma, 79
Treatment, 40, 42, 125; empirically supported, 41; outcome, 42; psychosocial, 40; studies, 78
Tricyclic antidepressant, 125
Twin studies, 170
Twins, 59; fraternal, 59; identical, 59

Undifferentiated somatoform disorder, 222, 226, 228–231
Urinalysis, 202

Venlafaxine, 126
Vulnerability, 120, 127, 128, 141–143, 149, 151; factors, 145–146, 150; constitutional, 170; personal, 170; to subsequent episodes, 148

Word-stem completion paradigms, 93